THE ALLERGY-FIGHTING GARDEN

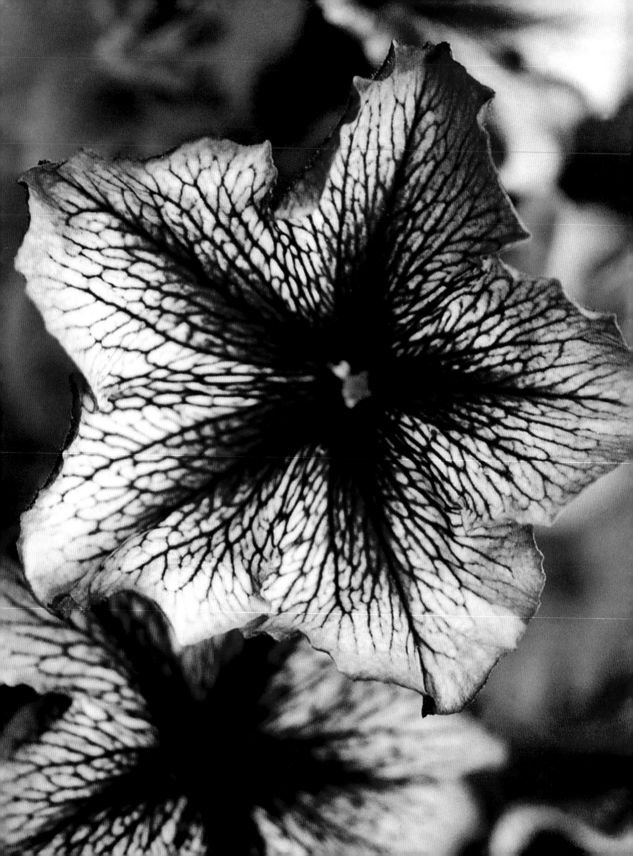

THE
ALLERGY-FIGHTING
GARDEN

Stop Asthma and Allergies
with Smart Landscaping

THOMAS LEO OGREN

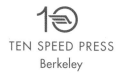

TEN SPEED PRESS
Berkeley

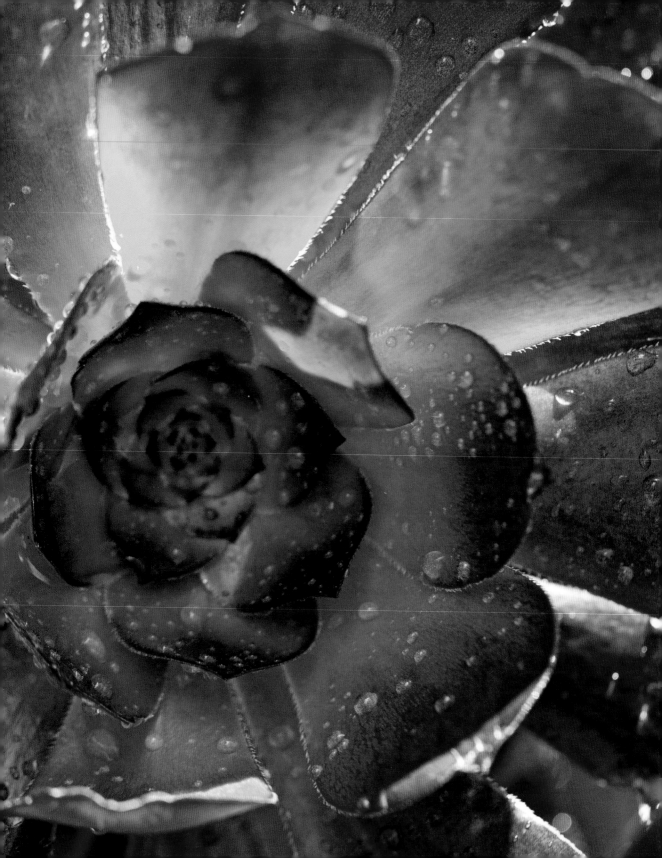

Contents

....

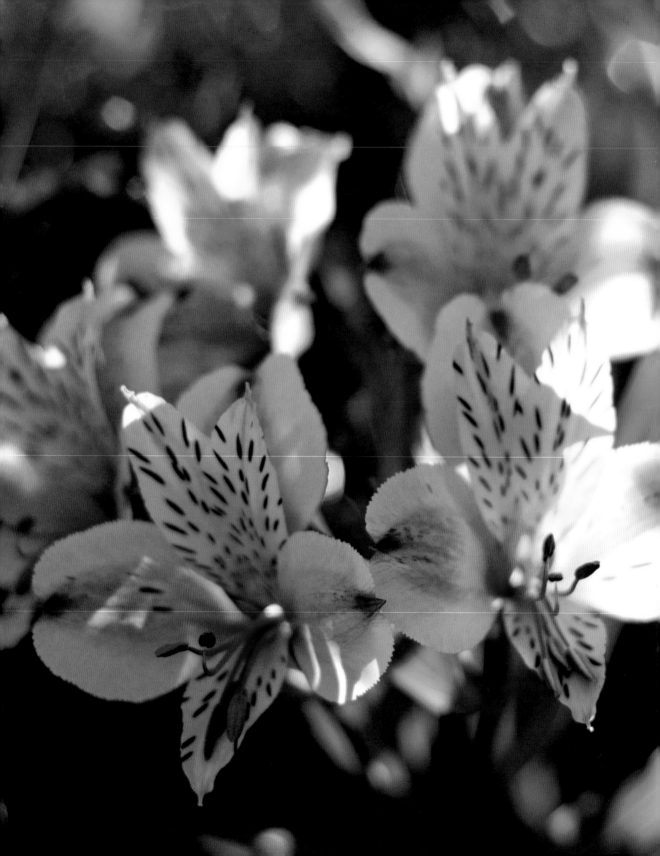

Foreword

....

Very rarely do we come across an idea that is both exceptionally good and revolutionary in its scope; the book *The Allergy-Fighting Garden* by Thomas Leo Ogren is such an idea.

I was a practicing allergist for more than fifty years. In the past I often advised people to avoid the "toxic" highly allergenic shrubs and trees, but my knowledge of botany was limited. Today, allergies are given short shrift in American medical schools. Students preparing for a medical career will receive only one or two lectures on the subject during a four-year course of intense study.

Allergies cause a huge amount of pain and suffering. There are many medical treatments for allergies, and none of them is perfect. All of them have side effects. The very best treatment for allergy is to avoid the offending substance. But when the state or city park department plants trees for shade, for example, they can end up causing intense suffering because of their poor choice of trees. Homeowners, too, unknowingly make poor choices and cause themselves years of allergy as they surround their houses with allergy-causing trees, shrubs, and lawns.

However, before this book, if you wanted to plant a landscape with allergy-free plants, you had few places to turn to for advice. Some landscapers knew that fruitless mulberries and olive trees caused allergy, but that was about it.

The Allergy-Fighting Garden is therefore a greatly needed book. Several things especially make this work so valuable. Ogren's allergy scale, assigning all plants a simple 1 to 10 allergy ranking, is a marvelous idea. All plants are not created equal. Certain plants cause no allergy, some cause very little, and some cause a great deal of suffering. Ogren's allergy scale addresses this problem head-on.

Another fine idea in this book is the reasoning about the dioecious species of plants. Dioecious (separate-sexed) plants cause far more than their share of allergies, because the male plants usually produce so much airborne pollen. These species, which include many

< Alstroemeria sp.

common plants such as willows, ash, and maples, are often described as the worst allergy offenders. What Ogren figured out here is that the flip side is also true. If the males are the worst, then the females are the best! This is a simple idea, perhaps, but up until now no one has really addressed it.

The Allergy-Fighting Garden should be on the shelf of every serious gardener. All allergy specialists would be wise to own a copy, and certainly the book should be in the library of every nursery and municipal park department. Perhaps most important of all, this text should be required reading for every college student of landscape design or horticulture. Ogren has made a valuable contribution to our good health, and now it is up to us to put the information to work.

DAVID A. STADTNER, MD

Introduction

For millions of people, allergies are no laughing matter. Allergies are not simply a bit of sneezing now and then; they are long days and nights of flat-out misery. Quite a few people have even died from severe reactions to allergenic pollen. In addition, there is now considerable data that demonstrate a powerful direct link between allergies and asthma—a very dangerous and often life-threatening condition. People with pollen allergies are more likely to develop food allergies and food intolerances. Pollen can cause rashes, sinus conditions, headaches, fatigue, irritability, and a number of other serious health problems that impact quality of life. It was recently reported in *Lancet*, a leading medical journal, that heart attack deaths rose 5 percent, heart disease deaths rose 6 percent, deaths from COPD (pulmonary/lung diseases) increased 15 percent, and pneumonia deaths jumped by 17 percent on days with peak pollen counts. The cost to the public in terms of drugs, doctors' visits, hospital care, and lost school and work days is many billions of dollars, and it keeps increasing. But the other cost, in terms of human misery, is even more tragic, especially when much of this suffering could be avoided in the first place.

Although there are a variety of factors that can contribute to allergies, pollen is *the* most common allergen to which we're exposed, and it is one that we can often control ourselves with the landscapes that surround our own houses, our schools, and the places where we work and play. I personally became involved in allergy-free gardening because my wife of forty-seven years, Yvonne, has asthma and allergies, and several times her asthma attacks almost killed her. Yvonne's asthma attacks occurred most often when her allergies were also at their worst, so when we bought a house in San Luis Obispo, California, I decided that I would re-landscape it so that nothing in our yard would trigger her allergies. First, I set out to buy some books on the subject, but found that there was nothing to buy. Because I had a background in horticulture, I began researching plants myself, one plant at a time, and in the process learned a great deal more about botany, medicine, pollen, and especially plant-flowering systems.

This book is a culmination of more than thirty years of research, and a combination of the best of my two previous books, *Allergy-Free Gardening* and *Safe Sex in the Garden*.

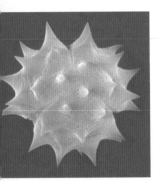

Single pollen grain,
Parthenium integrifolium

Fully revised, it contains hundreds of new and updated plant listings, plant rankings, and full-color photographs. Now with over 3,000 plant listings total, it is the most comprehensive resource available on the topic. As allergy and asthma rates continue to climb around the world, we can no longer afford to be passive. We must be proactive and use our gardens to fight back. The *Allergy-Fighting Garden* will help you do just that.

I'm often asked, did the relandscaping help your wife? Yes, it did. These days her allergies are much less intense, and I'm very, very pleased to say that she's been completely free of asthma symptoms for almost a decade now. It is my wish that with the simple advice and guidance in this book, you, too, can enjoy a healthier, happier life.

Erodium chamaedryoides >

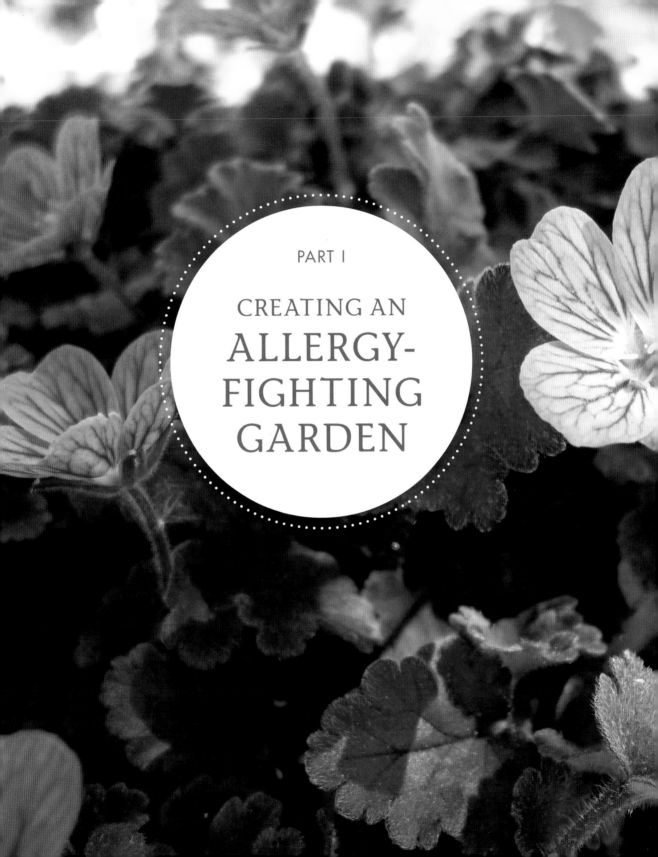

PART I

CREATING AN ALLERGY-FIGHTING GARDEN

ONE

Botanical Sexism
AND OUR CURRENT ALLERGY CRISIS

In the 1950s allergies affected only 2 to 5 percent of the people in the United States. By the 1980s more than 12 percent had allergies. By 1999 some 38 percent of the population suffered from allergies. The rates of both allergies and asthma continue to climb in almost all urban areas, usually at between 2 and 3 percent annually, and are now widely considered to be epidemic. In the U.S., asthma has become the number one chronic disease in children. In Canada, more than one person in three now has allergies.

What can account for this shocking increase?

In the early years of horticulture, most landscape plants were propagated by seed, and therefore male and female plants in the landscape were roughly 50-50, as naturally occurs in the wild. With the advent of powerful new rooting hormones, bottom heat, automatic mist and fogging systems, and controlled atmosphere greenhouses, clonal (asexual) woody plant propagation became much easier, quicker, and cheaper, and it allowed growers to produce separate-sexed (male or female) plants of their choosing.

In the 1940s the United States Department of Agriculture (USDA) started to recommend that when growing separate-sexed (dioecious) trees or shrubs from cuttings, budding, or grafting, that only male scion wood should be used. This, they said, would result in litter-free plants, as male plants make no seeds, seedpods, or fruit to fall on public sidewalks and create a "mess." What was missed was that these same male trees and shrubs would, of course, all produce allergenic pollen—a great deal of pollen. The pollen production of a single large male tree may easily be well more than ten thousand times greater than that of a perfect-flowered tree (one with both male and female parts in the same flowers, such as an apple or a plum tree). As time progressed, clonal trees and shrubs became the rule, not the exception, and more and more male plants were propagated, patented, sold, and planted in our cities.

The major shift came in the 1960s and 1970s when Dutch elm disease (DED) struck and killed off millions of American elm trees. At that time, the number one street tree in America for a hundred years had been the tall, stately, native American elm, *Ulmus americana*, which lined the streets of thousands of cities. DED struck first in the east, and then spread westward over the next decade. The trees that replaced the elms were more often than not these new, "improved" cultivars, male trees, many of which were developed by the USDA. They were first planted in massive numbers in eastern cities, and the eastern cities were the first ones to experience the sudden surge in urban allergies. Eventually, these replacement male trees were planted coast to coast, and as the ones in the west matured (and started to shed pollen), the west started to catch up with the east in the high percentages of people suffering from allergies.

The urban landscape before DED struck was, of course, a highly manipulated environment itself, but almost 100 percent of the street trees were seedlings, not asexually propagated clones. Manipulation of the environment is something that is done all the time in horticulture, and the old elm tree–lined streets were hardly good examples of environmental soundness. They totally lacked in biodiversity, which set the stage for their destruction by DED, but at least they had sexual balance.

Unfortunately, since the 1950s, it has also become common practice in many areas to cut down seedling-grown trees once it's determined that they're female—because they are deemed "messy." Seedling male trees are generally spared, left to grow old and large. This "unnatural selection" has taken a large toll on the females and has left us with ever more urban pollen, because female plants not only produce no pollen themselves, but they also trap and remove pollen from the air. In my own city of San Luis Obispo, California, I recently saw a yard where there were two yew pines (*Podocarpus gracilior*). The biggest tree was a female and produced large numbers of olive-size green and yellow fruits that fell on the lawn and the sidewalk in front of the house. The second tree, planted right next to the female tree, made no fruit, as it was a male. One day the homeowner had the large female tree cut down but left the male tree. Had he instead cut down the small male tree, the large female tree (with no pollinator) would have produced next to no fruit. Instead, now the male has all the room, it will soon enough grow much larger, and it will produce loads of pollen. There will be no female tree to trap this pollen, so it will drift around the immediate neighborhood, triggering allergies. This sort of thing is very common, in many places.

Between specifically planting large numbers of male clones and the systematic removal of female trees, we have created quite a situation. As is so often the case, when we manipulate large ecosystems and don't consider the consequences, we create a host of new problems. Dr. Robert C. Stebbins, professor emeritus of zoology at UC Berkeley, once told me, "This is what happens when those in charge do something on a very large scale and they never once stop and think about the ecology of what they're doing."

Today, the overuse of clonal male plants continues, and has, unfortunately, actually increased. Currently in the U.S., four out of five of the top-selling street tree cultivars are male clones. There continues to be considerable well-intentioned plans to "plant a million new trees" as well as huge pushes for more city trees, for additional "canopy," and again, it is mostly done with little regard for those with asthma and allergies. Landscapers, city planners, arborists, schools, and homeowners all want what they call low-maintenance or "litter-free" landscapes. But pollen is the invisible litterer. A typical pollen grain is about 20 microns in diameter, small enough to pass right through the

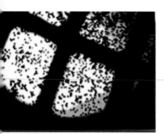

Pollen grain size in comparison to a window screen

tightest window screen. I once shook some pollen from a male yew onto a glass slide, placed a small square of window screen over the slide, and then looked at it with my microscope. I wanted to see how much protection, if any, a window screen actually provided. Although I knew what to expect I was nonetheless amazed at what I saw. I would estimate that as many as a thousand grains of this pollen could simultaneously pass through each tiny square in the window screen!

Pollen all over our sidewalks may not be as noticeable as seeds or fruit from female trees, but it is there, it is litter, and it makes millions of people sick.

If there has been one single purpose to my work it has been to reverse this unhealthy process. This hasn't been quick and it hasn't been easy; there has been huge resistance. Several years ago the *New York Times* asked me to write an opinion piece for them on New York's city trees and allergies. It kicked off quite a bit of debate and hundreds of readers sent me encouraging emails. Unfortunately, the people in charge of city trees dismissed the idea of using allergy-friendly city trees by claiming that "each tree only sheds pollen for a few days at most." This is not true at all; many city trees release allergenic pollen for months. Other trees release all of their pollen within a week or two, but the pollen falls on everything nearby and much of it remains allergenic for six months or longer, recirculating every time the wind blows.

However, there has been some progress. Legislation banning allergenic clonal male plants has started in some areas and is on the increase. Cities such as Albuquerque, New Mexico, have passed strict pollen-control ordinances that prohibit the sale or planting of the most allergenic of clonal male trees and shrubs. Likewise, Las Vegas, Nevada, banned the sale and planting of any more olive or male (fruitless) mulberry trees. Two major cities in Canada, Edmonton and Toronto, have already started to make a concerted effort to plant city trees that will not trigger asthma or allergies. In New Zealand, both Christchurch and Auckland have also shown that they wish to make their own cities as allergy friendly as possible.

In 2014, the California Department of Public Health released a Strategic Plan for Asthma, which strongly supports using more female trees, using more low OPALS-ranked trees and shrubs, not planting any more clonal male trees, and having a statewide pollen-control ordinance. Time will tell whether this ordinance will be enacted, but it is very encouraging. There have been several successful lawsuits over local pollen issues, and a respected university law review recently published an article on ways that parents can use the law to force school districts to use allergy-friendly landscaping.

My hope is that the people of the great city of New York, and any other city that still does not take the problem of allergies and asthma seriously, will fight back. No one expects a city to remove all their allergenic trees, but it is not unreasonable for them to stop planting any more highly allergenic trees. For more information on how you can effect change on a larger scale, see chapter 6. However, there is a great deal you can do right now, in your own garden, which is covered in the next chapter.

TWO

How to Fight Allergies
CLOSE TO HOME

You may wonder whether what you plant in your own yard can make any difference, because pollen can blow in from hundreds of miles away. But what you plant in your own yard most likely will make all the difference in the world. With pollen allergies, everything is in the actual dose received. If you have a headache and take two aspirin it will be just fine, but if you take twenty or thirty aspirin it will be terrible. It is the same thing with exposure to allergenic pollen; a small amount of pollen might well actually even be good for you, it would probably stimulate your immune system. But a very large overdose of pollen will quickly make many people ill. The closer you are to the source of the pollen, the greater your exposure will be.

A large pollinating tree will shed most of its pollen right next to the tree itself. The largest amount of this pollen will be found within a few dozen feet (or less) of the drip line of the tree. If the tree makes allergenic pollen, then those who live closest to this tree will get the biggest dose, the overdose. Yes, some of this pollen may drift on down the block, but exposure next to the tree may easily be well more than a hundred times greater than it would be a few houses away. Allergy researchers call this phenomena "proximity pollinosis."

You can understand proximity pollinosis by imagining cigar smoke. If someone is a block away from you, smoking a cigar, you might get exposed to a very small amount of secondhand smoke. However, your exposure would be so slight that you might not even notice. The opposite would be the case if you got onto an elevator and someone inside lit up that same fat, smelly cigar. Ah, now indeed you'd be exposed to it. This is locality, and this is the exact same principle that is at work with proximity pollinosis.

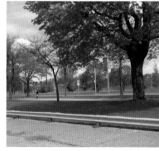

Male maple tree and pollen dispersal

Everyone Has a "Bucket"

It is well understood by many allergists that if someone is allergic to, say, six things, and three of them are removed, then the sufferer will often become symptom-free. This is an important insight. By creating an allergy-free yard, you will have eliminated the closest, most intense sources of what ails you. Even though your body will contact some allergens from outside your own area of control, your symptoms will probably diminish and sometimes they'll disappear. This leads us to the bucket theory of allergy.

When you get up in the morning and feel great, you have an "empty bucket." Then perhaps you absentmindedly run your hand over the top of the TV, kicking up a small dose of quickly inhaled dust. The dust goes "in your empty bucket."

At breakfast you may eat something you're allergic to and that, too, goes in your bucket. At this point you probably feel perfectly fine. You then inhale a dose of pollen from the bouquet of daisies on the table. This goes in your bucket, too. But there is still room in your bucket for a few more allergens and you still feel great. Your cat walks by and you inhale some cat dander. It goes in your quickly filling bucket, but still, you're all right.

Now you go outside to get the newspaper and a little puff of wind knocks a small cloud of invisible pollen from the seedless male tree overhead. You inhale this pollen-filled air, and those thousands of microscopic allergens go in your now almost-brimful bucket, all of a sudden overflowing it. Now you suddenly feel miserable.

It is usually the cumulative effect of multiple allergens that makes us feel lousy. The trick is to eliminate and avoid as many likely allergens as possible, to not let our buckets overflow. We need not eliminate all the allergens in our environments, just as many of them as we can. As with so many things, allergy is usually a question of degree. In the above case, with some safer trees in the garden, you might well have remained symptom-free.

Being symptom-free, by the way, should be the goal of all of those who have allergies or asthma; there is no real "cure" for these diseases. The best medicine for allergy is avoidance; avoid whatever triggers the allergy. With the right amount of avoidance, you'll remain symptom-free. As allergist David Stadtner, MD, has stated, "I have had many patients whose allergy symptoms improved by removing an offending tree or shrub near their home." Sometimes removing just one tree or large shrub can make a huge difference.

Finding the Best Plants

It is entirely possible to design a very good, low-pollen landscape by using the information in this book to select the best plants from those available at many quality nurseries and home garden centers. If you are buying plants at a nursery, especially trees or shrubs, don't buy them unless they are properly tagged. The tag should have the complete Latin name of the plant, with genus and species, and the plant's common name. For example, with the red maple tree commonly called "October Glory," the correct tag would read, in this precise order: *Acer rubrum* 'October Glory'. It also might be listed accurately but a tad differently, such as *Acer rubrum* c (or cv, or CV) 'October Glory'. The c or CV simply stands for "cultivar," which is the horticultural version of a cloned plant. You should always have in your hands a copy of *The Allergy-Fighting Garden*, so that you can compare the exact name of the plant in the nursery with the exact same plant in the book. If the plant is not named and ranked in the book, it's safest not to buy it. When looking over a tree or shrub in a container at a nursery, you'll have to compare the genus, the species, *and* the common name with what is listed in the book.

For years now I've been approaching large wholesale growers to see whether I could talk some of them into growing a collection of pollen-free plants or adopting OPALS tags (see chapter 9) on the plants they sell. This would make it very simple for shoppers to select the safest plants for them and their families. Unfortunately, to date there have been very few takers. One of the rare exceptions, so far, is the wholesale/retail grower and nursery Queux Patio Plants, on Guernsey, one of the Channel Islands. They are actively growing a large number of female plants. The owner of this nursery, Nigel Clarke, is totally committed to offering his customers the safest, healthiest, most allergy-free plants possible. His own nonprofit group, Green Legacy Guernsey, is committed to re-greening Guernsey, and doing so in a way that will not trigger allergies or asthma (see http://greenlegacyguernsey.org.uk).

There are already a number of places (some online) selling what they're calling "allergy-free plants," plants that are anything but. These should be approached with extreme caution. I have registered trademarks on both "allergy free gardening," and also on OPALS. No one is legally able to use these tags without permission, and I will not let people use the tags unless I am 100 percent convinced that the plants they're selling are exactly what they should be. If I can get more nurseries to agree to grow and sell pollen-free female plants, they will be listed on the SAFE Gardening website (www.safegardening.org).

Top-Grafting Sex Changes

If you are landscaping your yard from scratch and you follow the advice in this book on selecting low-allergy plants, you should be in good shape. But if you have an existing landscape, you will need to evaluate it to decide which plants can stay and which should be removed. In some cases, existing male trees can be top-grafted with scion wood from a female tree of the same species. This will affect a sex change. Some years ago I was talking to a midwestern city arborist about how his city had such an incredible number of male-cloned street trees. Most of these were recently planted, highly allergenic, male Chinese pistache trees. I told him that because these were fairly young trees, and because they were all deciduous, it would be a good idea to top-graft (or bud) them all over to female. He could do this in the winter when they were dormant. "You should give them all a sex change," I said.

The arborist shook his head and looked dismayed. "That is so California," he said. Perhaps it was, but I'd much rather graft a male tree to female than chop it down. I've top-grafted quite a few fruitless male mulberry trees. Every mulberry I grafted took. In one season those highly allergenic male trees were converted into allergy-free female trees.

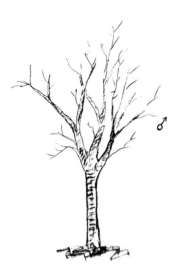 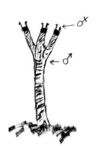 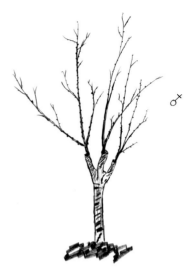

a. Dormant deciduous male tree before top-grafting.

b. Male tree cut back to three main branches and two scions of female wood cleft-grafted on each. (Two scions are used on each branch to increase the odds of a good take.)

c. Two years later, the strongest growing scion on each graft has been kept and the weaker one removed.

THE BIRDS AND THE BEES, AND THE BUTTERFLIES, TOO

Male trees produce no fruit for birds and small animals to eat, and they usually produce little or no nectar for butterflies, hummingbirds, and honeybees. The past three decades of sterile, litter-free landscapes have dramatically reduced urban food sources for many of nature's small creatures. As the sale of wind-pollinated, male cloned street trees expanded, it was accompanied by the decline in numbers of the cities' butterflies and honeybees. Deprived of major early-season food sources, many of these species simply starved. Allergy-free gardens and landscapes, with their reliance on female and insect-pollinated plants, may indeed be a bit messier. They will also bring us less allergy, less asthma, cleaner air, and more birds, honeybees, and butterflies.

Pollinator Plants, Bees, and Butterflies

The aim of an allergy-fighting garden is not to eliminate all pollen, but to strongly limit the amount of the most allergenic pollen. Most trees and shrubs in our yards and schools (but not necessarily all) should ideally be very low-pollen plants, or better yet, pollen-free female plants. We often don't need to be quite as careful with our smaller plants, the annuals and perennials, and actually it is beneficial on several levels to use many that are strictly insect-pollinated. It is good for our immune systems to be exposed to some pollen; this makes our bodies stronger. What isn't good is when we are overexposed to massive amounts of pollen.

Honeybees worldwide are in decline, but in urban areas that are rich in garden flowers they're often thriving. In my own gardens I always include flowering plants that attract and feed honeybees, bumblebees, butterflies, and other important pollinators; my many fruit trees always get well pollinated.

There are dozens of allergy-friendly plants that attract pollinators without causing allergies. Some of these make small amounts of large, sticky, not very allergenic pollen, and many others (especially among the mints, the mint relatives, and the salvias) are often pollen-free female plants. Female flowers make no pollen, but they almost always have very rich sources of nectar; female plants often use nectar to attract pollinators. I have long noticed that many all-female selections actually will outdraw pollinators. There are some very good books on gardening for pollinators, and on butterfly gardening, well worth owning. Attracting these creatures to your own garden will help the world, and it is just plain fun to see them working the flowers. Then, too, who doesn't appreciate seeing butterflies floating around in the garden?

A few of my favorite low-allergy, excellent pollinator plants:

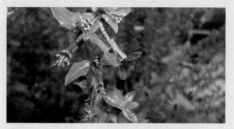

There are more than 250 species of **Cuphea** and all of them will attract pollinators, including hummingbirds.

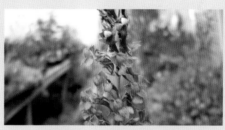

Linaria canadensis is an easy-to-grow, short-lived perennial with cute little blue, purple, or white flowers. In my yard, Linaria draws honeybees, native bees, bumblebees, and all manner of small (especially gray and blue) butterflies.

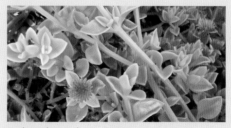

Red apple iceplant, *Aptenia cordata*, is only hardy to zone 8 (see Hardiness Zones, page 50), but it would be worth growing as an annual ground cover in colder climates.

Aptenia is a total honeybee magnet, produces no airborne pollen, and is super easy to root from cuttings. Aptenia will probably also winter over as a houseplant in colder zones.

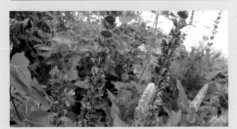

Salvia nemerosa is an attractive, small, easy-to-grow, winter-hardy perennial with nice purple flower spikes; it produces no pollen but lots of nectar, and it draws pollinators like crazy.

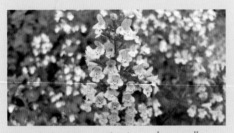

Nepeta nervosa, catmint, is another small, hardy, easy-to-grow perennial. It has fine little blue or white flowers and leaves with a wonderful minty smell. Nepeta is another total pollinator magnet in my garden and is almost never without some visitors.

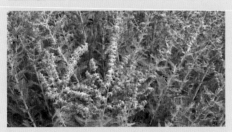

Russian sage, **Perovskia atriplicifolia**, is a hardy, tough perennial with small gray leaves, tolerant of all kinds of soils, and quite drought-resistant. In my garden it is a total honeybee magnet and also draws in small butterflies. With very low amounts of pollen but high amounts of nectar, Russian sage is a great addition to any allergy-friendly pollinator garden.

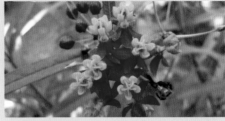

Asclepias species, the milkweeds; almost every garden should have a few of these beauties. There are hundreds of different milkweed species and all of them have merit. If possible, grow some that are native to your own area. Monarch butterflies are totally dependent on milkweed plants; they can lay and rear their young on no other species of plant. Milkweeds produce a white latex sap that is an irritant to the skin, and they're toxic to dogs, so keep these away from pets.

See **Asclepias** in the A to Z section of this book.

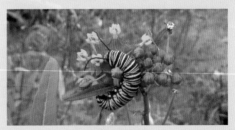

The caterpillar form of the monarch butterfly on Asclepias

THREE

Understanding Plant Sex
AND ITS IMPORTANCE IN ALLERGIES

Plant sex and allergies are intimately connected. Without an understanding of plant sex, we'll continue to suffer far too much.

In 1676 the English physician Sir Thomas Millington (*Anatomy of Plants*, 1682) first discovered that plants have a sex life. Botanist Christian Konrad Sprengel first wrote about dioecious (separate-sexed) plants and their abundant production of pollen in 1812. But in the puritanical climate of the early 1800s and in the late 1600s when Millington discovered plants' sex lives, it was considered lewd or obscene to speak or write of such things. Sprengel's work was largely ignored during his lifetime. Many botanical writers went to great lengths to avoid any words connected to sex, even avoiding using words such as *pollen*. Even the eminent plant geneticist Gregor Mendel (1822–1884) and the pioneering naturalist Charles Darwin (1809–1882) were both purposefully vague and obscure on floral sexual matters. As absurd as it sounds, I still find that many of the growers who propagate male plants today are not even aware that the plants are male. They simply think they are "seedless." Likewise, few of the landscapers and homeowners who buy and plant all these allergy-causing male trees and shrubs realize that they are male. Again, they think that they're just planting low-maintenance "fruitless" trees. They rarely think of the sex involved. Even most of our present-day botanists prefer to stick to the pristine PC terms *staminate* and *pistillate*, rather than simply using *male* and *female*. I, however, prefer to use the perfectly understandable words *male* and *female*. It would seem that the sexual revolution of the 1960s somehow was missed by many in botany and horticulture.

So, are all plants either male or female? No, not at all. Some of them are separate-sexed but by no means all of them. Let's explore the most basic flowering systems quickly. You probably won't remember all of this on first reading. That's fine. Just come back later and look it over if you get mixed up on the terms down the road.

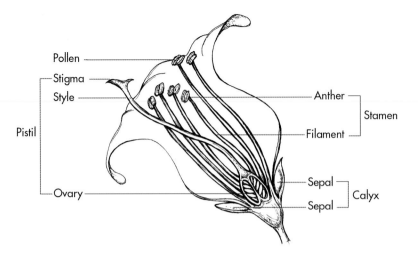

Pollen

Stigma

Style

Pistil

Ovary

Anther

Stamen

Filament

Sepal

Sepal

Calyx

Pistils and Stamens

The main female part of the flower is the pistil. On the tip of the pistil is the stigma, and it is here that pollen settles and sticks. Down at the base of the pistil are the ovaries (or ovules), where the seeds will eventually form. A separate-sexed plant that is all-female, one that has no male flowers on it at all, is what botanists call a "pistillate" plant. In all-female plants tips of the pistils (the stigmas) often have an almost feathery appearance.

The main male parts of a flower are the stamens. On the tip of each stamen is the anther, which holds a large collection of pollen grains. Pollen is the plant's equivalent of a male animal's semen. A flower that has only stamens and no female parts is called a "staminate" flower. Likewise, a separate-sexed (dioecious) plant that is all-male and has no female flowers is also called a staminate plant.

The goal of plants is to reproduce, and to do so, the pollen needs to get to the pistil. Female flowers (pistillate) on female trees or shrubs produce a negative (–) electrical current. Their stigmas are broad and sticky. Airborne pollen from male plants tumbles about in the air and picks up a positive (+) charge, and this pollen is light and dry. Because of the positive and negative electrical charges, the pollen and the stigmas (mutual attraction) are drawn to each other. Mother Nature saw to it that pollen would land, and stick, exactly where it was needed. Female plants are nature's best pollen traps, our most effective and potent natural air cleaners.

Today, though, most of the female plants are long gone from our urban landscapes. Female trees produce no pollen—zero; they are pollen-free trees, but they are scarce in most city landscapes. The pollen from the males floats about, seeking a moist, sticky, electrically charged target. We humans emit an electrical charge, and our mucus membranes—our eyes, skin, and especially the linings of our nose and throat—now trap this wayward pollen. We have become the targets. The farther that pollen needs to travel to find the female flower, the greater the chance that the pollen will accidentally end up in your nose instead. The distance that pollen is designed to travel depends on the type of plant—the shorter the distance, the less allergenic the plant; the longer the distance, the more allergenic the plant is likely to be.

Three Primary Types of Flowering Plants

There are three primary types of flowering plants: perfect, monoecious, and dioecious. **Perfect-flowered** plants (like a rose or an apple tree) have male and female parts in the same flower. This same system is also sometimes called bisexual, or hermaphrodite. The pollen doesn't have far to travel to reach the female parts, and they are usually pollinated by insects. As a result, perfect-flowered plants often cause fewer allergies. Some common perfect-flowered plants are most domestic strawberries, lilies, tulips, tomatoes, pears, roses, and magnolias. Unfortunately, some perfect-flowered plants are pollinated by both the wind and insects; a good example of this is goldenrod. Any time a plant is pollinated (even partially) by the wind, the potential for allergy increases greatly. Perfect-flowers can also be broken down into two groups, "perfect" and "complete." A complete flower has all the sexual parts; often a perfect flower that is not complete will be lacking some aspect of the flower, usually the petals. Next to actual all-female flowers, complete flowers represent (most of the time, but not always) the least allergenic choices.

Monoecious flowering plants have separate (unisexual) male and female flowers, both growing on the same plant. A good example of a monoecious plant is the pine tree. On the ends of the branches are clusters of male flowers (cones of pollen) and farther back in the tree are female flowers, which will turn into pinecones. Corn is another good example. The top of the corn plant, the tassels, are the male pollen-bearing flowers. Lower down on the plant, the ears of corn are actually clusters of female flowers. Other examples are begonias, cucumbers, cypress, birch, oaks, pecans, walnuts, and watermelons. Not all monoecious plants cause allergies, but many are wind-pollinated. Monoecious plants such as the Italian cypress, where the male parts are on the bottom of the plant and the female parts are on the top, are often highly allergenic because the pollen must be light and buoyant in order to float up to the female parts.

Dioecious plants are totally separate-sexed. With all dioecious plants, each individual plant will always be of just one sex, either a male, or a female, but not both. For example, with a dioecious red maple tree (*Acer rubrum*), one entire tree will be male, and another entire tree will be female. Males produce pollen, which makes them highly allergenic, while females do not. Females produce seeds or fruit. If a separate-sexed plant has seeds or fruit on it, it is always a female plant. If it never makes any seeds or fruit, it is probably (but not always) a male. A few examples of dioecious plants are asparagus, spider plants, red maples, box elders, junipers, yews, hollies, ash, poplars, date palms, poison ivy, kiwi vines, mulberries, willows, buffalograss, saltgrass, many species of bluegrass, some sedges, and pepper trees.

Other Flowering Systems

There are some other more complex and obscure flowering systems that are less common than the above systems, and I'll mention several of them here, briefly.

Androdioecious: These plants are either all-male individuals or bisexual, but they never make any plants that are all-female. Such species tend to be allergenic, and are often wind-pollinated. Some olive trees are androdioecious.

Gynodioecious: These plants are either all-female or bisexual, but they never produce any individuals that are all-male. Gynodioecious plants are almost never very allergenic and are often simply allergy-free plants. Catmints are good examples of this system.

Polygamous: These plants have both perfect-flowered flowers and single-sexed flowers on the same plant. A buckeye tree is a good example of polygamous flowering. On the tips of the flowering branches all the blooms are perfect-flowers, each individual flower complete with fertile female and male sex organs. However, 6 inches below the tips of the branch there will be many unisexual (one-sex) flowers, and with buckeye these will always be male-only flowers. The clusters of buckeye flowers are designed to be pollinated by both insects and the wind, and as a result, pollen from the male-only flowers indeed can become airborne and cause allergies.

However, sometimes a polygamous tree will have an assortment of perfect-flowers and unisexual all-female flowers. This is often seen with certain varieties of persimmons. A tree like this is almost always entirely insect-pollinated, will shed virtually no pollen, and so poses little allergy risk. This system, where there are perfect-flowers and unisexual female flowers (but no unisexual male flowers), is often found in the mints and salvias, and is always associated with low potential for pollen allergies.

CLONES AND CULTIVARS

Readers often get confused about the terms *clone* and *cultivar*. With trees, these words mean much the same thing. A cultivar is simply a cultivated variety, propagated (produced) asexually (without sex) by grafting, budding, layering, cuttings, or tissue culture. There are many cloned male trees and (fewer) cloned females ones.

Each cloned tree or shrub will normally have a Latin name, a common name, and a specific cultivar name. For example, take the red maple *Acer rubrum* 'Davey Red'. *Acer rubrum* is the Latin name. Red maple is the common name, and 'Davey Red' is the cultivar (clone) name. Every single tree of *Acer rubrum*, red maple, 'Davey Red' is cloned from the same original tree. In this case, the original tree was a female maple, so all of its clones are, too.

With shrubs, there are likewise many clonal selections (*selection* often being used to mean "cultivar") and most of these cloned shrubs are grown from cuttings. Nurseries prefer to grow trees and shrubs that are quick to root from cuttings, as this keeps their costs down.

Learning How to Tell the Boys from the Girls

I get a lot of email from people asking me how to tell the sex of a plant. "Am I supposed to turn it upside down and take a close look?" is one that I'm asked all the time.

No! It's not quite that simple.

Actually, though, with some species of plants it is very easy to determine the sex, but with others it takes someone trained in botany. One of the aims of this book, though, will be to make it a great deal easier for you to determine a plant's sex. And which sex is it we want to see used more in our gardens and landscapes? Females! More females. Feminists, we need you!

But before I get into how to tell the difference, let me give you a few examples of some confusion on this subject so that you can avoid mistakes. Some years ago I was asked to select the plant materials for a new low-pollen landscape that was being installed at the American Lung Association offices in Richmond, Virginia. The landscape designer had already installed a row of Himalayan junipers. Someone at the nursery where she bought these plants had told her that because they had berries on them, they were female. Now, most species of juniper are dioecious (separate-sexed) and berries are indeed an indication of femaleness in a separate-sexed species. However, Himalayan junipers are monoecious (both sexes on the same plant, remember?). I had to recommend that they pull up all of these plants, repot them, and return them to the nursery. They were replaced with female junipers.

In this same landscape, a dozen shrubs of yew, *Taxus* × *media* 'Densiformis', were used because, again, someone told the designer that this variety was always female. I did not recommend 'Densiformis' in my books then (nor do I now) because I had discovered that in the trade the variety is often confused. One nursery will sell a male version of it and another may sell a female one. The original 'Densiformis' yew had indeed been a female clone, but surety of this was no longer something gardeners could count on. In both these cases, the problem would have been avoided if a copy of *The Allergy-Fighting Garden* had been brought to the nursery and consulted to know with certainty which plants will be pollen-free and which will not be.

In the A to Z Plant Listings (page 52), the sex of a plant may not always be mentioned, but each plant variety will always have an OPALS ranking. A plant need not necessarily be female to be allergy-free, and a good OPALS ranking is always an indication of low potential to cause allergy or asthma. If you are able to purchase a plant that has an actual OPALS ranking (1 to 10) tag on it, then that is something you can trust.

I also advise talking to your nursery personnel and asking them about the sex of the plant in question. In the past few years quite a few retail nursery professionals have read my books themselves, many of them have heard me speak, and some have even taken classes from me. If you can find someone genuinely knowledgeable, he or she ought to be able to sex the plants for you.

Determining the Sex of Plants
Already Growing in Your Yard

If you or anyone in your family has allergies or asthma, in your own yards you may well want to remove the male plants and replace them with female ones.

Here you want to look for (and hopefully find) fruit, seeds, and/or seedpods. By "seeds" I mean seed such as the long, thin ones you would see on a female ash tree, or the winged seed on a female maple, or the hard nuts produced by a hazelnut bush. The term *seedpods* includes all those pod-forming shrubs, vines, and trees that produce seed-filled pods. These seed-bearing vessels may be long and fuzzy, such as the pods of a wisteria vine; long or smooth-sided, as found on a female honey locust tree; or flat and rounded, like the pods on a jacaranda tree. By "fruit" I mean any sort of plant-produced fleshy fruit or berry, not just edible fruits like apples or oranges. A rose hip is a fruit, as are the red berries of a hawthorn, pyracantha, or cotoneaster. Now, just because a plant has fruit on it doesn't mean that it is a female (it could be perfect-flowered or monoecious), *but* if it does have fruit or seeds or seedpods you can count on it that it is *not* a male plant.

But what if it is the wrong time of year and there are no fruits on any plants then? Must you then use a different strategy?

Many years ago a horticulture professor told me, when I asked him how to tell whether a plant was male, "Just look and see if it has any pollen on it." That advice was not nearly as good as it might have seemed. Male plants don't produce pollen all year-round. (Thank goodness!) Sometimes you just cannot tell the sex of a tree or shrub in your yard in late fall or during wintertime, when it is dormant. In this case, you may have to wait until springtime, when you can look at the actual flowers.

Male flowers will indeed have pollen, but bear in mind that pollen is not always that easy to see, nor is it always bright yellow. I've seen pollen that was white, gray, green, brown, red, and even purple. Nonetheless, once a tree is blooming, it is entirely possible to sex it.

Some of the Gender Giveaways of Common
Separate-Sexed Landscape Plants

Below is a list of some of the more commonly sold and used landscape shrubs, trees, and ground covers that are dioecious (separate-sexed). Within these species are the male plants you'll most want to avoid, and also the finest pollen-free female plants available. Here's what to look for to tell those boys from the girls.

Ash trees have small flowers that look like the winged seeds that eventually appear, if the tree is female. Female ash trees usually produce many seeds that often persist long into the season, still hanging on the trees. Also, every single ash tree that has been grafted (look for the graft mark low on the trunk) will be a male.

Female **cedar** trees (Cedrus species) produce large, fat, rounded cones that stand upright on the branches. The cones on male cedars are much smaller, much less than half as large as the cones on the female cedar trees. Do not confuse cedars with junipers, as is often done. They're two totally different species of plants.

Some types of currants, such as the hardy, deciduous shrub **Alpine currant**, only produce the small, bright red fruits on the female bushes.

Desert olive (*Forestiera neomexicana*) female trees and shrubs produce the small, blue to black olivelike fruits. Don't buy these unless they have fruit you can see, or if they are tagged OPALS #1 ranked female plants.

Fringe tree (Chionanthus species) females make small, olivelike, hard green fruits that turn almost black by fall. Males make no fruit at all.

Gold dust plant (*Aucuba japonica*) females produce thumbnail-size bright red fruits. Males make none. Only buy ones with the red fruit on them.

Hardy rubber trees (*Eucommia ulmoides*) and **tallow** trees (Sapium species) and other separate-sexed landscape trees, such as **Hovenia**, **Mallotus**, **Sapindus**, **Idesia**, and **Cudrania**, also make their small, long-lasting small fruits on only the female trees.

Holly (Ilex species) are all dioecious, so only female hollies make berries. Sometimes these need a male pollinator somewhere near to set a good crop of red berries, but not always. Some female hollies set a large crop of berries without any pollination at all. This fruit that sets without being pollinated is called parthenocarpic fruit. Any holly with any fruit is a female plant.

Junipers (Juniperus species), which are some of the very most common landscape shrubs and trees in the world, are mostly separate-sexed, but not all of them. When buying junipers, you only want female plants. You do not want junipers that have both sexes on the same plants (monoecious junipers) and you certainly don't want separate-sexed male junipers.

Of the many species of junipers that are dioecious (separate-sexed) only the female plants have the round, blue-green juniper berries. But with the monoecious juniper species, all of them have berries. In much of Utah, almost all the wild juniper trees are monoecious. They all have berries there. But in most other areas, only the female trees or shrubs have fruit.

When buying junipers to plant, be sure to take a copy of *The Allergy-Fighting Garden* along with you and carefully compare the data. If you have a large juniper in your own yard, and it has fruit on it, that's a very positive sign. But if you suspect it might be a monoecious species, you'll need to check and see whether you can find the small, numerous, brown male pollen "cones," which are born on the tips of the branches. If you're still confused on this one, pick a piece of it and take it to your county

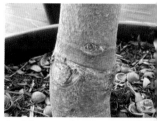

Graft line on ash tree

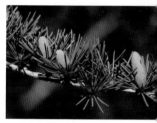

Female cedar tree

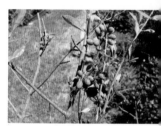

Forestiera, female

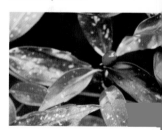

Aucuba japonica, female

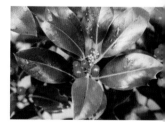

Ilex, female

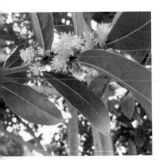

Laurus nobilis, male

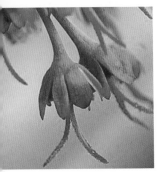

Acer rubrum, female

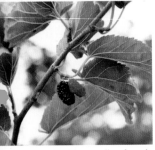

Morus alba, female

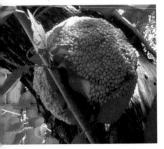

Maclura pomifera, female

agriculture agent and see whether he or she can identify it for you. If all else fails, email me a photo and we'll get to the root of it eventually.

If you have allergies, one thing you don't need is a pollinating juniper in your own yard. I have posted a clear photo of a monoecious juniper on my website, www.allergyfree-gardening.com. On this same website you can also find photos of numerous male and female flowers of a great many species.

Kaffir plum trees (*Harpephyllum caffrum*), common in mild-winter areas, only have the olive-size red fruits on female trees. Males make nothing but pollen.

Mature female **bay laurel** trees (*Laurus nobilis*) make small, green and then turning black, olive-like fruits that persist on the trees for many months. Male trees are fruitless. Most trees now sold, such as 'Saratoga', are clonal males.

Kentucky coffee tree (*Gymnocladus dioicus*) females make the big, dark seedpods. The male trees are much more popular because they don't make the big, messy seedpods, but they're the ones with the pollen.

Female **red maple** or **silver maple** trees (Acer species) in bloom have small flowers that look a great deal like the winged seeds they eventually turn into. These female flowers will always be paired in twos. This is also true for **box elders**, which are actually a type of maple tree, and it is also true for some of the other separate-sexed maples such as Devil's Maple or Horned Maple, and the Ivy-Leafed Maple.

Mirror plant (Coprosma), of which there are a great many species, forms small, soft, bright red berries on female plants only. Many female mirror plants can make viable fruit even if they are never pollinated by a male plant.

Female **mulberry** trees produce large crops of fruits much favored by kids and birds (and me). Male mulberry trees, sold as "fruitless" mulberry, produce huge amounts of very allergenic pollen. Weeping mulberry trees used to always be female forms that were top-grafted onto a standard seedling rootstock (or grafted onto a cutting-grown male mulberry). Now, however, nurseries are selling a male weeping mulberry tree called 'Chaparral', and it is a male tree you do not want. Weeping *Morus alba* 'Pendula' will always be a female, pollen-free tree.

Osage orange trees (*Maclura pomifera*) make big, baseball-size, round orange fruits only on the female trees. Male osage orange trees make no fruit, but a great deal of very allergenic pollen. These trees are related to mulberries. There are several clones sold that are thornless, but unfortunately, they're male trees.

Oso Berry, **Silverberry**, and **Bear Berry**, attractive, cold-hardy shrubs, are all separate-sexed and only form their small red or silver fruits on the female plants.

Female **palm** trees and female **pepper** trees will usually hang on to some fruit almost all year long. All pepper tree species and some species of palms are dioecious (separate-sexed). If you have any species of pepper tree or, for example, a Phoenix palm, a Bismarck palm, or Windmill palm, and it has any fruit on it at all, you're in luck. It's a female tree. Keep in mind, though, that many palm trees are monoecious; see the A to Z section of this book for the actual species of palm tree you're considering. There are a great multitude of different palm species.

Persimmon trees (Diospyros species) are almost all sold as dioecious (separate-sexed) trees. Many of these, such as 'Fuyu', will be female trees that can produce good crops of seedless fruit. Any fruiting kind of persimmon will be a female tree. Persimmon trees, by the way, can be exceptionally attractive during all seasons of the year, and they should be used more often in the landscape. Most cultivars of persimmon can make fruit without a pollinating male tree.

Pistache trees (Pistacia species) of all species are dioecious and females will form clusters of small, persistent fruits, often bright red colored. Males produce none. All budded or grafted trees of Chinese pistache will prove to be males . . . avoid them.

Podocarpus. See yews and yew pines.

Sassafras trees (*Sassafras albidum*) produce small black fruits only if they're female. These trees will spread in the wild from roots that sprout. Sometimes an entire hillside will be covered with sassafras trees all of the same sex, essentially clones of each other. So if you have a male sassafras tree in your yard, be on the alert!

With landscape shrubs such as **Shiny Xylosma**, **Griselinia**, **Osmanthus**, and **Laurel Snailseed** (*Cocculus laurifolius*), the female plants may form small, rounded black fruits. Male plants of these species never make any fruits or seeds.

Smoke tree (Cotinus species), and its other poison ivy–related relatives like **African sumac** and the **varnish** trees, produces clusters of small, round, long-lasting, usually translucent watery fruits, only on the female plants. The fruits on a female smoke tree are normally tiny, and if you squish one in your fingers, there will be a single hard seed inside of it.

Wax myrtle (Myrica species) bushes make clusters of the small sweet-smelling, waxy berries only if they're female. The exception to this is the Pacific wax myrtle, *Myrica californica*, as these can be all-female, all-male, or monoecious. With this species it is best to buy either an OPALS-tagged fruiting plant or one that actually has fruit on it when you buy it.

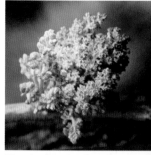

Pistacia chinensis, female

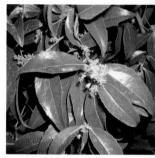

Xylosma, male

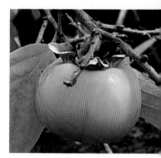

Diospyros, female

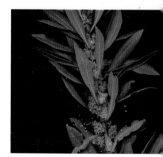

Myrica, male

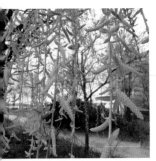

Salix, male

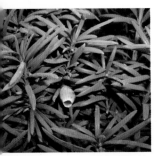

Taxus, female

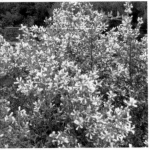

Baccharis pilularis, female

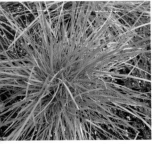

Poa fendleriana

Willows and **poplar** (Salix species and Populus species, respectively) are all dioecious. Their flower clusters, long, often drooping catkins (and this includes all the cottonwoods, popples, and aspens), have hundreds of tiny stamens, each tipped with a minute cluster of bright yellow pollen, if the tree is a male. Female flowers on willows and poplars look quite similar but lack the bright yellow-tipped stamens. So-called "pussy willows" are grown for their attractive flowers (catkins), and these shrubs or small trees may be either male or female plants, but males are far more commonly used because they make the most attractive flowers.

Poplars and willows that produce "cotton," that fluffy material that blows all over the place in spring, are female trees. The "cotton" is actually just masses of fluffy seeds and it is often mistakenly blamed for causing allergies. Certain cultivars of willow and poplar will always be either male or female, and for these you should first consult the OPALS rankings in the A to Z plant section of this book.

Yews (Taxus species) and **yew pines** and **fern pines** (Podocarpus species) are separate-sexed. Female yews will set marble-size, hard to miss, bright red fruits. Female Podocarpus make round, marble-size, hard greenish blue fruits that eventually turn a light yellow color. Males of all Podocarpus and yew species produce copious amounts of pollen that is both highly allergenic and quite poisonous.

With some of the less common separate-sexed shrubs such as the beautiful yewlike **Cephalotaxus**, and the stiff-leafed evergreen **Torreya**, once again it is only the females that produce the grape-size, red, round fruits. With Cephalotaxus, unfortunately, in the trade almost all plants sold are clones, and all of these are males.

With the landscape ragweed relatives, the ground cover **coyote brush** (Baccharis species), and the flowering shrub **Olearia**, the female plants make large amounts of fluffy, cottonlike seeds. The "litter-free" male plants just produce that "invisible litter," allergenic pollen.

There are many other separate-sexed plants; some are vines, some are houseplants, some are cactuslike succulents, some are trees, and some are grasses. In all of these dioecious species only the females form seeds or fruits. With dioecious grasses, such as many of the **bluegrass** species (Poa), **saltgrasses** (Distichlis spicata), or **buffalo** grasses (Buchloe dactyloides), it sometimes really does take an expert to tell the boys from the girls. But with most of the other species, you can usually do it yourself.

FOUR

Allergy-Blocking Hedges

One of the best things you can do to protect yourself and your family from allergenic pollen is to plant a tall allergy-free hedge on the windward side of your property. The more room you have, the taller and wider the hedge can be. On a very large property it would make good sense to plant a row of female trees, and then next to the trees, plant a row of allergy-free shrubs to form a tight hedge. The actual plants you would want to use for these protective hedges will differ, depending on the size of the property and the area's plant zone of winter hardiness. Almost any hedge of this kind will stop incoming pollen, but ideally you would want one that would eventually get to 6 feet tall, or taller.

The ideal protective hedge is one that is naturally healthy, disease-free, and bug-free; it should be something that is attractive, easy to grow, and fairly fast growing. The very most important thing about a protective hedge is that it should be made up of plants with low OPALS-rankings; it should ideally be an all-female hedge, or at least one that when it flowers sheds very little pollen. Native plants, if you can get them in a low-pollen or female form, are often excellent choices, because they generally thrive in their native areas. Some other things to consider:

Wind direction: In most areas there will be a prevailing wind, or most of the breeze or wind will generally come from one direction. I live a dozen miles from the Pacific Ocean, and here the prevailing wind is from the west. In each geographical area it may well be different. If the prevailing wind in your area is from, for example, the west, then ideally you'd want your hedge to go on the furthermost western side of your property.

Pollen travel: Prevailing winds sometimes pick up pollen from far away, but almost always they catch pollen from all the allergenic plants close by in your own neighborhood. A tall hedge planted on the side of your property, one that will act as a wind block, will also catch, trap, and stop a great deal of pollen, mold spores, dust, and other allergenic particulates from coming into your yard. Besides stopping incoming pollen, the right tall protective hedge will also provide for privacy, block wind, and shut out considerable outside noise.

Ocean properties: If you're one of the very lucky people who live right next to the ocean, you don't need a protective hedge on the ocean side, as the air that comes off the ocean is about as pollen-free as any you can find. Still, even in a choice spot like this, it makes very good sense to have a protective hedge on the side of your property that is between you and the inland side.

Protection from traffic-caused air pollution: Anyone who lives close to a very busy street or worse, to a busy highway or freeway, would certainly benefit from a tall protective hedge between them and the traffic. There is a well-documented strong link between shortened life spans and proximity to heavy traffic. If you live very close to a freeway, consider moving at the first opportunity. If you can't move, and if you have the space, do consider planting a tall protective hedge to block some of this negative vehicular influence.

Keeping your hedge clean: Many times a hedge like this will also stop dust, smoke, and other forms of air pollution, and when your hedge is in a polluted urban and/or dusty place, these plants do need to be cleaned regularly. The best way to clean a big hedge is with a garden hose and a nozzle. The entire hedge should be hosed down, top to bottom, as often as needed. This could be weekly, but in most areas a monthly good hosing down will help keep it clean.

Full sun or shade: If the hedge is to grow in an area that is shaded, it is of key importance that only plants that have good shade tolerance be used. Shrubs without shade tolerance, if planted in the shade, may grow but they won't thrive, and soon they may be weak, and will then attract insect pests and eventually mildew and other mold spores.

How big, how tall: Ideally, a protective hedge is one that does not need to be sheared or pruned all the time. Each type of tree or shrub will eventually grow to a certain size, and it's always smart not to plant things that might end up getting far larger than the space you're planning to grow them in. For example, you could use female cottonwood trees, planted closely together, as a tall, protective hedge. Of course, over time these, would grow into huge trees, and unless you had a great deal of room, it just wouldn't be practical. It would be better to plant something that over time will grow to a size your yard can handle.

Very tall hedges: Big tall hedges can be used where there is ample room and space. Female willows and female poplars (aspen, cottonwoods, and poplars) can be planted from potted plants, bare-root plants, or direct-stuck dormant cuttings. Perhaps the best selection for this type of hedge is the female selection *Populus* 'Thieves Select'. This tall, narrow, fast-growing selection is winter hardy in all zones. *Bambusa oldhamii*, timber bamboo, can work well in mild winter areas.

To be avoided: Privet hedges (Ligustrum species) are very common and many of them need to be sheared and topped back several times a year. Privet is a poor choice for a protective hedge because they produce considerable allergenic pollen. Other common but poor choices, because of their allergy potential, are male yews, male junipers, male willows, any kind of cypress (including Leyland cypress), olive trees, desert olive (unless it is a female clone), and arborvitae. Russian olive trees are often used as big hedges, but they are quite allergenic and should be avoided. 'Lombardy' poplar trees are also commonly used, but all of them are male clones and allergenic. Lilac bushes can make a tall hedge, but the smell of the flowers will bother most perfume-sensitive individuals.

Excellent Choices for Hedges

Here are some suggestions for plants that work well as allergy-blocking hedges.

Dodonaea viscosa 'Naomi', purple hopseed bush, is a tall, erect female plant, very bushy, and evergreen in zones 9 and 10. Fast-growing and insect- and disease-free, it makes a dense tall hedge if planted on 4-foot centers. 'Naomi' is a selected female shrub or small tree, is pollen-free, and is resistant to urban smog. Without any pruning it can reach 15 to 18 feet in height, and 6 to 8 feet wide, but the sides can be sheared and kept to 4 feet wide or less.

Coprosma 'Big Glossy Girl' is a fast-growing, evergreen shrub or small tree, native to New Zealand. 'Big Glossy Girl' is a pollen-free female selection and if planted on 3-foot centers will quickly make a thick, glossy green hedge. Best in zone 10 and does very well near the ocean. 'Big Glossy Girl' can be sheared and kept to almost any size, but is easily held to 8 to 10 feet tall and 3 to 4 feet wide. Needs full sun.

Griselinia littoralis 'Lillian Grace' is a new, soon-to-be released variegated female shrub for zones 9 to 10. 'Lillian Grace' is exceptionally handsome and disease- and insect-free, grows quickly, and is very drought-tolerant once established. It can be sheared if need be and will make a sturdy 10-foot-tall by 6-foot-wide hedge.

Griselinia littoralis 'Green Girl' is a green-leafed female selection, similar to 'Lillian Grace' but with somewhat smaller all-green leaves, and it grows a bit faster. Of the two Griselinia selections, 'Green Girl' may have a bit more winter hardiness, and may grow better in hotter inland locations. Very drought-tolerant once well established. *Note:* Almost all other forms of Griselinia sold in the U.S. are males and to be avoided.

Pittosporum tenuifolium 'Susan' is an easy-to-grow, attractive, evergreen, pollen-free female selection that makes a fine 8- to 10-foot-tall hedge in zones 9 to 10. Drought-tolerant once established, it grows best in full sun, but will tolerate some light shade.

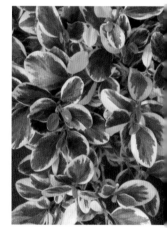

Griselinia

Pittosporum tenuifolium 'Tall Girl' is a fast-growing, pollen-free female selection that will quickly get to 12 feet tall if given adequate water when young. Planted on 3-foot centers, 'Tall Girl' will make an attractive protective hedge that requires little care. Leaves on 'Tall Girl' are smaller than those of 'Susan', and the stems of the new wood are almost black in color.

Rhamnus alaternus 'Italian Girl' is a fast-growing, pollen-free female selection that will quickly get to 12 feet tall if given adequate water when young. Planted on 3-foot centers,

'Italian Girl' will make an attractive protective hedge that requires little care. Leaves are glossy and attractive, and these female plants may make some small red berries that birds like. 'Italian Girl' will take a good amount of shearing if needed, and can easily be held to a height of 8 to 12 feet, and a width of 3 to 4 feet. Hardy to 12°F, zones 7 to 10, 'Italian Girl' is very drought-tolerant once established. Good choice for spots where the hedge must go into both full sun and shade, as it is shade-tolerant.

Laurus nobilis 'Guernsey Girl' and 'California Girl' are two pollen-free, evergreen, female tree/shrub selections of the noble bay laurel tree. In Europe, 'Guernsey Girl' would be the preferred cultivar, and in the U.S., 'California Girl' would work best. Both of these selections may make a few attractive fruits the size of a small olive, but neither is a messy tree and they work well near sidewalks. Long-lived, easy to grow, moderate growth rate, with dark green large leaves that are aromatic when crushed. Both of these cultivars will grow in either sun or shade, and they are tolerant of shearing. Ultimate size of these as hedges (depending on the amount of yearly shearing) could be as small as 6 feet tall and 3 feet wide, or they could be allowed to grow much taller and wider if desired. Best in zones 8 to 10, either of these plants will also work as a houseplant in a sunny exposure. Drought-tolerant, either cultivar will make a tall, dense hedge if planted on 3- to 4-foot centers; they are also excellent as stand-alone trees. (Not to be confused with the California bay laurel tree, *Umbellularia californica*, a moderately allergenic species not well suited as a hedge plant.)

Podocarpus gracilior 'Rachel Carson' fern pine is a very attractive, pollen-free, fast-growing female tree or shrub. Very suitable as a stand-alone large evergreen tree, 'Rachel Carson' is also highly adaptable to close planting as hedge material. Best in zones 9 to 10, it is very drought-tolerant once established. 'Rachel Carson' is unusual because although it is female, it rarely makes any fruit. Excellent for a dense, glossy green, easily grown hedge, especially where a good deal of height is needed. The width of the hedge can be sheared and kept to as little as 3 to 4 feet wide. Hedges, if never topped, could exceed 20 feet in height. Good choice also as a fairly quick privacy hedge between two closely spaced two-story houses, with plants set on 3- to 4-foot centers.

Podocarpus macrophyllus 'Pearl Buck' is a pollen-free, nonfruiting female tree or shrub, smaller in potential size than *Podocarpus gracilior* 'Rachel Carson'. Leaves of 'Pearl Buck' are gray-green in color. Slower growing than 'Rachel Carson', it also requires less annual shearing to maintain a size of 8 feet tall and 4 feet wide.

Ribes alpinum 'Northern Girl' currant is a very useful, tough, easy-to-grow, very hardy, pollen-free, fruiting female hedge plant suitable for the coldest plant zones, best in zones 3 to 7. Planting on 2-foot centers will result in a dense, 6- to 8-feet-tall hedge that can be kept sheared to 4 to 5 feet wide. Attractive glossy green leaves with little bright white flowers are followed by small cute red berries that are not messy and are appreciated by numerous species of songbirds. Deciduous, and needs adequate soil moisture to thrive.

Myrica pensylvanica 'Northern Girl' bayberry is a tough, winter-hardy native shrub suitable for informal tall hedges in northern climates. 'Northern Girl' is a heavily fruiting, pollen-free female selection; the small bluish fruits are clustered on the stems and are eaten by numerous songbirds; they are also the main source for bayberry wax for scented-candle making. Average water needs, the plant is drought-tolerant once established. Deciduous in winter, 'Northern Girl', when planted on 2-foot centers, will make a 6- to 8-foot-tall hedge. A good plant for sandy or poor soil areas, will do best only in acid or slightly acid soils. Zones 2 to 7.

Myrica pensylvanica 'Myriman' is a male, pollen-producing plant. If one 'Myriman' plant is used for each six female plants, a good set of fruit will be ensured. Do not plant 'Myriman' by itself or it could trigger allergies. As a small part of a female hedge, though, it will present no allergy potential.

Myrica pensylvanica 'Myda' is another female selection of northern wax myrtle (bayberry) that is very winter hardy, fruits heavily, and can also be used as an informal hedge plant. 'Morton' (Silver Sprite), a new female fruiting selection, forms a dense, broad oval mound with gray-green leaves. Unfortunately, it grows to only 5 feet tall.

Myrica cerifera 'Southern Girl' wax myrtle (bayberry) is another tough, useful, fruiting female native shrub selection. Adapted best to the U.S. southeastern states, 'Southern Girl' will grow in zones 6 to 10, but will do best in acid soil with adequate moisture. Similar to all the forms of wax myrtle, 'Southern Girl' does not need fertile soil to grow and thrive. Planted on 2-foot centers, it will make a 6- to 10-foot-tall informal hedge. Tolerant of shearing, it is best used where it can grow in a less formal form. The fruit is also used in making fragrant wax myrtle candles. Southern wax myrtle, if not topped, can get more than 20 feet tall; the species is less drought-tolerant than other Myrica species. Deciduous in winter.

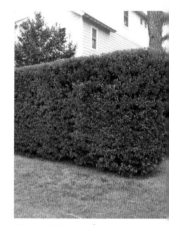

Myrica, Wax myrtle

Myrica californica 'California Lady' is a heavy fruiting selection of native, western wax myrtle. Evergreen, 'California Lady' does best in zones 8 to 10. Adaptable to shearing, a fairly fast-growing hedge can be had by planting on 2- to 3-foot centers. Tolerant of heavy clay soils, 'California Lady' is very drought-tolerant once established. In coastal areas it should only be planted in full sun, but in hotter inland areas it can tolerate more shade. Small waxy fruits are eaten in winter by songbirds, especially by the yellow-rumped warblers. 'California Lady' is not an all-female plant, but because the female flowers on it are quite fertile and pollen production from its male flowers is fairly low, it can still be recommended for a tall protective hedge. Size can be held to 6 to 12 feet tall by 3 to 5 feet wide.

Feijoa sellowiana, pineapple guava, is a fruiting shrub or small tree for zones 8 to 10 that can be used quite well as a tall, protective, low-allergy privacy hedge. Although the perfect flowers of the Feijoa will produce some pollen, the production is not great and the plant has a low (good) OPALS ranking of 3. Planted on 2- to 3-foot centers, one-gallon plants will quickly grow into a hedge of around 8 to 10 feet tall and 4 to 5 feet wide. Feijoa is easy to grow, disease- and insect-resistant, and once well established, quite

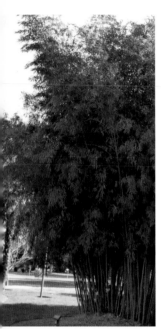

Phyllostachys bambusoides

drought-tolerant; the plants also make large numbers of very delicious guava-like fruit. Fruit will be quite a bit larger if the plants are irrigated regularly.

There are hundreds of different species and cultivars of bamboo, and many of the taller ones are very suitable for a tall hedge. Likewise, there are different species of bamboo for almost every climate, but if you live in a cold winter climate, you must pick a species that can take the cold. An ideal bamboo would be one that is hardy and fast-growing, and that grows to a height that you want. Do some basic research on bamboo before deciding which one to use. Most bamboo species are monocarpic, which means they only bloom once in their lifetime (and then go to seed and die); as such, they have very little allergy potential.

With any bamboo cultivar, no one can say with certainty how long it will live—it could be a few years, or it might last for a hundred. Because it blooms so infrequently, bamboo is almost never an allergy problem, and the right bamboo can make a top-quality, very fast-growing privacy hedge that will also protect from pollen of other species. *Note*: Most bamboo is either "clumping" or "running." With running bamboo, you must put in a root barrier on both sides of the bamboo, or else it could quickly spread into areas where you don't want it. There are relatively inexpensive heavy plastic root barrier materials to use, and these should go down 2 feet deep into the ground to keep the bamboo in check.

Ilex species (holly), especially 'Nellie Stevens', can make a very good evergreen hedge in zones 6 to 8. 'Nellie Stevens' grows fast, is a fruiting female tree, and forms a dense, long-lived tall hedge. With some shearing it can be kept to around 6 to 8 feet in width; height may eventually get to 20 or more feet tall. The leaves are shiny and attractive, but they are prickly.

Forestiera pubescens and *Forestiera neomexicana* (desert olive) is a native, multibranched, deciduous shrub or small tree, 8 to 15 feet tall, with smooth, gray bark, arching branches, somewhat spiny branchlets, and light green leaves. Male desert olive plants are allergenic, but the soon-to-be released cultivar 'Desert Girl' is a fast-growing, pollen-free female plant. The tiny blue, olive-like fruits are enjoyed by wild birds and not messy. 'Desert Girl' is tough and insect- and disease-free, and will grow in almost any soil type. Once established, it is extremely drought-tolerant. It will grow in the hottest deserts, the mountains, or in most urban areas. Plants given more water will grow taller, faster. Probably not best for low pH (acid) soils. Zones 4 to 10.

A great many Taxus species (yews) sold are male clones and these are very allergenic. Nonetheless, if you find a yew with small red berries, it is a female. A newer female cultivar, suitable for tall hedges in zones 5 to 8, is *Taxus* × *media* 'Hicks Select'. This pollen-free cultivar will eventually grow to around 10 to 12 feet tall, and the width can be clipped to a very narrow 2 feet or so if desired; tolerant of shade but grows faster in full or partial sun. Slow to moderate growth rate.

Atriplex lentiformis, quailbush, is a separate-sexed gray-leafed shrub species native to the southwestern deserts of the U.S. Tough and easy to grow, male plants are quite allergenic, but females are pollen-free. Look for the female selection 'Quail Girl'. Seeds (on female plants) are readily eaten by quail and other wildlife. Not a plant for a formal, clipped hedge, it can nonetheless be a useful hedge plant in desert areas where little else will grow and thrive. Unpruned, it will eventually get to 8 feet tall, and as wide.

Grayia spinosa, hopsage bush, is another tough, native desert shrub that is separate-sexed. Female plants make reddish hoplike seedpods that are very attractive. Hopsage will only grow in soil that is neutral to alkaline, but it grows wild from the deserts to the mountains of the southwestern U.S. In each area the plants often look quite different. If used as a wild hedge, it can grow to 6 feet tall and around 4 feet wide. Plants that are pruned once a year will be bushier and have more attractive foliage. Once established, it's extremely drought-tolerant. The leaves are small and gray colored. Look for the female cultivar 'Hopsage Sally'. Zones 6 to 10.

Juniperus scopulorum 'Wichita Blue' is 10 to 18 feet tall, 4 to 6 feet wide, and grows in zones 5 to 9. 'Wichita Blue' is a compact, conical, evergreen shrub that makes a good thick hedge. Most 'Wichita Blue' plants are female and make berries, but occasionally the form has been mixed up in the trade. If possible, buy one with an OPALS #1 tag on it. Fast-growing and moderately drought-tolerant once established.

Fruiting pear trees often grow tall and narrow, and can be planted close together to form a hedge. Apple and plum trees can also be planted close and used as an informal hedge. In zones 10 and 11, banana trees or giant bird-of-paradise plants can be used to make a tall hedge/screen. Rose of Sharon can be used for an informal, relatively tall hedge, and the double-flowered forms are often pollen-free. Certain tall species of viburnum can be used for hedges, but many evergreen forms are not shade-tolerant.

FIVE

Eliminating
ALLERGY-CAUSING MOLD SPORES

Tiny mold spores cause plenty of allergies. Often our gardens are full of molds, but luckily there are many things we can do to eliminate allergy-causing mold spores. All molds produce tiny reproductive spores and the trick is to find ways to get rid of the molds themselves.

Location

What we plant, and where, has a large influence. I continually see the flat-out dumb practice of planting tall evergreen trees and shrubs on the south sides of houses. In the winter the sun is low on the horizon and we get most of our light, and warmth, from the sunlight that shines from the south. Our warm morning light comes from the east, and it is never a good idea to block that with tall evergreens either. The best place for tall evergreens is on the north side of our houses. There they can act as a windbreak and not rob us of any needed winter sunlight.

A house with tall evergreen trees on the southeast side is one that will always be cold, and damp, in the winter months. And cold and damp is exactly what mold thrives on.

I was once at a store, standing outside waiting for a friend to finish up inside. It was a cool wintry day and I was in the full, deep cold shade of a very large Canary Island pine tree. I walked over about thirty feet and stood in a spot in between the trees where the sun was shining through. There it was nice and warm. To my left was the big pine shading that store, and just to my right was another huge evergreen tree, a *Ficus retusa*, the Indian laurel fig.

The big fig cast a shade even deeper, and colder, than did the pine. I looked down at the sidewalk to my left and right, and sure enough, you could see mold growing in the cracks and along the edges. The north side of the trees, where I was, also had a good deal of mold growing on the tree leaves themselves.

Deciduous trees are perfect for these locations. In the hot summer they will be all leafed out and will cool down the buildings behind them. In the cold winter months they will be bare of leaves, and the low sunlight will come through and warm things up. In this day and age of exploding energy costs, it is just plain ignorant to plant evergreens where they don't belong. For stopping mold spores, planting deciduous trees on the southeastern exposure is the only way to go.

Mulches

Many people seem unclear on just exactly what mulch is. Very simply, mulch is anything that covers the soil. It can be made of old leaves, straw, rocks, bark, gravel, boards, bricks, even plastic.

Mulch holds down weeds and cuts down on summer water loss. Earthworms often thrive under mulch, and in general mulches usually help plants grow better. Mulches are almost always a very good idea, but when it comes to mulches and molds, they aren't all created equally. Bark is a very good material on which to grow mold. Newspaper mulches not only look trashy, but they also grow lots of mold. Gravel mulches are good because they don't encourage mold growth. I like smooth gravels and river gravel. Flat stones and pavers work well for this too, and in the right spot, they look good as well.

The one spot where mulches are less effective is in those cold, always shaded areas. Here mulch will keep the soil from ever warming up. Everywhere else, though, mulch is useful.

Airflow

In every place there are prevailing winds. The breeze generally blows mostly from one direction. Many landscapes are so plugged up, so crowded, that the breeze simply can't penetrate the mess. A landscape with no airflow is one where molds will thrive. Molds grow best in conditions with poor air circulation.

If your own yards are overgrown and choked for lack of fresh air, then get out the pruning saw and start thinning them out. Clean, fresh air, free to move about, equals less mold and fewer mold spores.

Sunlight

Bright light and fresh air are the enemies of mold. Many landscapes have huge trees that let in little light. Consider hiring a tree trimmer to thin out some of the branches overhead. Open the trees up so that the sunlight can come through. Perhaps it would be a good idea to actually remove a tree or two if they're growing too close together. Let the light shine!

When planting any new tree, always consider the shade that it will cast when it is full grown. Certain trees always develop very thick canopies while others will be light and airy.

Watering and Irrigation

Perhaps as important as any other single mold factor is the watering. Too little water makes for weak plants that attract insects. Too much water will also always produce weak plants.

Automatic irrigation systems, on timers, are responsible for a great deal of mold growth. Allergists in desert areas often find very high mold spore counts in the middle of the summer! Much of this is being directly caused by irrigation systems that are not being monitored closely enough. Often they are set to irrigate lawns that are already still soggy from the last watering. Overwatered lawns will quickly become mold factories and will shower everyone near them with an abundance of mold spores.

Insects and Disease

Plants that are not being grown correctly will usually get infested with insects. The insects secrete "honeydew" and on this very nutrient-rich gooey substance, molds grow quickly. The molds then start producing spores and pretty soon there is a serious allergy situation in the landscape. The insect dander itself is highly allergenic and just adds to the problem. Buggy plants often look dirty and this is because they are covered with honeydew, mold, and yuck! They *are* dirty. Clean, healthy plants are what we want in our yards.

Why are the plants covered with insects? Well, if a tree is native to the cold, damp forests of Japan or Minnesota, it just won't thrive in a place like Los Angeles. It certainly might grow in Los Angeles, though, and that's the problem. It will grow there, but it won't thrive. Because it doesn't have the conditions it needs, it will always be somewhat weakened, and pests always prey on the weak. Remember, insect pests equal mold spores.

If an area is very deficient in fertilizer, the plants there won't thrive. As they grow weaker, insects start to prey on them. However, if plants are getting far too much fertilizer, they will also become weak.

If a tree is a type that needs regular water in the summer but never gets it, again it may become weak and soon be a target for whiteflies, aphids, scale, spider mites, and mealybugs.

If shrubs or trees are native to an area with acid soil and you're growing them in alkaline soil, sure enough they'll probably become bug infested. The reverse is also true.

If a tree is simply not tolerant of urban smog and it is planted right smack in the middle of a great metropolis, it will almost always draw pests and become an allergy problem.

If a row of shrubs are all the kind that love bright sunshine, but someone has planted a fast-growing tree over them, perhaps a pine, and now the whole row of shrubs is growing in deep shade, if they live, they will certainly become an insect magnet. I know of a hedge just like this near where I live. A large old hedge of lantana, now shaded by a big pine, is literally covered top to bottom in whiteflies and mold. It is growing right outside the back entrance to a health clinic!

There are many other cultural reasons for plants not to thrive and any one of them can result in weak plants and mold. Judicious use of natives is often one of the very best ways to avoid many of these weak plants and mold problems. However, make sure the "natives" you buy are endemic to your own particular area. Also, make sure you're not getting a bunch of male (pollen-producing) clones. Unfortunately, many of the native trees, shrubs, and ground covers sold now are male clones.

WILD SONGBIRDS

One of the easiest and most cost-effective things we can do to limit mold spores in our yards is to attract large numbers of songbirds that mainly eat insects. Wild birds have extremely high metabolism rates, and when they're not asleep, they're probably eating. Birds that are attracted to seed feeders will also eat a sizable number of insects each day, but for the most bang for the buck, we want to attract birds whose diets are almost all insects. These birds are only rarely attracted to seed feeders, but they are almost all drawn in by suet feeders. Suet feeders (usually made of strong, coated wire) can be filled with blocks of suet and hung from a strong nail on a large branch of a tree. Hang them where the feeding birds cannot be caught by wandering cats. Blocks of suet can be bought for around a dollar a block, and in my own yard a new block of suet lasts for five to seven days. Replace as soon as it is gone. The uncooked fat from a roast of beef can also be used in place of prepared suet.

You can also attract these birds by keeping a birdbath full of fresh water. Birdbaths (which birds also drink from) are especially good in drier climates. I always place a large rock in the middle of my birdbath, in case a bird falls in and can't get out. A bird can climb up on the rock to escape. Too many birdbaths have overly slick sides, and many a songbird drowns this way, hence the rock in the middle. Clean the bath with a brush and replace the water once a week.

Apartment-style swallow and or purple martin houses, placed on the top of a very tall pole, are also extremely effective. Likewise, in many areas several species of bluebirds will use bluebird houses to nest in, and bluebirds are not simply beautiful—they also almost entirely eat insects. Wrens will also use wren houses, and wrens, too, are insect-eating friends of the garden.

One can attract beautiful warblers, orioles, and tanagers, all of them insect eaters, by hanging a grape jelly feeder in a tree in the yard. There's a photo of a simple, easy-to-make grape jelly feeder on my own website, www.allergyfree-gardening.com. These birds are also fun to see in our yards.

While you're at it, please do consider treating yourself to a decent pair of binoculars (8 x 42 power is best) and a good bird book. Keeping a count of the different species of birds that come to your own yard can add huge pleasure and satisfaction to your gardening. "Birding," as we who do it call it, has become one of the great pleasures of my life, right up there with gardening. Consider making a "yard list" of all the different species of wild birds that show up in your own yard. The more birds you get, the healthier a place your garden will be.

ANTS, APHIDS, AND SCALE

Ants will protect aphids and scale from their natural predators. When the aphids and scale have ruined one part of a plant, the ants will move them to another fresh spot.

Frequently, we can't seem to get rid of the insects because there are so many ants on the trees. To kill the ants I use a slow-acting but effective mix of powdered sugar and borax. Look for boxed borax in grocery stores where they sell laundry products. Mix the sugar and borax in a 50-50 ratio. Sometimes I like to flood the area under where the ants are thick with a hose and then when they're all over the place, I sprinkle the sugar and borax mix. *Note*: Do not put more than a handful of borax directly under a young tree, as the boron in it can be toxic to the tree roots.

A few types of ants don't much care for sugar, so for these try mixing cornmeal and borax. This bait mix will also kill some other garden pests such as slugs, earwigs, and roaches. I have also had fairly good luck killing ants with a mix of nondairy creamer and borax. Cockroaches inside the house cause plenty of allergies and the best way to kill them is with a mix of boric acid and powdered sugar as a bait. Sprinkle this powder down where the roaches will walk through it. You can buy boric acid in almost any drugstore. These baits are cheap, are safer than other poisons, and they work.

Out in the yard don't put these baits where a dog will eat them. Sometimes it works well to hide them under old boards or flat rocks.

I have also had luck at controlling ants in fruit trees by spraying the trunks of the trees with the a homemade insecticide-fungicide (see page 35). If you are just going to spray the trunk, and not the leaves, then you can double the amounts of soap and vegetable oil used. If you can keep the ants from climbing up the tree trunks, often this will control them, and will also help control the scale they protect. This is especially effective on citrus trees.

PLANT DISEASES AND SPORES

Many plant pests are not insects but fungal-type diseases, such as mildew, rust, black spot, scab, and leaf blight. These organisms also produce allergenic airborne spores. The very best way to avoid these diseases and their spores is by planting disease-resistant plants. The second most valuable approach is to keep plants growing cleanly and strongly. Insect-attacked plants will often later be attacked by fungus diseases, and vice versa. Healthy plants go a long way to keeping our air clean.

Certain plants, if grown in the wrong area, can almost be counted on to harbor disease. Evergreen viburnum growing in the shade will certainly get moldy and full of mildew. Crape myrtle trees grown in an area that doesn't have hot summers will almost always have mildew. Wax myrtle trees or shrubs grown in too much shade often get moldy.

A cold, wet spring frequently brings out a huge flush of both mildew and anthracnose on the leaves of California sycamore trees. In areas with cool, foggy nights and warm days, rust will surely grow on any roses, hollyhocks, or snapdragons that are not rust-resistant. Most roses grown in too much shade will quickly mildew. Actually, almost any plant that thrives in full sun will run into problems in too much shade.

INSECTICIDES AND FUNGICIDES

When you see a plant covered with insects or fungus, fight the urge to get out the chemical sprays. Many chemical sprays will themselves trigger allergies. They may also weaken your immune system.

A shrub full of insects can often be helped immensely by just blasting off the bugs with a strong jet of water from the garden hose. Spider mites on plants can also often be brought under control with this same stiff spray of water.

Many insect pests can be killed with a simple, nontoxic homemade spray of vegetable oil, water, and liquid dish soap. For a gallon of water add 2 tablespoons of vegetable oil and 2 to 4 tablespoons of soap and shake it well before using. I like Ivory Liquid.

For fungus diseases, spray them with a mix of baking soda and water. I use from 2 to 6 tablespoons of baking soda per gallon of water, depending on how bad the infestation is. This often needs to be repeated all summer long. The baking soda will also kill some aphids. If you like, you can just add some baking soda to the insecticide mix of soap and oil and have an all-around safe, organic insecticide-fungicide spray mix.

Do not expect these homemade sprays to be just as effective as the most powerful chemical killers. Often they're not. But they do work, and they are much safer and a whole lot less likely to cause allergies.

INTEGRATED PEST MANAGEMENT

The theme of integrated pest management (IPM) is that we are not looking to eliminate insect pests—just control them. Using beneficial insects such as ladybugs, mealybug destroyers, tiny parasitic wasps, and green lacewings is always worth a try. It would be worthwhile for any gardener interested in allergy control to read a book or two on organic pest control.

A Note about Ferns

Ferns don't produce mold spores, but they do produce fern spores. Often these spores from the ferns can be just as allergenic as the mold spores. Fern spores usually shoot out and land fairly close to the fern. Small ferns growing in a shady part of the garden rarely trigger much allergy. But people love to grow ferns in hanging baskets, and then they often hang these over patio chairs and tables—right where people will be sitting.

When these overhead ferns cast off their miniscule spores, they land directly on the unsuspecting victim underneath. Hanging-basket ferns are fine, but watch where you hang them!

Tree ferns are handsome creatures, but again we need to watch where we plant them. All too often they are planted right next to front doors where, with their added height, they can shower spores on the people coming and going. Another consideration with tree ferns is that they have millions of tiny reddish brown, needle-sharp hairs on their trunks. These little fern hairs can make you itch and they can also cause irritation of the throat and nose when they're inhaled. Plant tree ferns back away from most human traffic.

No matter what you do, think twice before you plant. Plants make our world a far better, kinder place, but let's plant smart. A small tree or shrub we plant today may be around long after we're gone ourselves, and it pays to take some extra time, and put some extra thinking and effort, into making the healthiest selections. To your good health, and good gardening!

SIX

Fighting Allergies
IN YOUR NEIGHBORHOOD AND CITY

It makes total sense to make our own gardens and yards as allergy-free as possible, to cocoon ourselves and our families as much as possible. It makes great sense to plant female trees and shrubs, pollen-free lawns, and protective hedges. Nonetheless, we do not always stay at home, and for the biggest possible impact, we also need to get our schools, workplaces, states, cities, and counties on board.

The highest pollen count ever recorded in the U.S. (60,000 grains of pollen per cubic square yard of air space) came from a site in Las Vegas. Last year I tracked down this site, very curious to see exactly what was planted there. The pollen-collecting site turned out to be right smack in the middle of an elementary school. I counted a total of twenty-three fully grown trees at this school, many of them right in the schoolyard. Of those twenty-three mature trees, twenty-two were "fruitless" males.

On another occasion, I visited two elementary schools at the request of parents to evaluate the school landscapes. Of twenty-six trees at one school, I found twenty-one that were highly allergenic male trees. Out of seventeen trees at the second school, fifteen were extremely allergenic male mulberries. I found no female trees at either school. Springtime pollen levels at these two schools must be incredible. Sadly, these schools are in no way exceptions.

To become part of the solution, write letters or send emails to magazine and newspaper editors, talk to your own landscapers or gardeners, talk to the people at schools and nurseries, ask horticulture and landscape design professors to teach this, talk to your doctors about it, and talk to your friends. If your children's school or your company is considering landscaping, offer to be on the landscaping committee or give a copy of this book to whoever is. I encourage anyone who doesn't already belong to join a garden club or to become a Master Gardener. These are wonderful, smart, enthusiastic, friendly, socially responsible people. They help tremendously to make our world a friendlier and more beautiful place. Whenever possible, please support all proposed sensible local pollen-control ordinances.

There is now a new national nonprofit organization, the Society for Allergy Friendly Environmental (SAFE) Gardening, the purpose of which is to promote the concepts of safe gardening, safe landscaping, and low-pollen and allergy-free plants for urban plantings. SAFE will also be pushing hard to get more growers on board and to make a larger assortment of allergy-free, OPALS-ranked plants available to the consumer at the retail level. For advice on how to jump-start a pollen-control ordinance in your own city or county, visit the SAFE Gardening website at www.safegardening.org.

In addition to SAFE Gardening, in Canada there is another new nonprofit organization, Healthy School Yards, which is devoted entirely to the idea of promoting allergy-free schoolyards all across Canada. The organization's Allergy Free School Yard Initiative is largely the work of horticulturist Peter Prakke. So far this organization has already convinced the largest Catholic school district in Ontario to agree to go allergy-free in all future school landscapes. In addition, it has been instrumental in getting a large number of new "Bravery Parks" (each one named for a Canadian soldier killed in Iraq or Afghanistan) to be landscaped with OPALS. For more information, visit healthyschoolyards.org.

For all of you with allergies, or those of you with loved ones who have allergies, asthma, or other breathing problems, you have the ability to make a change in the world. You deserve air that isn't filled with excessive amounts of pollen. The trees, shrubs, and lawns the city, state, parks, and counties plant have a profound effect on your health. Your taxes pay for the planting and upkeep of these trees and shrubs; you have every right to insist that those in charge always seriously consider your family's health when they're choosing plants for landscapes.

If all else fails, you might have the law on your side. In a just-published law journal essay called "Regulating Pollen," lawyer Brian Sawers argues that the trespass law can be used to sue if a neighbor's tree is swamping your own yard with allergenic pollen. Sawers thinks the best place for lawsuits on pollen issues will turn out to be schools. If parents want a school to replace the most allergenic trees or shrubs and the school refuses to do so, there may now be a legal way to force them to do it. To read this very interesting and well-written essay, visit www.minnesotalawreview.org/headnotes/regulating-pollen.

Aeonium sp. >

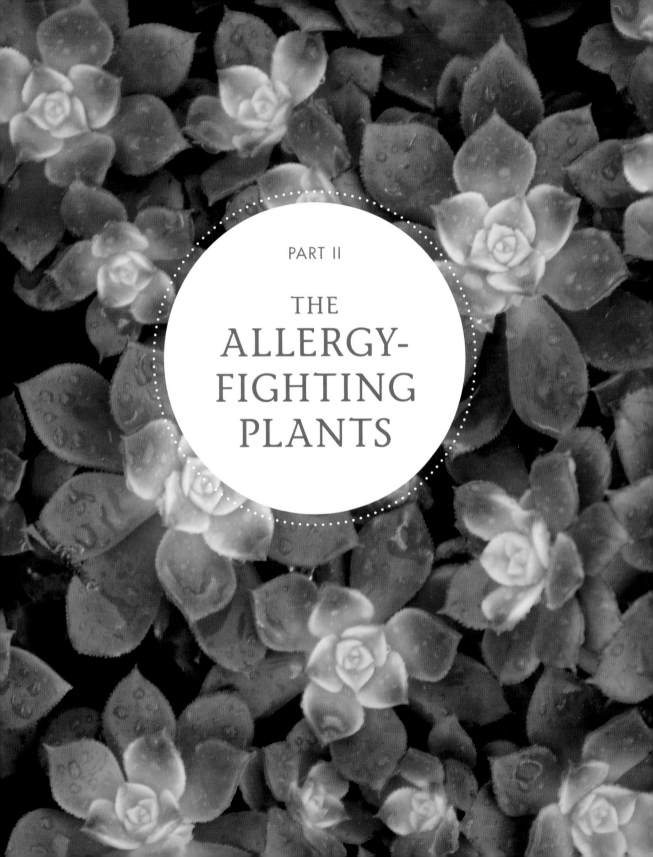

PART II

THE
ALLERGY-
FIGHTING
PLANTS

SEVEN

Understanding OPALS

OPALS is an abbreviation of Ogren Plant Allergy Scale. On occasion, OPALS is also said to stand for Ogren Pollen Allergy Scale. This is the numerical scale I created more than twenty years ago that has been used to allergy-rank each plant listed in this book's A to Z section. Many different factors went into the ranking process:

- The amount of pollen produced, if any

- The potency of the pollen

- How much of the year the plant is in bloom

- The size of the actual pollen grains

- The specific gravity of the pollen grains

- How sticky or dry the grains are

- Whether the tree is perfect-flowered, monoecious, dioecious, or polygamous

- Whether the sap causes dermatitis

- Whether the smell of the flowers bothers people

These and other factors were weighted and compiled and became the foundation of the OPALS scale. With OPALS, plants are ranked on a scale of 1 to 10. A plant ranked 1 is the least allergenic and a plant ranked 10 is the most allergenic.

OPALS ranks each plant against other plants of the same type. For example, all perennials are ranked only against other perennials. The shrubs are ranked according to other shrubs. And trees are ranked only against other trees. Note that a tree ranked 8, for example, has far more potential for allergy than a perennial also ranked 8. This is simply because the tree is so much larger.

How to Use OPALS

Some people tell me that they want to move to an area where most of the landscapes would average out to 1 or 2 on the scale. "Good luck!" I tell them, for there is no such place, yet, unfortunately. Nonetheless, if some creative big developer wished to do so, it is now possible to landscape an entire large development that would all be OPALS ranked 1, 2, or 3. Such a neighborhood would be a delightful place for those with allergies. The best thing people can do to make their own place as allergy-free as possible is to cocoon their house and yard (see chapter 2). The next best thing is to get involved in this at the city level, to try and influence your own city council to enact a ban on the planting of any more highly allergenic trees in your neighborhood (see chapter 6).

Factors Used to Build OPALS

More than 130 possible factors are used to develop allergy rankings for plants. Each factor is either a positive factor or a negative one. All factors are not weighted the same, because some are more important than others. Almost all plants have a combination of positive and negative factors that are computed to determine its OPALS ranking. Below are some of the positive and negative factors used in building OPALS.

SOME POSITIVE FACTORS

These are the things we want to find, factors that mean a plant has less potential to cause allergy:

- Perfect-flowered (The pollen doesn't need to travel far.)

- Self-fertile (Any fruit tree that is self-fertile can and will pollinate itself and is probably not very allergenic.)

- Large petals (These attract pollinating insects, indicating less reliance on wind pollination. Anything that attracts pollinating insects is good, because pollen transported by insects, rather than the wind, is much less available to cause allergies.)

- Brightly colored petals (These attract pollinating insects more than lighter pastel colors.)

- Flowers with rich nectar sources (Nectar attracts pollinators.)

- Flowers where the male parts are deep inside the flower, as in a snapdragon (The pollen is less exposed.)

- Polygamous with separate female flowers (A plant like this, gynodioecious, has both perfect flowers and separate-sexed female flowers, and thus it has low pollen production and has an excellent chance of attracting and trapping almost all of its own pollen.)

- A light, pleasant scent (It will draw pollinating insects.)

- Disease resistance (It will have fewer pest insects and less disease, thus less insect dander and mold. Insect dander is not a problem associated with pollinating insects, such as honeybees. Dander is a definite problem from plant-predatory, sucking pest insects such as mealybugs, whiteflies, scale, or aphids. Any botanical plant feature that limits pest insects is beneficial.)

- Female only (Female plants have no pollen.)

- Pollen-free but not strictly female (Again, per allergy, no pollen is always a plus. Some clonal plants never bloom and are stuck in a stage of permanent juvenility, and this is a plus.)

- Flowers colored red, orange, blue, or pink (These colors attract the most pollinators, indicating little reliance on the wind.)

- Large flowers (Bigger flowers rely more on insect pollinators.)

- A very short bloom period (Less time available for pollen production.)

- Blooming only on old wood (The flowers, if allergenic, can often be pruned away before they bloom.)

- Not in the same genus or family as any highly allergenic plants (There is much less chance of interspecies cross-reactive allergenic responses. Certain plant families are rife with allergenic members.)

- Sticky pollen (It cannot travel easily in the air.)

- Pollen grains that are heavy and have a high specific gravity (Heavy pollen sinks faster and travels poorly in air.)

- In perfect-flowered plants, a ratio of one pistil to five stamens (Fewer stamens means less pollen per flower and also that a larger percentage of each flower's pollen may be trapped by that flower.)

- From a family of plants where a great many individuals can be expected to be functionally female (As found in many of the mint, catmint, and salvia relatives. Even though they are seedlings, many plants will be pollen-free female individuals.)

- Having the ability to set seed through apomixis (Apomictic plants are normally low-pollen producers and can set viable seed even if they are not actually pollinated.)

- Brightly colored sepals (This is another good indication of insect pollination. The sepals are underneath the petals, and colorful sepals add to the attraction of the petals.)

- Monocarpic (These plants only bloom once in their entire life cycle, and then they die, thus there is no pollen exposure until the final year. Many species of bamboo are monocarpic.)

- Not blooming until very advanced in years (Plants are pollen-free for a longer period of time in the landscape. This factor is of less importance if the plant is known to live for a great many years.)

- Monoecious plants with female flowers on the same plant that are always abundant and also receptive at the precise same time the male flowers of that plant are releasing pollen (A plant like this is designed by nature to trap its own pollen.)

- Monoecious plants with all the male flowers positioned above the female flowers (A great example is the corn plant, where the tassels on the top have the pollen, and the ears of corn are collections of female flowers. The pollen is heavy and gravity will bring it down to the female flowers.)

- Pollen grains with an odd shape that is not well designed to stay airborne for long

There are many other plus indicators I use, things that make a plant less likely to trigger allergies, but this ought to give you a good idea of what constitutes positive factors used to form OPALS rankings.

SOME NEGATIVE FACTORS

These are the things that contribute to the allergy-causing potential in any plant. The more of these negative factors any plant has, the worse will be its OPALS rank. Not all negative factors are weighted the same; some are more negative than others.

- The plant belongs to a family of plants well known to cause allergies (Prime examples are the cashew, olive, spurge, and sunflower families. Here there is often exceptional potential for interspecies cross-reactive allergenic responses.)

- May cause skin rash from contact with sap, flowers, or leaves (This is self-explanatory.)

- Skin rash, when caused, is long lasting (Certain plant-triggered cases of allergic dermatitis may persist for months, or in a few cases, for years.)

- Skin rash, when caused, is severe and may cause permanent scarring (Sap from certain plants is not just allergenic but also dangerous.)

- Very long bloom period (Certain trees, like many eucalyptus species, bloom for many months in the year, greatly increasing the pollen exposure around them.)

- Blooms on new wood, wood grown in the current season (Even if hard pruned, it will still bloom. The flowering is thus difficult to control by pruning or shearing.)

- Pollen grains are light and dry, with a low specific gravity (This pollen will travel easily in the air.)

- Pollen grains are smaller than 30 microns (Smaller pollen can be inhaled deeper into the lungs, and it may also travel farther in the wind. Very small grains are more capable of triggering asthma.)

- Pollen grains are completely round (Round pollen travels well in the air.)

- Pollen grains with sharp spines (This type of pollen can cause skin rash, dry skin, and irritation of the nose, eyes, and throat. Sharp-spined pollen can also cause irritation simply from mechanical action rather than allergic response. Skin may be easily irritated by this itchy pollen and when rubbed or scratched, it has a sandpaper effect, resulting in a rash or dry, flaky skin.)

- Pollen grains are produced in large quantities (This is never a plus with allergy control.)

- Pollen may cross-react with common food allergies or intolerances (Food allergies are on the increase and cross-reactions with certain pollen types are common.)

- Male cultivar (Cultivars are cloned plants, asexually propagated, and all male clones produce large amounts of pollen and trap none.)

- Has a strong fragrance, known to trigger allergies (Certain floral smells are well documented for provoking allergies.)

- Has a disagreeable odor from its flowers or leaves (Different odd plant odors can trigger allergic responses. These odors are actually composed of tiny allergenic airborne oils. You can't see them but they are perfectly real.)

- Stamens are exserted, exposed (These pollen-bearing stamens are more easily accessed directly and from the movement of the air. These will be more likely to shed pollen.)

- In perfect-flowered plants, ratios of thirty or more stamens per stigma (Less pollen will be trapped per flower and more will be produced; this is a strongly negative factor.)

- A polygamous plant with unisexual male flowers, androdioecious (The male-only flowers will produce windborne pollen.)

- Small, light yellow, off-white, or greenish-colored flowers (Many of the most highly allergenic flowers are colored this way, which is unattractive to most pollinators.)

- Flowers lacking petals (They are far less attractive to pollinators and more likely to have pollen that will move freely in the air.)

- Flowers lacking sepals (Again, this usually means that a flower will be less attractive to insect pollinators.)

- Flowers lacking both petals and sepals (Unattractive to pollinators, this is a very strong sign of high allergy potential.)

- Flowers that are numerous and small (This is the typical arrangement with most highly allergenic plants.)

- Monoecious flowered (Production of unisexual male flowers usually is associated with airborne pollen.)

- Monoecious flowered with male flowers below the female flowers (In monoecious plants this is an additional strong negative. A good example of this is an Italian cypress, where the female flowers are on the top of the plant, and the male pollen flowers are on the bottom two-thirds. The cypress pollen must go *up* in order to pollinate. This system always involves large amounts of airborne pollen.)

- Pollen well known to cause asthma (Pollen of some species, such as castor bean or olive, frequently triggers serious bouts of asthma; this is a strongly negative factor.)

- Lacks nectaries (No nectar makes the flowers much less attractive to insect or animal pollinators and thus more reliant on the wind.)

- The plant is poisonous (More often than not, a poisonous plant will produce pollen that is also poisonous. If the plant is also male, then this is an exceptionally negative factor.)

- Pollen grains that are high in tannic acid (Certain plants—in particular, oaks and acacia species—produce pollen very high in tannic acid. Dry, airborne tannic acid has been linked to cancer, allergy, and asthma.)

- Any plant known to be entirely reliant on the wind for pollen dispersal (More pollen will be exposed.)

- Any plant that in my own testing proves to be pollinated by both insects and the wind, amphiphilous plants (These may not be as allergenic as entirely wind-pollinated plants, but nonetheless, there will be considerable exposure to their pollen.)

- Plant spores or sharp hairs that could cause skin, eye, bronchial, lung, or nasal mechanical irritation (Certain plants, such as the sycamore tree, have minute, sharp material on their leaves or stems that can go airborne and cause allergy or asthma when inhaled. In some cases, this will be more significant than their pollen.)

- Monoecious plants whose female flowers are few in numbers, relative to numbers of male flowers (Less pollen will be trapped and more will be in the air.)

- Monoecious plants whose female flowers are not receptive at the precise same time that its male flowers are releasing their pollen (This plant, even though it produces female flowers, can trap none of its own pollen.)

- Nonnative allergenic invasive plants, known to spread quickly and to naturalize (These are domesticated plants that can easily spread into wild lands, and are then very difficult to eradicate. Landscape plants that naturalize often cause a wide array of problems. They often upset the natural balance, forcing out native species of both plants and animals. Invasive allergenic plants that may naturalize, such as Casuarina, are exceptionally troublesome.)

- Plants that produce considerable more volatile organic compounds (VOCs) than they consume (VOCs worsen air quality and contribute to smog. Smog in turn makes pollen more allergenic.)

There are numerous other factors used to allergy-rank plants, but these are the most basic factors I have used; they should give you a good idea of how it is done and what I look for. Again, it should be stressed that plants ranked 1 to 5 are all considered to be of fairly low allergy potential.

Examples of OPALS

Note: 1 is least allergenic and 10 is most allergenic.
In each of the ten examples below, one particular plant or plant species is used to illustrate each degree of ranking. Reasons are given, positive or negative, or often both, to explain (roughly) how each ranking was determined.

OPALS RANK 1: 'Autumn Glory' red maple (*Acer rubrum* 'Autumn Glory'). 'Autumn Glory' is a female tree, traps pollen from male trees, produces no pollen itself, does not have spores or sharp hairs, has no sap or smell that causes allergies, is winter-hardy, is disease-resistant, is widely adapted, and doesn't cause allergies.

OPALS RANK 2: Petunia hybrids. A very limited number of people may, on rare occasion, react to the smell of petunia flowers, and the flowers do produce a small amount of pollen. On the plus side, the pollen grains are large, sticky, and heavy; the petals are large and brightly colored; the plants are insect-pollinated; the stamens are hidden deep inside the flowers; the ratio of pistils to stamens is good; and the plants are not known to trigger any skin allergies. All in all, petunias are of very low allergy potential and perfectly safe.

OPALS RANK 3: Pinks, carnations, dianthus species. These present very little opportunity for pollen allergy, are not closely related to families of highly allergenic plants, are insect-pollinated, are both perfect-flowered and complete-flowered, have brightly colored large petals, have full sets of sepals, and have sticky pollen that is heavy and moderately large. Occasionally, certain species, such as clove pinks, can trigger some minor allergy from their fragrance, and people who frequently handle Dianthus (usually carnations) as cut flowers on rare occasions get dermatitis from the sap. All told, the carnations, pinks, and Dianthus are allergy-friendly, safe garden plants.

OPALS RANK 4: **Night-blooming jasmine** (*Cestrum nocturnum*). This plant is perfect-flowered; has large, sticky pollen; is insect-pollinated; has rich nectar sources; and is not known to cause skin rashes. But, Cestrum also has a powerful fragrance that can trigger allergies, especially if it is planted too close to bedroom windows. The pollen, while not plentiful, is nonetheless poisonous. The flowers are also numerous and small. A substance that is poisonous (toxic) will negatively affect anyone who ingests or inhales it. Pollen that is allergenic will usually affect only those with susceptible allergies. Planted in the right place, Cestrum should cause next to no allergy problems; in the wrong place, it could.

OPALS RANK 5: **St. John's wort** (Hypericum species). This is perfect-flowered; has large, brightly colored petals and full sets of sepals; has rich nectar sources; and is not in a family with numerous highly allergenic relatives. However, Hypericum has numerous male stamens, fully exserted stamens, produces considerable pollen, is pollinated by both wind and insects, and causes often fatal photodermatitis in animals that eat it. Not a pet-safe plant, but overall, not a plant with large potential for allergy. Contact allergic dermatitis is possible from Hypericum.

OPALS RANK 6: **Female Chinese tallow tree**. This tree is disease-resistant where adapted, produces no pollen, and will trap pollen from male Sapium trees. The sap and VOCs from the stems and leaves, however, give it the potential to be a strong allergen. The tree is in a family well known to have many highly allergenic members (Euphorbiaceae), and potential for cross-reactive allergy, especially to the sap, is considerable. People with an allergy to latex have an even greater chance of reacting to Sapium. Male Sapium trees are ranked much worse, 10.

OPALS RANK 7: **Boxwood** (Buxus species). Boxwood is imperfectly flowered and the flowers produce considerable pollen per flower. On the plus side, boxwood plants are often sheared hard each year, and this will remove much of the flowering. On the negative side, boxwood pollen is a known allergen, and it is rarely possible to prune away all the flowers. The flowers are off-white in color, very small in size, very numerous in number, all the stamens are exserted, and the ratio of pistil to stamens is quite high. On the plus side, these are rarely very large landscape plants. Contact with boxwood leaves and flowers can trigger itch or rash for some.

OPALS RANK 8: **Most species of Eucalyptus**. These trees grow very large and are often in bloom for eight to ten months of the year. Eucalyptus pollen is not exceptionally allergenic; however, exposure to this pollen is very common, and this increases allergy to it. Eucalyptus species ranked 8 make abundant pollen and most of it is amphiphilous, pollinated by both insects and the wind. The scent of the leaves can trigger allergies for some. Pollen grains of Eucalyptus are large and often form clumps, a strong plus factor, but more often than not these same clumps of pollen will have large numbers of tiny insects living on them. The insects (and their allergenic dander) will be inhaled along with the pollen. The insect-dander on the pollen is probably more allergenic than the pollen itself.

OPALS RANK 9: **Primrose tree** (*Lagunaria patersonii*). This tree is perfect-flowered and insect-pollinated; it has nectar sources and large, brightly colored flowers. Negatives of this tree are that it has many stamens, all of them exserted (extended from the flowers), and the flowers are numerous. The bloom period is quite long, and the tree produces extremely large numbers of minute, needle-sharp stinging hairs that can cause asthma if inhaled, skin rash, and severe irritation to the eyes when contacted. Almost all of the hazards from this tree are highly localized, or confined to the immediate area surrounding the tree.

OPALS RANK 10: **Male Brazilian pepper tree** (*Schinus terebinthifolius*). Males are commonly used because they are seedless, fruitless, and thus "litter-free." This tree produces large amounts of highly allergenic pollen every year and blooms for a long period of time. Although insects often visit it, it also produces airborne pollen. The flowers are tiny, pale yellow, extremely numerous, and all imperfect, unisexual, and male. The odor of the flowers is odd and strong, attracting flies, and may cause allergy for some. The odor of the leaves is odd, and the VOCs from the crushed leaves can trigger inhalant allergies. The sap or simple contact with the leaves or flowers of these trees can cause persistent, delayed-reaction skin rash that is very similar to that triggered by its relatives, poison ivy and poison oak. Crushed leaves from this tree produce volatile oils that can trigger skin allergies. Fumes from the wood can cause severe allergy or asthma if it is burned. The species itself is highly invasive in some areas.

Male Brazilian pepper trees are large and long-lived and bloom profusely at an early age. Allergies to the pollen and odors of this tree and all male members of the Schinus family are well documented and common. The trees are widely planted and are in the cashew family, known to contain some of the most highly allergenic trees, shrubs, and vines in the world. Schinus may cross-react with any of its relatives: varnish tree, mango, poison oak, poison sumac, and poison ivy. Pollen allergy to Schinus may also trigger cross-reactions with mango, cashew, and pistachio nuts.

EIGHT

Using the A to Z Plant Listings

All plants are listed in alphabetical order with their scientific name, genus first, in italics. If the plant listed is of a particular species, the exact species name is given following the genus. If a whole group of plants is discussed, only the genus is given. A few genera have only one species: *Ginkgo biloba* is a good example. In many other genera, there are many different species. Eucalyptus, for example, has hundreds of different species. In this text, where there are long lists of different species of the same genus, the genus is abbreviated using only its first letter. Thus, in a list of maples (*Acer*), the text reads: *A. argutum*, *A. rubrum*, *A. saccharinum*, *A. tataricum*, and so on. If there are two botanical names for the same plant, one name will be listed after the other in parentheses, for example, *Emblica officinalis* (*Phyllanthus emblica*). After the scientific name, the common name or names by which the plant is known are listed, also in alphabetical order.

Cultivated Varieties

In addition to genera and species, there are hundreds of thousands of cultivated varieties, or cultivars, known to horticulture. An example of this is the domestic apple, *Malus domestica*, of which there are more than 7,000 cultivars. Where a cultivar is listed, the exact name of the cultivar will always be enclosed in single quotation marks. Thus, for the apple tree *Malus domestica* 'McIntosh', *Malus* is the genus, *domestica* is the species, and 'McIntosh' is the cultivar.

Hybrids

When hybrids are discussed, the female plant (the seed parent) is listed first. A hybrid cross between a red maple and a silver maple is listed as *Acer rubrum* × *saccharinum* when the seed parent is red maple (*A. rubrum*) and the pollen parent is silver maple (*A. saccharinum*).

Cross-Referencing of Names

Every attempt has been made to cross-reference common names with scientific names. For example, *Aptenia cordifolia* is a ground cover plant with little red flowers. However, it is quite possible that you only know the plant by its common name, red-apple iceplant. If you look up red-apple iceplant in the text, it will direct you to *Aptenia cordifolia*.

OPALS Allergy Index Scale

A plant with a ranking of 1 or 2 has very little potential for causing allergy. If the plant has a rank of 3 to 5, it may have low potential to cause pollen allergy unless directly sniffed, but it also may have other dangers, such as the potential to trigger a skin rash from contact, strong odors that could irritate odor-sensitive people, or toxic qualities. Always read the full plant description carefully and take note of any warnings.

Plants that rank from 1 to 5 are considered low-risk plants, but the allergy potential does rise as the number increases. So while there is little wrong with having some 5s in the garden, or perhaps even a 6 or a 7, you wouldn't want to plant too many of them. Plants with allergy rankings of 9 to 10, the worst, can often cause both hay fever and asthma. They may well also trigger skin rashes. A plant ranked 10 is known to cause the worst kind of allergy and to have the potential to affect a large number of people.

The best plants (those with an OPALS ranking of 1 or 2) are marked with a ✪ symbol. The worst plants (those with an OPALS ranking of 9 or 10) are marked with a ◗ symbol.

Hardiness Zones

An attempt has been made to give a cold-hardiness rating to each plant, and each plant is described as perennial, annual, shrub, vine, ground cover, or tree. Plant hardiness zones used in this book are based on the standard United States Department of Agriculture (USDA) 1 through 13 zoning system. The USDA Plant Hardiness Zone Map appears on page 240. In this system, the coldest areas (mountaintops, most of Alaska) are zone 1. Zones 10 to 13 are the warmest, frost-free zones and exist only in southern areas, close to the oceans, or in the tropics. The actual hardiness (to cold) of a species is affected by its size, age, type of soil, exposure to wind and drought, and many other factors. Often a plant can be grown successfully one zone colder than its normal range if all other conditions are favorable.

Gardeners sometimes confuse the terms *hardy* and *tender*. In horticulture, a hardy plant is one that can withstand a great deal of frost and cold. A tender plant, on the other hand, cannot take either extreme cold or frost. See the Glossary for detailed explanations of the botanical and horticultural terms used in this text.

Poisonous Plants

In this text, I have included references to poisonous plants, including plants such as the varnish tree, which are poisonous to the touch, and also many others that are poisonous only if eaten. Many plants that are poisonous if eaten do not necessarily cause allergies, and the ranking of a plant reflects only its allergy potential. Being poisonous does not by any means make a plant an allergy problem; still, it is good to know which ones could be dangerous.

TO MY READERS

If you discover a plant-related allergy that I may have overlooked, please contact me and share the information. I am always on the lookout for additional data and I value your input. I also welcome letters and email, and I will try to answer them all in a timely fashion. All new useful information will eventually find its way into the next edition of *The Allergy-Fighting Garden*. My email address is tloallergyfree@earthlink.net.

NINE

A to Z Plant Listings
WITH OPALS ALLERGY RANKINGS

Allergy Index Scale: 1 is Best, 10 is Worst.
✪ for 1 and 2   ❧ for 9 and 10
No matter what the ranking, always read the full plant description carefully and take note of any warnings.

AARON'S BEARD. See *Hypericum.*

Abelia. 4
Evergreen flowering shrubs hardy in plant zones 8 to 10. There are numerous species of Abelia and all have many small, white flowers, often tinged with pink. Easy to grow, all Abelia thrive in full sun to partial shade. The many flowers attract large numbers of honeybees and release little pollen. Abelia is a honeysuckle relative; individuals allergic to honeysuckle (see Lonicera) may experience cross-allergic reactions, although allergy to Abelia is much less common. In a few cases, skin rash caused by contact with the leaves has been noted.

Abeliophyllum distichum. 6
WHITE FORSYTHIA. A deciduous flowering shrub, hardy to zone 5. An olive family member. Dormant branches are often cut and brought into the house to bloom. This is not advisable if you have allergies.

Abelmoschus esculentus. 3
OKRA. A common vegetable with handsome flowers that resemble Hibiscus, to which it is related. The plants need good soil, ample water, and warmth to bear well. The prickly leaves are known to cause contact skin rash.

Abies. 2 ✪
ALGERIAN FIR, BALMIES, BALSAM FIR, CORK FIR, FIR, GRAND FIR, NIKKO FIR, NOBLE FIR, RED FIR, SANTA LUCIA FIR, SILVER FIR, SPANISH FIR. Large, slow-growing evergreen, coniferous trees with classic "Christmas tree" shape. There are more than forty species; some are hardy to zone 1. Most firs do not grow well in hot, dry areas or in hot, smoggy cities. One species, *A. nordmanniana*, the Nordmann fir, from Asia Minor and Greece, grows well in most areas of California if supplied with plenty of water. All true firs produce pollen, but it has a waxy covering and rarely causes allergy.

Abronia. 1 ✪
SAND VERBENA. A perennial native of coastal areas, sand verbena grows best in sandy soil and is tolerant of seaside conditions. Large clusters of white, pink, or red tubular, sticky flowers on low, spreading plants.

Abrus precatorius. NOT YET RANKED, AVOID
ROSARY PEA. A vine with pealike flowers producing attractive scarlet, black-spotted seeds, occasionally used as beads. These seeds are extremely poisonous; one seed can kill a child.

Abutilon. 3
CHINESE LANTERN, FLOWERING MAPLE. Tall, evergreen vinelike shrubs hardy only in the mildest climates. Easy to grow; many different varieties with a wide array of colors.

ABYSSINIAN BANANA. See *Ensete.*

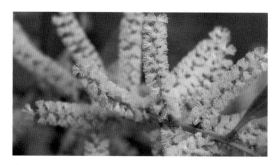

Acacia. SHRUBS 8, TREES 10 🌂
AUSTRALIAN WILLOW, BLACKWOOD ACACIA, GOLDEN
WATTLE, MIMOSA, MULGA, RIVER WATTLE, SILVER
WATTLE, WHITETHORN. (Pictured above.) Common
evergreen shrubs and trees from warm areas all over
the world, especially Australia. Hardy in zones 8B to
13, they are far too common in California and Florida.
Acacia trees cover themselves with thousands of little
yellow flowers in early spring. Easy to grow and fast
growing, they cause plenty of allergies. Acacia leaves are
poisonous; the pollen is high in tannic acid, a possible
carcinogen.

ACACIA, SMOOTH ROSE. See *Robinia*.

Acaena. 2 ☉
SHEEP BUR. Small, low-growing perennials from New
Zealand. Not hardy in cold winter areas, they are grown
for their pale green leaves. After flowering, they produce burrs, which stick to clothes.

Acalypha. MALES 7, FEMALES 1 ☉
CHENILLE PLANT, COPPER LEAF. A tender houseplant with large leaves and long, drooping clusters of
chenille-like flowers. Acalypha is a separate-sexed
species, however, and virtually all of the plants sold
in the United States, Canada, and Europe are female
clones, which cause no allergy.

Acanthophoenix. 6
BARBEL PALM. Subtropical palm trees. Monoecious
trees; on existing trees, if possible, cut off branches
with male flowers before the flowers open and shed
pollen. Zones 10 to 13.

Acanthus mollis. 1 ☉
BEAR'S BREECH, SNAIL'S TRAIL. A big, shade-loving
perennial with large leaves; hardy to zone 3 if mulched
heavily in fall. Bear's breech often thrives where nothing
else will grow. Tall spikes of white or purple flowers.
Must be protected from snails and slugs.

ACEITUNO. See *Simarouba*.

ACER GENUS

Acer. INDIVIDUALLY RANKED
MAPLE. A large group of deciduous trees and large
shrubs. Various maples are hardy in all zones. Maples
do well in most areas, but few are well suited for desert
landscapes, because all require plentiful water. Many
cause allergy, but some species are among our very
finest choices for allergy-free landscapes. Some maple
species are separate-sexed; other species are not. Where
the sex of the trees is not constant, it is not possible to
rank the cultivars individually; these are marked "not
ranked." They are not recommended for planting in
allergy-free gardens.

Note: There are other, less often used maples than
those listed here. None are recommended for the allergy-
free garden.

A. argutum. 7
POINTED-LEAF MAPLE.

A. buergeranum. 6
TRIDENT MAPLE.

A. campestre. 6
HEDGE MAPLE.

A. cappadocicum. 6
CAUCASIAN MAPLE.

A. carpinifolium. MALES 8, FEMALES 1 ☉
HORNBEAM MAPLE.

A. circinatum. 5
VINE MAPLE.

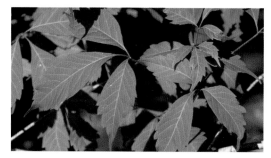

A. cissifolium. MALES 8, FEMALES 1 ☉
IVY-LEAFED MAPLE. (*Acer cissifolium*, male, pictured
above.)

A. crataegifolium. 6
HAWTHORN-LEAF MAPLE.

A. davidii. 6
DAVID'S MAPLE.

A. diabolicum. MALES 8, FEMALES 3
HORNED MAPLE. Tiny stinging hairs on the seeds cause rash.

A. distylum. 6
LIMELEAF MAPLE.

A. × *Freemanii.*
Freemanii maples are natural hybrids of red maple and silver maple.

A. × *F.* 'Armstrong'. 5
A tall, broad, hardy tree with some pollen.

A. × *F.* 'Autumn Blaze'. 7

A. × *F.* 'Autumn Fantasy'. 1 ✪
No pollen. Female.

A. × *F.* 'Celebration'. 8

A. × *F.* 'Celzam'. 8

A. × *F.* 'Indian Summer'. 1 ✪
Fast-growing, big tree; great scarlet fall color and no pollen.

A. × *F.* 'Jeffersred'. 7

A. × *F.* 'Marmo'. 8

A. × *F.* 'Morgan'. 1 ✪

A. × *F.* 'Scarlet Sentinel'. NOT RANKED

A. ginnala. 4
Small tree with fragrant flowers.

A. glabrum. MALES 8, FEMALES 1 ✪
ROCK MAPLE, SIERRA MAPLE.

A. griseum. 6
PAPERBARK MAPLE.

A. japonicum. 5
JAPANESE MAPLE. Many kinds.

A. macrophyllum. 8
BIGLEAF MAPLE. The numerous seeds of this species have tiny stinging hairs that cause contact rash. Plenty of pollen here, too.

A. mandshuricum. 7
MANCHURIAN MAPLE.

A. negundo. MALES 10 ◐, FEMALES 1 ✪
ASH-LEAFED MAPLE, BOX ELDER. Fast-growing, deciduous trees with leaves more like the ash than the maple. Some box elders cause severe allergy; the female trees cause none at all.

A. negundo 'Auratum'. 1 ✪
No pollen.

A. negundo 'Aureo marginatum'. 10 ◐
A male tree.

A. negundo 'Baron'. 10 ◐
A male clone.

A. negundo 'Rubescens'. 1 ✪

A. negundo 'Variegata'. 1 ✪
VARIEGATED BOX ELDER. A handsome female tree with unusual colored leaves and no pollen.

A. negundo 'Violaceum'. 10 ◐
A male clone.

A. oblongum. 7
EVERGREEN MAPLE.

A. opalus. 7
ITALIAN MAPLE.

A. palmatum. 5
JAPANESE MAPLE. There are several hundred named cultivars of this small, handsome, deciduous tree. All cause rather limited allergy.

A. paxii. 5
EVERGREEN MAPLE. Not hardy in cold areas.

A. pensylvanicum. MALES 7, FEMALES 1 ✪
STRIPED MAPLE. Grows well only in shade.

A. platanoides. 8
NORWAY MAPLE. A large, common urban tree. There are many varieties sold; all can cause allergy.

A. pseudoplatanus. 8
SYCAMORE MAPLE. A very common, widely adapted, large, monoecious deciduous urban tree.

A. rubescens. 6
TENDER MAPLE. From Taiwan.

A. rubrum.
RED MAPLE, SCARLET MAPLE. A large group of handsome trees that grows fast and likes plenty of water. They vary in allergenic potential.

A. rubrum 'Autumn Flame'. 8
A male tree.

A. rubrum 'Autumn Glory'. 1 ✪
Very good orange fall color, female and no pollen.

A. rubrum 'Autumn Spire'. 9 ◐
A male tree.

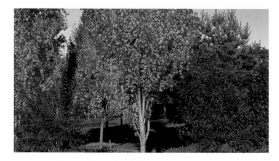

A. rubrum 'Bowhall'. 1 ✪
(Pictured above.) Pyramidal form with good orange-red fall color and female, no pollen.

A. rubrum 'Columnare' ('Pyramidale'). 8
A male tree.

A. rubrum 'Davey Red'. 1 ✪
Good fall color; female, can withstand more cold than most—hardy into zone 2.

A. rubrum 'Doric'. 1 ✪
Brilliant deep red fall color and female, no pollen.

A. rubrum 'Embers'. 1 ✪
Vigorous tree with a broad crown, great fall color, female, and no pollen.

A. rubrum 'Festival'. 1 ✪
A female tree.

A. rubrum 'Firedance'. 8
A male tree.

A. rubrum 'Flame'. *See* 'Autumn Flame'.

A. rubrum 'Franksred'. *See* 'Red Sunset'. 1 ✪
A female tree.

A. rubrum 'Karpick'. 8
A male tree.

A. rubrum 'Landsburg'. *See* 'Firedance'.

A. rubrum 'Northwood'. 8
A male tree.

A. rubrum 'October Brilliance'. 8
A male tree.

A. rubrum 'October Glory'. 1 ✪
Good lawn tree that does not cast a dense shade; dependable bright red-crimson fall color and no pollen. A fine female tree.

A. rubrum 'Red Skin'. 1 ✪
Very good fall color and female, no pollen.

A. rubrum 'Red Sunset'. 1 ✪
Thick leaves that turn a reddish maroon color in fall; female, no pollen in spring.

A. rubrum 'Schlesinger'. NOT RANKED

A. rubrum 'Shade King'. NOT RANKED

A. rubrum 'Sun Valley'. 9 🍃
A male tree.

A. rubrum 'Tiliford'. 9 🍃
A male tree.

A. saccharinum. MALES 9 🍃, FEMALES 1 ✪
SILVER MAPLE. The silver maples make up a large group of common, fast-growing deciduous trees, hardy in all zones. They will often grow where other maples will not. Their fast growth leads to weak wood, and large broken branches are common. Most varieties should be avoided in the allergy-free landscape, especially 'Silver Queen' and 'Skinner's Cutleaf Silver Maple', both of which are male.

One silver maple can be recommended, however. *A. saccharinum* 'Northline' is a variety that produces no pollen, grows slower than most, has a wide-spreading habit, and is among the hardiest of all maples. 'Northline' turns a bright yellow color in the fall.

A. saccharum. 7
SUGAR MAPLE.

A. tataricum. 5
TATARIAN MAPLE.

A. tataricum ginnala. 5
AMUR MAPLE.

ACEROLA. See *Malpighia glabra*.

Achillea. 4
YARROW. Several species of hardy, easy-to-grow, yellow- or white-flowered perennials. They grow best in full sun and are often used for dried flowers.

Achimenes. 1 ✪
ORCHID PANSY. Small tender perennial with many varieties and a wide range of colors.

Ackama. 7
Several species of small trees native to New Zealand; occasionally used in zones 10 to 12.

Acmena smithii. 5
LILLY-PILLY TREE. Small, evergreen tree with small pink flowers, edible berries. Hardy only in zones 10 to 13.

Acnistus australe. 3
Tall perennial for zones 7 to 10 that bears pendulous, trumpet-shaped lavender flowers.

Acoelorrhaphe wrightii. 1 ✪
EVERGLADES PALM, PAROUOT PALM, PAUROTIS WRIGHTII. A shade-loving palm native to Florida and hardy in most southern states.

Acokanthera. 9 ◗
AFRICAN WINTERSWEET, BUSHMAN'S POISON. Two species of poisonous evergreen shrubs with fragrant white or pink flowers, occasionally used as a hedge or foundation plant in zones 10 to 12. The sap can cause severe skin rashes. Seeds and fruit are extremely poisonous if eaten.

ACONITE. See *Aconitum*.

Aconitum. 4
ACONITE, MONKSHOOD. Common, poisonous, hardy, easy-to-grow perennial for moist, shady areas. Aconitum is one of the most highly poisonous plants and even a few leaves or flowers, if eaten, could be fatal.

Acorus gramineus. 5
Grasslike perennial hardy in most zones. Used as ground cover in rock gardens.

Acrocarpus fraxinifolius. 3
PINK CEDAR. A briefly deciduous tree for zone 10. Not a true cedar but a member of the legume family. Small red flowers appear in spring on this fast-growing tree. Not good in windy areas.

Acrocomia. 5
GRU-GRU PALM. Hardy only in coastal areas of zone 10 and zones 11 to 13, this palm has small, sweet, edible fruits.

Actinidia. MALES 5, FEMALES 1 ✪
KIWI. Several species. One, *A. arguta*, is hardy. The plants are sold as male or female. To get fruit you need both. The males can cause some allergy; the females have no pollen and cause no allergies.

Actinorhytis. 7
Tropical and subtropical palms. Zones 10 to 13.

ADAM'S NEEDLE. See *Yucca*.

Adansonia digitata. 3
BAOBAB TREE. Native to Africa, with a very thick, unusual barrel-shaped trunk. A medicinal plant with many uses. Frost-tender but can be grown in a container as a houseplant. Zones 11 to 13.

Adenium obesum. 5
Tender, odd-shaped shrub mostly grown in containers. Sap can cause rashes.

Adiantum. 3
MAIDENHAIR FERN. Ferns do not have pollen but produce spores that can cause allergies. The maidenhair is one of the better ferns, because it produces only small amounts of spores.

Adromischus. 1 ✪
PLOVER EGGS. Desert succulent grown for its thick leaves.

Aechmea. 2 ✪
AIR PINE. A bromeliad; tender except in warmest zones.

Aegopodium. 3
BISHOP'S WEED. A very hardy, perennial ground cover that grows well in the shade; a good substitute for ivy. May get weedy. Possible contact skin allergy potential.

Aeonium. 1 ✪
Large group of easy-to-grow tender succulents for zones 9 to 13, or houseplants elsewhere.

Aeschynanthus (Trichosporum). 2 ✪
BASKET PLANT, LIPSTICK PLANT. Houseplants grown for their unusual foliage.

Aesculus. 6 TO 7
BUCKEYE, HORSE CHESTNUT. Large, deciduous, flowering trees. There are many kinds of Aesculus, none especially good for the allergy-free landscape. Has poisonous seeds and pollen that is occasionally fatal to honeybees.

Aethionema. 2 ✪
STONECRESS. Small, hardy, flowering perennial that grows best in sandy soil with a high pH.

AFRICAN BOXWOOD. See *Myrsine*.

AFRICAN BREAD TREE. See *Treculia*.

AFRICAN CORN LILY. See *Ixia*.

AFRICAN DAISY. See *Arctotis*; *Dimorphotheca*; *Osteospermum*.

AFRICAN EVERGREEN. See *Syngonium podophyllum*.

AFRICAN LINDEN. See *Sparmannia africana*.

AFRICAN RED ALDER. See *Cunonia capensis*.

AFRICAN SUMACH. See *Rhus*.

AFRICAN VIOLET. See *Saintpaulia ionantha*.

AFRICAN WINTERSWEET. See *Acokanthera*.

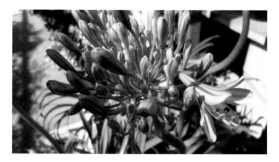

Agapanthus. 2 ✪

LILY-OF-THE-NILE. (Pictured above.) Large, easy-to-grow perennial with white or blue flowers. Most Agapanthus are evergreen and none is hardy too far from the coast. Lily-of-the-Nile makes a good container plant outdoors. Possible skin rash from sap.

Agapetes serpens. 1 ✪

An evergreen shrub for the cool areas of zones 9 and 10, with showy red hanging flowers in spring. Does best in moist, acid soil.

Agastache. 3

GIANT HYSSOP. A group of about thirty species of tall perennials, some native to the United States. *A. cana* is grown in zones 9 to 13 for its dense clusters of rosy pink flowers. Members of the mint family, these plants are attractive to butterflies and bees.

Agathis robusta. MALES 8, FEMALES 1 ✪

DAMMAR PINE, QUEENSLAND KAURI. Tall, narrow evergreen tree with bright green leaves; hardy only in zones 9 to 12. It needs fertile soil and ample water to thrive. Occasionally substituted for Podocarpus.

Agave. 4 TO 6

CENTURY PLANT, RHINO'S HORN. Big, bold succulents hardy only in the warmest areas, or grown as houseplants for sunny rooms. Some Agave species grow far too large for the average landscape, and many have stiff leaves tipped with very sharp, dangerous spines. Do not use the spine-tipped species near walkways or where children play. Plants may not flower for many years and then usually die after blooming. The attractive *A. attenuata*, or rhino's horn, is spineless and makes a fine and unusual houseplant for a sunny room. The sap of certain Agave, especially *A. americana* (century plant), can cause severe contact skin rash. Landscapers removing old century plants often contract this blistering rash. All parts of some species of Agave are poisonous.

Ageratum. 2 ✪

Summer annual for all zones, bearing pink, white, or, most popular, blue flowers.

Aglaomorpha. 4

A tropical fern used in the greenhouse and as a houseplant. Ferns should be used with care as hanging plants, because they may drop spores.

Aglaonema. 5

A rather common tropical evergreen perennial houseplant that has some limited potential to be allergenic when in bloom. Can grow outside in zones 10B to 13.

A. modestum. 2 ✪

CHINESE EVERGREEN. A common, easy-to-grow houseplant that has been found by the National Aeronautics and Space Administration (NASA) to be especially good at cleaning up, or "scrubbing," indoor air pollution.

Agonis flexuosa. 5

AUSTRALIAN WILLOW, PEPPERMINT TREE. Medium-size evergreen type of myrtle tree, many selections with very dark, almost brown, leaves; hardy in zones 9 to 12.

Agrimonia eupatoria. 10 ◐

AGRIMONY. Native, tall hardy herbs sometimes grown in shady herb gardens for medicinal uses. Several species, most with small yellow flowers and fuzzy or hairy leaves. This plant can cause severe skin rashes.

AGRIMONY. See *Agrimonia eupatoria*.

Agropyron. 6

QUACKGRASS, WHEATGRASS. Hardy grasses that grow well in the Rocky Mountain area and are the cause of some allergy. One species, *A. repens*, commonly called quackgrass, is a low-pollen-producing species and as such it may have value in lawns of the future. In general, the wheatgrasses do not usually produce highly allergenic pollen, making them a genus of grass that deserves further attention for their potential as a lawn grass.

Agrostemma githago. 4

CORN COCKLE. Annual herb grown for its purple flowers. The black seeds are poisonous.

Agrostis. 9 ◐

BENT GRASS, REDTOP. Hardy lawn grasses, which must be kept mowed very low to avoid flowering.

Ailanthus. MALES 7, FEMALES 1 ✪

STINK TREE, TREE-OF-HEAVEN. A weedy tree with malodorous flowers that produce plenty of allergenic pollen. These trees are more appreciated in their native

China, hence the name tree-of-heaven. Here they grow in waste places where other trees fail. This is said to be the tree in the book *A Tree Grows in Brooklyn*, by Betty Smith. *Ailanthus altissima* 'Betty Smith' is a new, soon-to-be-released, winter-hardy, fast-growing female selection.

Aiphanes. 6
Tropical and subtropical palms.

AIR PINE. See *Aechmea.*

Ajuga. 1 ✪
CARPET BUGLE. A hardy, blue-flowered ground cover perennial, Ajuga thrives in moist shade and is a good substitute for ivy.

Akebia quinata. 4
FIVE-LEAF AKEBIA. Fast-growing perennial vine native to Japan. Akebia is hardy only in zones 9 and 10; it bears attractive leaves and small, edible fruits.

AKEE TREE. See *Blighia sapida.*

ALASKA YELLOW CEDAR. See *Chamaecyparis.*

Albizia julibrissin. 6
MIMOSA, SILK TREE. A hardy Japanese native common in California; it thrives in areas with high summer heat. Zones 9 to 13. Leaves are poisonous.

Alcea. 2 TO 3 ✪
HOLLYHOCK. This old-fashioned tall perennial is hardy in all zones. The doubles are occasionally hard to find but worth the effort. The large, bristle-covered leaves occasionally cause contact skin rash for those with sensitive skin. Hollyhock flowers produce a rather abundant low-allergenic pollen; these flowers should never be directly sniffed. The double-flowered varieties have a better allergy ranking. Use rust-free varieties.

Alchemilla erythropoda. 4
DWARF LADIES MANTLE. A low-growing hardy ground cover perennial in the rose family that is easy to grow and widely adapted. Plants are used in natural medicine for many things and this sometimes does cause allergy. Good garden plants, native to Europe. Zones 3 to 9. Full sun in northern areas and shade in southern. Parts of the plant are used to stop flow of blood from cuts.

ALDER. See *Alnus.*

Aleurites fordii. 9 ✦
TUNG OIL TREE. A small- to medium-size evergreen tree for zones 9 to 12. Both pollen and sap are allergenic, and simple contact with the leaves could severely affect certain individuals, especially those with an allergy to rubber products. The seeds are poisonous and fatal to people and livestock.

ALEXANDER PALM. See *Ptychosperma.*

ALEXANDRA PALM. See *Archontophoenix.*

ALGERIAN FIR. See *Abies.*

ALGERIAN IVY. See *Hedera canariensis.*

ALKALI GRASS. See *Zigadenus.*

Allium. 2 ✪
CHIVES, FLOWERING GARLIC, FLOWERING ONION, GARLIC. Hardy and easy-to-grow bulbs, Alliums do best in full sun in rich, moist soil. Some of the ornamental garlics and onions have a disagreeable odor when crushed.

Alloplectus (Hypocyrta) nummularia. 1 ✪
GOLDFISH PLANT. Attractive small indoor potted plant that needs warmth and humidity to thrive.

ALLSPICE, CAROLINA. See *Calycanthus floridus.*

ALMOND. See *Prunus communis.*

Alnus. 9 ✦
ALDER. Large, hardy deciduous shade trees that grow incredibly fast when given enough moisture. Alder-caused allergies are very common and well known. Alders bloom extremely early in spring, occasionally as early as late December in zones 9 and 10. They shed a great deal of bright yellow, highly allergenic pollen.

Alocasia. 1 ✪
ELEPHANT'S EAR. A tender perennial grown for its large, bold leaves. It is used outdoors only in the warmest coastal zones. Zones 10 to 13.

Aloe. 1 ✪
Perennials and several species of small trees that are hardy outdoors in zones 9 and 10, and popular as houseplants elsewhere. Members of the lily family, they are easy to grow.

Alopecurus. 8
FOXTAIL GRASS. Common forage grasses.

Aloysia triphylla. 3
LEMON VERBENA. Shrubby perennial in zones 9 and 10, prized for its fragrant leaves.

Alpinia. 2 ✪
GINGER. Easy-to-grow perennial in warm coastal areas.

Alstroemeria. 4
PERUVIAN LILY, SOUTH AMERICAN LILY. Alstroemeria is an easy-to-grow perennial for zones 4 to 11. It

produces showy flowers during much of the year. The flowers are very long lasting when cut. The pollen is exposed but presents few problems unless directly inhaled. The leaves occasionally cause an allergic skin rash, so use caution when handling them or working around them in the garden.

Alternanthera ficoidea. 5
Shade plant grown as an annual in most zones, and used like Coleus, for its attractive leaves. Do not let it flower; keep the blooms clipped off because the flowers may be allergenic.

ALTHEA. See *Hibiscus*.

ALUMINUM PLANT. See *Pilea*.

Alyogyne huegelii. 3
BLUE HIBISCUS. A common tall perennial subshrub in warm coastal areas. Blue, hibiscus-like flowers on a plant hardy to 20°F. The flowers attract hummingbirds.

Alyssum. 5
A low-growing perennial for all zones, with yellow, heavily fragrant flowers. The strong smell may bother some people. Contact with Alyssum flowers and leaves may irritate the skin. In the garden, use it sparingly.

ALYSSUM, SWEET. See *Lobularia maritima*

AMARACUS. See *Origanum majorana*.

AMARANTH. See *Amaranthus*.

Amaranthus. 6
AMARANTH, LOVE-LIES-BLEEDING. Tall annuals grown in all zones for their long, drooping reddish flowers. They are closely related to common weeds known to cause much allergy.

Amarcrinum. 2 ✪
A tall, fragrant lily, easy to grow in mild winter areas. Most sold are hybrids.

AMARYLLIS. See *Hippeastrum*.

Amaryllis belladonna (Brunsvigia rosea). 2 ✪
BELLADONNA LILY, NAKED LADY. Hardy in zones 8 to 11 if protected in winter. Naked lady has big pink trumpet-shaped flowers that are borne when the plant has no leaves. Leaves grow after the flowers have bloomed. Clumps of naked lady may last for many years. Some may find the unusual, sweet fragrance too strong when used in the house as a cut flower.

AMAZON VINE. See *Stigmaphyllon*.

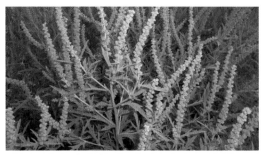

Ambrosia. 10 ◐
RAGWEED. (Pictured above.) Some native and others accidental imports, ragweeds thrive where people have neglected the land. They grow almost worldwide, but are most common in the midwestern United States. Ragweeds are also found in Eastern Europe and in parts of France. Most of the United Kingdom is free of Ambrosia.

On land untouched by human hands, ragweeds are rarely found. These and many of the worst allergenic weeds flourish only where people have disturbed the soil and natural vegetation, and then left it in a disturbed state. Nature abhors bare ground and soon covers it with weeds. Ragweeds are common in burned-out soils, waste, and dump areas, and wherever the ecosystem is out of balance.

One of the principles of sustainable agriculture is that the soil should always be covered, either by plants or by mulch. Bare soil, exposed to the destructive effects of wind, rain, and sun, is soil being destroyed. If the cultural conditions are changed so that soil can sustain its fertility, friability, organic matter, earthworms, and all the other microorganisms that keep it healthy, then ragweeds, cheeseweeds, and tumbleweeds quickly disappear.

To get rid of ragweed, chop it down before it can bloom and reseed. More important, work toward sustainability of the soil.

Farmers often spray ragweeds with an herbicide containing 2,4-D (the same chemical as in dandelion killers). The sprayed ragweeds quickly wilt and become highly attractive to livestock. Cattle in particular have frequently been poisoned with 2,4-D after grazing on recently sprayed weeds.

Amelanchier laevis. 3
SERVICE BERRY, JUNEBERRY, SHADBUSH. A group of shrubs, small trees, and ground covers hardy to zone 3. Service berry is among the first flowering trees to bloom in early spring and puts on a show of bright white blossoms, followed by small fruits that look and taste

much like wild blueberries. Birds are very fond of these fruits—as am I. These should be used much more often than they are.

Ammophila. 9 🖋

BEACHGRASS. Several species of imported grasses used to stabilize beaches. Once established, they often crowd out less aggressive native species and produce allergy.

AMOMYRTUS. See *Luma apiculata.*

Amorpha fruticosa. 4

INDIGOBUSH. Very large shrubby native perennial hardy to zone 4. Fruits eaten by wild birds and flower spikes visited by bees and butterflies. Interesting large leaves, easy to grow, may become invasive in Washington State, where it is not native. In the Fabaceae family, related to peas.

Ampelopsis brevipedunculata. 2 ✿

BLUEBERRY CLIMBER. A deciduous vine for sun or shade, hardy in all zones; it grows strong and fast and needs good support. The fruits resemble blueberries and are attractive to birds. Ampelopsis is a good substitute for English ivy.

Amsonia illustris. 5

OZARK BLUESTAR. Native perennial for wild gardens in zones 5 to 9; small blue star-shaped flowers and shiny leaves. Member of the Dogbane family, almost all of which are at least slightly suspect for allergies. Sap is poisonous and is a potential dermatitis agent; handle with care.

AMUR CHOKECHERRY. See *Prunus maackii.*

AMUR CORK TREE. See *Phellodendron*

AMUR MAPLE. See *Acer tataricum ginnala.*

Amyris madrensis. 3

Native Texas shrub sometimes used in landscaping in zones 9 to 11. Small fragrant flowers, glossy green leaves, very heat- and drought-tolerant.

Anacardiaceae.

CASHEW FAMILY. Large group of more than 600 species of trees and shrubs, mostly evergreen but some deciduous, many with poisonous properties. This family of plants accounts for more cases of allergy than any other, and includes genera such as Astronium, Cotinus, Harpephyllum, Laurophyllus, Lithrea, Mangifera, Pistache, Rhodosphaera, Rhus, Schinus, Semecarpus, Smodingium, Spondias, and Toxicodendron. Individually ranked. In this group are poison ivy, poison oak, cashew, pistachio nut, mango, and pepper trees.

Anacardium occidentale. 10 🖋

CASHEW. A large, spreading evergreen tree to 40 feet, grown as an ornamental in zone 10. It is native to tropical America and widely grown in tropics and subtropics; commercially in India. It is notable for its milky allergenic sap, yellowish pink flowers, and 3-inch-long edible red fruits called cashew apples, the seeds of which are cashew nuts. Zones 11 to 13.

Anacyclus depressus. 3

A perennial hardy in all zones with daisylike flowers on a low-growing, spreading plant. It grows best in lighter soils.

Anadenanthiera. 5

YOPO TREE. Mimosa-like tropical tree with psychoactive properties. Not well implicated in allergy, but it is possible that the pollen also might have some of these psychoactive properties.

Anagallis. 3

PIMPERNEL. Low-growing perennials or annuals for full sun in all zones. The small flowers are scarlet or blue. Plants are poisonous.

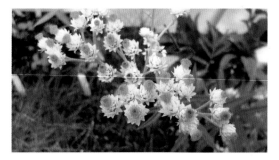

Anaphalis. MALES 6, FEMALES 1 ✿

PEARLY EVERLASTING. (*Anaphalis margaritacea*, female, pictured above.) A perennial grown as a cut flower and for long-lasting dried flowers. Avoid its use in the landscape and as a dried flower. Anaphalis is separate-sexed, but is not usually sold sexed. *Anaphalis margaritacea* 'Pearly Girl Everlasting' is a soon-to-be-released new female, pollen-free cultivar propagated by rhizomes.

Anchusa. 2 ✿

BUGLOSS. Hardy annuals or perennials similar to forget-me-nots (Myosotis) but on much larger plants. It thrives in full sun and dry soil, where it produces its clusters of bright blue flowers in abundance.

Andrachne. MALES 7, FEMALES 1 ✿

A native shrub occasionally used in landscaping in south-central areas of the United States.

Andromeda. 2 ✪

BOG ROSEMARY. A hardy rock garden evergreen shrub with pale pink flowers for wet areas. See also *Zenobia*.

Andropogon. 6

BEARDGRASS, BIG BLUESTEM GRASS. A common grass that is the cause of some grass allergies.

Androsace. 2 ✪

ROCK JASMINE. A low-growing hardy perennial.

Andryala aghardii. 2 ✪

A small, low-growing yellow-flowered annual for rock gardens.

Anemone. 3

WINDFLOWER. Grown from seed, divisions, or tubers, Anemones are attractive garden flowers in all zones. In the garden these flowers present little allergy problem, but as cut flowers they are suspect. Anemone leaves and flowers are poisonous.

ANEMONE, BUSH. See *Carpenteria californica*.

Anemopaegma chamberlaynii. 2 ✪

YELLOW TRUMPET VINE. Hardy only in zones 10 to 13; a good flowering vine for mild areas.

Anemopsis californica. 2 ✪

YERBA MANSA. A common western wildflower for wet places. The flowers look like small coneflowers with white petals (actually bracts). The leaves of yerba mansa are long and wide. As a wildflower it ranges from California to Texas and has long been used by inhabitants of the Southwest as an old folk remedy plant. The root is used to make a tea said to help relieve asthma.

Anethum. 3

DILL. A garden annual, easily grown from seed.

ANGEL TRUMPET. See *Brugmansia*; *Datura*.

Angelica. 6

Biennial for all zones that thrives in rich, moist soils. Contact with the leaves of Angelica may cause skin rashes.

ANGEL'S HAIR. See *Artemisia*.

ANGEL'S TEARS. See *Narcissus*; *Soleirolia soleirolii*.

Angophora costata. 5

GUM MYRTLE. Evergreen tree for zones 9 and 10.

Anigozanthos. 2 ✪

KANGAROO PAW. Tender evergreen native perennials for light soils with full sun and good drainage. Best in zones 9 to 12; very drought-tolerant. Fuzzy flowers (on long stems) come in many colors, especially bright orange, pink, and red tones.

Anisacanthus. 2 ✪

DESERT HONEYSUCKLE. A perennial shrub for mild winter areas of zones 8 to 10. It bears bright orange flowers much of the year.

ANISE. See *Foeniculum*; *Pimpinella anisum*.

ANISE TREE. See *Illicium anisatum*.

Annona cherimola. 3

CHERIMOYA. A small, deciduous tree for warm coastal areas of zone 10. It has large attractive leaves and big, green, delicious fruits. Cherimoya is easily grown from the large black seeds. The leaves and stems of Cherimoya are quite poisonous.

Anredera (Boussingaultia). 5

MADEIRA VINE. Evergreen vines hardy to zone 8, or in colder zones if the tubers are dug and stored over winter. Anredera is notable for its heart-shaped leaves and clusters of fragrant white flowers.

Antennaria. MALES 5, FEMALES 1 ✪

LADIES'-TOBACCO, PUSSY TOES. A group of small deciduous perennial herbs, native to North and South America, and to North Europe and Asia. A few species are hardy in all zones. Dioecious (separate-sexed) plants, especially *A. dioica*. The male plants are smaller than the females and in some species, male plants are unknown. Not usually sold sexed, but look for selected females. Possible ground cover plant; quite drought-resistant.

Anthemis. 5

CHAMOMILE, DOG FENNEL, MARGUERITE DAISY. A daisylike perennial that is hardy in all zones. Tea from chamomile is known to trigger allergy. Has been known to cause skin rash from contact with the leaves.

Anthoxanthum. 10 ✎

SWEET VERNAL GRASS, VERNAL GRASS. A European grass introduced and naturalized in the United States and the cause of widespread allergy, especially early in the spring.

Anthriscus. 3

CHERVIL. An annual herb for all zones, chervil grows best in partial shade.

Anthurium. 2 ✪

Houseplants.

Antiaris. 10 ⬙

Tropical trees or shrubs. Sap used for poison arrows.

Antidesma. MALES 9 ⬙, FEMALES 1 ✿

CHINESE LAUREL. An evergreen tree, zone 10.

Antigonon. 2 ✿

CORAL VINE. Deciduous vine for zones 9 and 10, bearing long clusters of red flowers. It does well in desert areas and should be mulched in colder areas.

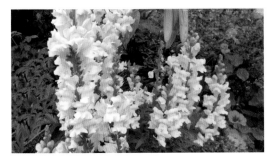

Antirrhinum majus. 1 ✿

SNAPDRAGON. (Pictured above.) A hardy annual for all zones that thrives in cooler weather. Many sizes and colors are available.

Aphanamixis. MALES 9 ⬙, FEMALES 1 ✿

Seldom-seen, dioecious trees, zones 10 to 13.

Aphananthe. 8

MUKU TREE. Several species of fast-growing elm-related trees from Korea, eastern China, and Japan, occasionally used in landscaping in the United States. Hardy to zone 6, the muku tree is one of the few elm relatives that has separate male-only flowers, and because of this it releases large amounts of pollen into the air. Elm allergy is common and often severe.

Aphelandra. 2 ✿

Houseplant with big, striped leaves that does best in filtered light.

Apium graveolens. 4

CELERY. There are many documented examples of allergy to eating celery, as well as numerous examples of skin rashes caused by contact with leaves in sensitive individuals. Celery is related to certain common allergenic weeds, such as Queen Anne's lace, and cross-reaction allergies are common, especially during the fall peak of the ragweed bloom. Persons with ragweed allergies would be wise to avoid eating celery in the late summer and fall months. Carrot allergy may arise with already existing celery allergy.

Apocynum. 4

DOGBANE. A hardy perennial herb. The sap may cause rash in sensitive persons. Poisonous.

Aponogeton distachyus. 2 ✿

CAPE PONDWEED, WATER HAWTHORN, WATER LILY. Aquatic plants for lakes, ponds, and small pools.

APPLE. See *Malus*.

APRICOT. See *Prunus armeniaca*.

Aptenia cordifolia. 1 ✿

RED-APPLE ICEPLANT. Low-growing evergreen perennial for zones 9 and 10. It bears small red flowers and is very easy to grow from cuttings inserted directly into the soil.

Aquilegia. 1 ✿

COLUMBINE. Hardy perennials for all zones, columbines are good garden and woodland flowers. Poisonous.

ARABIAN TEA. See *Catha edulis*.

Arabis. 1 ✿

ROCKCRESS. A hardy perennial for all zones, often used as a rock garden plant. Easy-to-grow, attractive flowers are usually white or pink.

Arachis hypogaea. 3

PEANUT. Annual legume needing a warm summer, sandy soil, and a long growing season to produce well. All parts of the plant are edible, but allergy to eating peanuts is common and often severe. Allergy to pollen of peanuts, however, is quite rare.

Aralia. 5

A group of often spiny, deciduous shrubs or small trees with big, bold leaves. Hardy to zone 5.

ARALIA, FALSE. See *Dizygotheca*.

ARAR TREE. See *Tetraclinis*.

Araucaria. MALES 7, FEMALES 1 ✿

BUNYA-BUNYA, MONKEY PUZZLE TREE. Large group of nonnative evergreen trees; some hardy into zone 5. *A. heterophylla*, the Norfolk Island pine, is often grown as a houseplant tree. Kept in a container, most Araucaria will never bloom or cause allergies. Planted in the ground, however, they are not good choices for allergy-free landscapes.

Most species are separate-sexed and, in the future, female-only plants may be available. Because young Araucaria trees do not bloom, a small Norfolk Island pine can be a good substitute for a real pine Christmas tree for those with odor and perfume allergies to pine.

Araujia. **3**
WHITE BLADDER FLOWER. Easy-to-grow, woody vine for zones 8 to 10.

ARBOR SANCTA. See *Melia.*

ARBORVITAE. See *Platycladus*; *Thuja.*

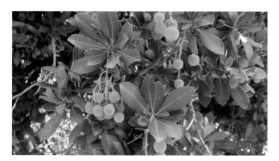

Arbutus. **3**
MADRONE, STRAWBERRY TREE. (Pictured above.) Several species of native trees and shrubs hardy to zone 4. Attractive bark, small to medium size, and attractive fruits make these popular landscape choices. Drought-tolerant.

Archontophoenix. **6**
ALEXANDRA PALM, KING PALM. Hardy only in warmest areas of zones 9 and 10, these are handsome palms that unfortunately cause some allergy. On existing trees, if possible, cut off the male branches each year before the flowers open and release pollen.

Arctocarpus communis. **2** ✪
BREADFRUIT. Grown mostly in the West Indies, Polynesia, and eastern India, the breadfruit tree is a large evergreen with huge leaves and giant, bland fruits. The seeds are roasted and eaten like chestnuts. A low allergy risk.

Arctostaphylos. **2** ✪
BEARBERRY, KINNIKINNICK, MANZANITA. Evergreen shrubs and increasingly popular ground covers. Hardy into zone 5, manzanita is native to the dry areas of the West. Easy to grow in well-drained soil, they do best in full sun. Many varieties have been developed for use as ground covers, and all of these are good choices where adaptable.

Arctotheca calendula. **4**
CAPE WEED. Gray-leafed ground cover for zones 9 to 12, Cape weed spreads fast in full sun and is soon covered with yellow daisylike flowers.

Arctotis. **4**
AFRICAN DAISY. An annual and a perennial that is easy to grow. It is available in many colors. Some double forms are pollen-free.

Ardisia. **3**
SPICEBERRY. Evergreen shade-loving shrub or ground cover that requires ample moisture to grow well.

Areca. **6**
BETEL NUT PALM. Tropical and subtropical palms.

Arecastrum romanzoffianum. **6**
QUEEN PALM. Occasionally sold as *Cocos plumosa.* Monoecious; if possible, cut off male branches before the flowers open and shed pollen.

Arenaria. **3**
SANDWORT. Hardy perennial ground cover occasionally used as a lawn substitute. Good in rock gardens.

Arenga. **3**
TROPICAL AND SUBTROPICAL PALM TREE. Monocarpic, they only bloom once, then die after blooming.

Argemone. **2** ✪
PRICKLY POPPY. Annual or biennial for all zones. Very drought-tolerant, tall plant with prickly stems and big, showy white poppy flowers. Native to dry areas in the desert. *A. mexicana* has orange flowers. Poisonous.

Arikuryroba schizophylla. **6**
Small subtropical palm trees, occasionally grown in Florida.

Arisaema triphyllum. **2** ✪
JACK IN THE PULPIT. Hardy, shade-loving small perennial for zones 3 to 8, native to the eastern U.S. and Canada, best in rich moist soils with lots of organic matter. Roots are poisonous.

Aristolochia. **3**
BIRTHWORT, CALICO FLOWER, DUTCHMAN'S PIPE VINE. Hardy in most zones and easy to grow, Aristolochia thrives in either full sun or deep shade. The odd-shaped flowers resemble a curved tobacco pipe. Very poisonous.

Armeria. **1** ✪
SEA PINK, THRIFT. A low-growing evergreen perennial native to coastal areas. Hardy in all zones. Very good plants for edging flower gardens. Easy to grow and often in bloom with many pink, red, or rose-colored flowers.

Armoracia rusticana. **2** ✪
HORSERADISH. Easy-to-grow, very hardy perennial grown for its pungent roots, which are used as a

condiment. 'Variegata' is a fancy-leafed cultivar with some extra color.

Arnica. 8
Relatives of *Senecio*. A group of about thirty species of hardy perennial herbs and flowers. The pollen of Arnica species is highly allergenic, especially for anyone already allergic to the ragweeds, to which Arnica is closely related. Many species are capable of causing severe allergic skin reactions. All species are poisonous if eaten.

Aronia arbutifolia. 2 ⊙
RED CHOKEBERRY. Deciduous shrub native to the eastern United States and hardy to zone 4. Easy to grow and tolerant of wet soils, it has attractive autumn color and red berries that attract birds.

Arrhenatherum elatius. 3
TALL OATGRASS. A meadow grass, used mostly for pastures. For a grass species, it produces little pollen and is unimportant in causing allergy. This grass may find greater use as a lawn grass in the near future. There is a clump-forming variegated type of oatgrass sold as an ornamental grass, and it is much less allergenic than most ornamental grasses now sold.

ARROW GRASS. See *Triglochin*.

ARROW ROOT. See *Zamia*.

ARROWHEAD VINE. See *Syngonium podophyllum*.

ARROWWOOD. See *Viburnum*; *Zamia*.

Artemisia. 7 TO 9 ◗ DEPENDING ON SPECIES
ANGEL'S HAIR, DUSTY MILLER, OLD MAN, SAGEBRUSH, SOUTHERNWOOD, TARRAGON, WORMWOOD. Many species of evergreen or deciduous shrubs or woody perennials, hardy in all zones. Artemisias are close relatives of ragweeds, and many people have strong allergic reactions to all of them, both from their odors and from their abundant pollen. Many more species of Artemisia are being used now, due to the popularity of native landscaping.

Artemisias are often called sage and as such are occasionally used in cooking. However, true culinary sage is actually a type of Salvia and is not related to Artemisia. Many species of Artemisia are poisonous if eaten, including their seeds, flowers, and leaves. Certain types of Artemisia are used in herbal medicinals; use Artemisia very carefully, if at all. If you are allergic to the ragweeds, it would be wise to avoid any contact with the Artemisias.

One species, *A. absinthium*, a fragrant herb, was used to flavor a liqueur called absinthe. Popular in the late 1800s, many people, including the painter Vincent van Gogh, were addicted to absinthe. Van Gogh's heavy absinthe consumption is said to have caused much of his famously erratic behavior. Absinthe was made illegal in France in 1912 and in the United States in 1915; however, it recently seems to be making a comeback and is again used in mixed drinks.

ARTICHOKE. See *Cynara*.

ARTILLERY PLANT. See *Pilea*.

Arum. 4
BLACK CALLA. Large-leafed perennials, hardy to zone 6. Grown mostly as curiosity plants, some Arum bear very malodorous flowers. Recently, a giant arum with a 6-foot-tall purple flower bloomed at the Huntington Gardens in Los Angeles. Huge crowds came to see this corpse flower. The smell of the flower was compared to that of a rotting carcass. The smell alone could cause allergy for some. Don't plant this one too close to the house. Poisonous.

Aruncus sylvester. MALES 8, FEMALES 1 ⊙
GOATSBEARD. Tall white-flowered perennial with ferny foliage that grows best in moist, shady spots. Some new female cultivars may be available. Best in zones 4 to 9.

ARUNDINARIA. See *Bamboo*.

Arundo donax. 8
GIANT REED. Hardy perennial for all zones. Arundo may quickly become invasive.

Asarina antirrhinifolia. 2 ⊙
Tall annuals with colorful flowers that resemble snapdragons.

Asarum. 1 ⊙
WILD GINGER. Hardy, attractive, big-leafed perennials that produce red flowers on low-growing plants. Gingers require ample moisture and rich soil to thrive.

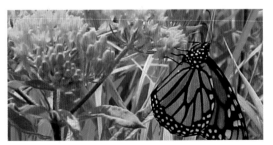

Asclepias. 3
BUTTERFLY WEED, GOOSE PLANT, MILKWEED. (*Asclepias tuberosa*, pictured above.) Hardy in full sun in all

zones. Monarch butterfly larvae depend, 100 percent, on these plants for survival; I always plant some in my own gardens just for the butterflies. Milkweed flowers may also draw wasps (which then eat the eggs of the butterflies). *A. tuberosa* is hardy in zones 3 to 9, native, and has bright orange flowers. *A. syriaca* is native, hardy in zones 3 to 9, and good for monarch butterflies (as are all milkweeds). *A. incarnate*, native, zones 3 to 12, has fragrant pink flower clusters; good pollinator plants. The many species of this genus are toxic if eaten; cattle in particular are often poisoned from eating milkweed.

ASH. See *Fraxinus*.

ASH-LEAFED MAPLE. See *Acer negundo*.

ASH, MOUNTAIN. See *Sorbus*.

Asimina triloba. 3
PAW PAW. Small, large-leafed, deciduous native fruit tree for moist areas of zones 5 to 8. The bland, custard-like fruit are borne on attractive trees.

Asparagus. MALES 6, FEMALES 1 ☻
Ornamental and edible perennials. Ornamental asparagus is not nearly as hardy as the edible variety. Asparagus fern, not a true fern, is a popular houseplant. These are complete-flowered and ranked lower for allergy, at 3. The edible asparagus is separate-sexed, and most commercial varieties are males. People living near fields of asparagus are at risk from the pollen of the mature plants. People who handle a great deal of cut asparagus can get skin rashes, and this is fairly common in asparagus canning plants. Some people also report allergic reactions to eating asparagus. 'Mary Washington' is a mostly female clone. The 'Knight' series is almost all male plants.

ASPEN. See *Populus*.

Asperula azurea. 3
A hardy blue-flowered fragrant annual grown from seed.

ASPERULA ODORATA. See *Galium odoratum*.

Asphodelus albus. 3
A white-flowered lily.

Aspidistra elatior. 1 ☻
CAST-IRON PLANT. An evergreen perennial, hardy to zone 7 and grown as a houseplant elsewhere. It will grow well in deep shade and needs little care.

ASPIDIUM. See *Rumohra adiantiformis*.

Asplenium. 4
BIRD'S-NEST FERN. Houseplants or outdoors in mild areas in shade with plenty of moisture. Spores from ferns can cause allergies, but usually the spores do not travel far from the parent plant. Unless used in overhead hanging baskets, most ferns do not present much of a problem in the allergy-free garden. (See also *Fern*.)

ASSYRIAN PLUM. See *Cordia*.

Astelia. 3
Large tufted, grasslike, strap-leafed clumping perennials for zones 9 to 10.

Aster. DOUBLES 2 ☻, SINGLES 4
Hardy perennials for all zones, asters are common garden flowers in a wide array of colors. Some make fairly large shrubs. Asters have a bad name in allergy studies and single-flowered asters do not make good cut flowers for the allergic household. Nonetheless, not all asters produce the same amounts of pollen. A few plants in a large garden should not present much of a problem. Fully double-flowered varieties have far fewer exposed pollen parts, and some are actually pollen-free.

ASTER TREE. See *Olearia*.

Asteriscus maritmus. 4
Easy-to-grow, mound-forming perennials with yellow flowers. Full sun in zones 8 to 10.

Asterogyne. 5
Tropical and subtropical palms.

Astilbe. 4
Shade-loving perennials hardy in all zones, they are long-lived in cold-winter areas. Astilbe needs rich, moist soil to thrive.

Astrantia. 3
MASTERWORT. Shade-loving, large-flowered perennial or annual from seed.

Astrocaryum. 6
PALM. *A. mexicanum* grows in parts of zones 10 to 13.

Astronium. MALES 9 🍃, FEMALES 1 ☻
Numerous species of small allergenic trees native to South America, occasionally found planted in zones 9 and 10. In particular, *A. balansae*, a 30-foot evergreen tree with long compound leaves like sumac, is often used in landscaping.

Athrotaxis. 8
Evergreen coniferous tree from Tasmania used in zones 9 to 12. Related to Cryptomeria, these cause allergy.

Athyrium. 5
LADY FERN. Hardy fern for moist, shady areas. Grows to 4 feet.

ATLAS BROOM. See *Cytisus*.

ATLAS CEDAR. See *Cedrus atlantica*.

Atriplex. MALES 9 🍃, FEMALES 1 ✿

DESERT HOLLY, QUAILBUSH, SALTBUSH. Native desert perennials or large shrubs. Easy to grow and drought-tolerant, male shrubs cause allergies. Female plants are easy to grow from cuttings and root quickly. 'Desert Girl' is a soon-to-be-released female *Atriplex lentiformis* cultivar that is fast growing, is hardy to zone 7, needs little care, and is pollen-free.

Attalea. 7

Tropical and subtropical palms.

Aubrieta. 2 ✿

Hardy, low-growing perennial for rock gardens or along rock walls.

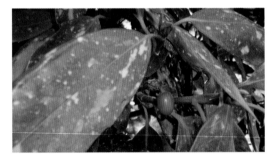

Aucuba japonica. MALES 6, FEMALES 1 ✿

GOLD DUST PLANT. (*Aucuba japonica*, female, pictured above.) A small group of Asiatic evergreen shrubs hardy in zones 5 to 10 and used as a greenhouse plant in colder climates. Aucuba grows well in deep shade and has large, toothed, often variegated leaves. These are separate-sexed plants; males cause allergies, females do not. Look for named varieties or those already producing large red berries. The varieties 'Aureo-maculata', 'Fructu Albo', 'Longifolia', 'Nana', 'Pictura', 'Serratifolia', and 'Sulphur' are all females and have excellent allergy rankings. The variety 'Crotonifolia' is a male and should be avoided. 'Variegata' can be either male or female. Don't buy 'Variegata' unless it is tagged as a female or has red fruit. 'Guernsey Gold' is a selected, easy-to-grow, female form and is pollen-free.

Aulax. 2 ✿

Three species of South African evergreen shrubs with white or yellow flowers.

AURICULA. See *Primula*.

Aurinia saxatilis. 3

BASKET OF GOLD. Hardy perennial for all zones. May winter-kill in cold areas if not mulched. Bright yellow flowers are borne on low-growing plants ideal for the rock garden.

AUSTRALIAN BLUEBELL CREEPER. See *Sollya heterophylla*.

AUSTRALIAN BOTTLE PLANT. See *Jatropha*.

AUSTRALIAN BUSH CHERRY. See *Syzygium*.

AUSTRALIAN FUCHSIA. See *Correa*.

AUSTRALIAN PINE. See *Casuarina*.

AUSTRALIAN WILLOW. See *Acacia*; *Geijera parviflora*.

Austrocedrus. MALES 9 🍃, FEMALES 1 ✿

CHILEAN INCENSE CEDAR. Shrubs or small trees for zone 8, where summers are cool. Separate-sexed (dioecious) plants, but not yet sold sexed. Females are excellent choices for the allergy-free garden.

AUTUMN CROCUS. See *Colchicum autumnale*.

Avena. NOT YET RANKED

OATS. A common grain that may cause allergy but usually less so than corn, wheat, or barley. Wild varieties cause more allergy.

Averrhoa. 1 ✿

Two species of small Asian evergreen fruiting trees, occasionally found in zone 10 in Florida.

AVOCADO. See *Persea americana*.

Azadirachta indica. 7

NEEM TREE. A semitropical tree for zones 10 to 13, with legumelike compound leaves and small white flowers with many exposed stamens. The source of the natural insecticide, neem; the pollen from this species is also a major source of pollen allergies in its native India.

AZALEA. See *Rhododendron*.

Azara. 4

Large, shade-loving evergreen flowering shrubs for zones 9 and 10. The flowers are small, yellow, and very fragrant; it may not be a good choice for those sensitive to odors.

Azoria vidalii. 2 ✿

Hardy perennial for shady, moist spots; bears large, bell-shaped flowers on erect stalks. Needs protection in most cold-winter areas.

AZTEC LILY. See *Lilium*.

Allergy Index Scale: 1 is Best, 10 is Worst.
✺ for 1 and 2   ❦ for 9 and 10
No matter what the ranking, always read the full plant description carefully and take note of any warnings.

BABASSU. See *Orbignya*.

Babiana. 2 ✺
BABOON FLOWER. South African native for zones 4 to 10; grown from corms. It bears spring-blooming flowers of red, blue, lavender, and white.

BABOON FLOWER. See *Babiana*.

BABY BLUE EYES. See *Nemophila*.

BABY'S BREATH. See *Gypsophila*.

BABY'S TEARS. See *Soleirolia soleirolii*.

Baccharis pilularis. MALES 9 ❦, FEMALES 1 ✺
COYOTE BRUSH, DESERT BROOM. Hardy in zones 6 to 10. Perennial shrubby ground cover or large loose bush. Coyote brush is closely related to ragweed, and allergies are common and often severe. Most varieties of Baccharis ground cover sold are all-male cultivars and are especially potent. Coyote brush became a very popular ground cover in California during the drought years of 1987–1995 because it is very drought-tolerant; allergy to this plant is on the rise. All plants are poisonous.

BACHELOR'S BUTTON. See *Centaurea*.

BACHELOR'S BUTTON, YELLOW. See *Polygala*.

Bacopa. 2 ✺
Many species of low-growing, prostate perennial plants that make excellent, long-lasting, easy-to-grow hanging baskets for full or partial shade. Hardy to zone 8, but used as an annual in all colder zones. Many new colors and hybrids now available. Bacopa is also used as a medicinal plant.

Bactris. 5
SPINY-CLUB PALM. Small palms from tropical America.

Bacularia. 6
Tropical and subtropical palms.

Baeckea. 4
Large evergreen shrubs to 5 feet tall, quite drought-tolerant. Best in zones 9 to 10.

BAHIA GRASS. See *Paspalum*.

Balaka. 6
Tropical palms.

BALD CYPRESS. See *Taxodium*.

BALLOON FLOWER. See *Platycodon grandiflorus*.

BALM-OF-GILEAD. See *Cedronella*; *Populus candicans*.

BALMIES. See *Abies*; *Populus balsamifera*.

BALSAM. See *Impatiens*.

BALSAM FIR. See *Abies*.

Bamboo. 2 ✪

GIANT GRASSES. Many people are allergic to grass pollen, and allergies to bamboo pollen are not unusual in the tropics; however, most bamboo does not flower when grown in the United States (except Hawaii). (I had a planting of golden bamboo, a 3-foot-tall variety, that grew for many years and never flowered.) There are many varieties of bamboo and most can be cut to the ground every year; they will regrow without flowering. Some of the more exotic and expensive species, such as black bamboo, are usually kept confined to a large pot. See chapter 4.

BAMBOO PALM. See *Rhapis*.

BAMBURANTA. See *Ctenanthe*.

BANANA. See *Musa paradisiaca*; *Ensete*.

BANANA SHRUB. See *Michelia*.

BANANA YUCCA. See *Yucca*.

Banksia. 3

Large group of evergreen trees and shrubs mostly grown in Australia.

Baptisia australis. 2 ✪

WILD INDIGO. Tall perennial for full sun, hardy in all zones. Spikes of indigo blue flowers resemble sweet peas. *B. alba* and *B. australis* are both native species, as is the yellow-flowered *B. bracteata*. Good pollinator plants.

BARBADOS CEDAR. See *Cedrela*.

BARBADOS CHERRY. See *Malpighia glabra*.

BARBADOS NUT. See *Jatropha*.

BARBASCO. See *Jacquinia*.

BARBEL PALM. See *Acanthophoenix*.

BARBERRY. See *Berberis*.

BARLEY. See *Hordeum*.

BARREL CACTUS. See *Echinocactus*; *Ferocactus*.

BARREL PALM. See *Colpothrinax wrightii*.

BASEBALL PLANT. See *Euphorbia*.

BASIL. See *Ocimum*.

BASKET FLOWER. See *Hymenocallis*.

BASKET OF GOLD. See *Aurinia saxatilis*.

BASKET PLANT. See *Aeschynanthus*.

BASSWOOD. See *Tilia*.

Bauhinia. 4

ORCHID TREE. Medium-size evergreen or deciduous flowering tree for zones 9 to 11. The flowers resemble orchids. Easy to grow from seed. Poisonous.

Baumea articulate. 6

JOINTED TWIG RUSH. A tall, grasslike Australian perennial sedge that will grow in standing water.

BAY. See *Laurus nobilis*; *Umbellularia californica*.

BAY LAUREL. See *Umbellularia californica*.

BAY, RED. See *Persea borbonia*.

BAY STAR VINE. See *Schisandra*.

BAYBERRY. See *Myrica*.

BEACH ASTER. See *Erigeron*.

BEACH NAUPKA. See *Scaevola*.

BEACH WORMWOOD. See *Artemisia*.

BEACHGRASS. See *Ammophila*.

BEAD PLANT. See *Nertera granadensis*.

BEAD TREE. See *Melia*; *Pithecellobium guadalupensis*.

BEANS. See *Phaseolus*.

BEARBERRY. See *Arctostaphylos*; *Rhamnus*; *Salix*.

BEARD TONGUE. See *Penstemon*.

BEARDGRASS. See *Andropogon*; *Polypogon*.

BEAR'S BREECH. See *Acanthus mollis*.

BEAR'S FOOT FERN. See *Humata tyermannii*.

BEAR-TONGUE LILY. See *Clintonia*.

Beaucarnea recurvata. MALES 6, FEMALES 1 ✪

BOTTLE PALM, PONYTAIL. Tall succulent with large, woody base. Hardy only in zone 10. Separate-sexed but not usually sold sexed. Only female plants will make seeds.

Beaumontia grandiflora. 2 ✪

EASTER LILY VINE, HERALD'S TRUMPET. Evergreen vine for zones 9 and 10 with large, fragrant, trumpet-shaped white flowers with bright green veins. Needs good soil and plenty of water. Flowers on old wood only, so do not prune too heavily. Protect from wind.

BEAUTY BUSH. See *Kolkwitzia amabilis*.

BEAUTYBERRY. See *Callicarpa bodinieri giraldii*.

BEE BALM. See *Monarda*.

BEE GUM. See *Nyssa*.

BEECH. See *Fagus.*

BEEF PLANT. See *Iresine herbstii.*

BEEFWOOD. See *Casuarina.*

BEETLEWOOD. See *Ostrya.*

BEETS. See *Beta vulgaris.*

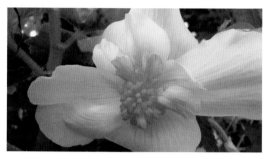

Begonia. FIBROUS 4, TUBEROUS 2 (SEE EXCEPTIONS) ✪
(Pictured above.) Annual and perennial shade-loving flowers. Begonias from seed are called fibrous begonias. Tuberous begonias are grown from fleshy tubers. Begonias are all monoecious, but the male flowers are often situated above the female blooms. The petals are large, richly colored, and attractive to insects.

The small fibrous begonias shed more pollen than the larger tuberous kinds. In large-flowered begonias, the female flowers are often single while the males are usually fully double. Fibrous begonias are not high-allergy plants, but they expose the gardener to more incidental pollen than would impatiens. Good for hanging baskets in all but the hottest areas.

Exceptions: Many tuberous begonias (especially the hanging varieties) now have functional female flowers, and male flowers with many petals and no pollen parts at all. These would rank OPALS 1. Recently the nursery trade has been producing a new kind of begonia, usually sold in 4- to 6-inch pots, and these are all-male plants. This is an unfortunate trend, and these plants would have an OPALS ranking of 7. One of these male begonias is called 'Sparks Will Fly', and I suspect we'll soon be seeing more like it, alas.

Belamcanda chinensis. 2 ✪
BLACKBERRY LILY, LEOPARD FLOWER. Rhizomatous perennial, hardy in all zones, bearing stalks of orange-red flowers. The seeds resemble blackberries.

BELLADONNA LILY. See *Amaryllis belladonna.*

BELLFLOWER. See *Campanula.*

Bellis perennis. 3
ENGLISH DAISY. Low-growing perennials hardy in all zones.

BELLS OF IRELAND. See *Moluccella laevis.*

BELLY PALM. See *Colpothrinax wrightii.*

BELOPERONE. See *Justicia.*

BENJAMIN BUSH. See *Lindera.*

BENT GRASS. See *Agrostis.*

Bentinckia. 6
Tropical palms.

Berberis. 3
BARBERRY. Deciduous and evergreen spiny shrubs, some hardy in all zones. A useful plant, easy to grow in tough landscape situations. Poisonous.

Bergenia. 2 ✪
Evergreen shade perennial hardy in all zones. Its large, cabbagelike leaves and small pink, rose, or white flowers are susceptible to snails and slugs.

Berlandiera. 4
CHOCOLATE DAISY. A hardy perennial native to the southwestern states of the U.S. Hardy in zones 4 to 10, an easy-to-grow attractive yellow-flowered plant that attracts pollinators. Good for poor, dry soils.

BERMUDA GRASS. See *Cynodon dactylon.*

BERMUDA PALM. See *Sabal.*

Bertholletia excelsa. 1 ✪
BRAZIL NUT, CREAM NUT, PARA NUT. A large, evergreen tree from tropical South America and the West Indies, grown for its seeds. Not grown in the United States, except in the mildest parts of zone 10. Trees have very large, 20-inch-long, leathery leaves and creamy white flowers. Fruits are round, 5 inches in diameter; the large seeds are the Brazil nuts of commerce. The trees are entirely insect pollinated and are not known to cause allergy. They are fairly easy to grow from seed.

BE-STILL PLANT. See *Thevetia.*

Beta vulgaris. 1 ✪
BEETS, SWISS CHARD. Garden vegetables. Beets should always be harvested long before they flower (if left to flower, they are no longer edible). The flowers may cause allergies, but this is rare, because most are never allowed to bloom. Beets have a very good allergy ranking under regular culture.

Allergy to sugar beet flowers is common and growing in incidence as the acreage of this crop is increased. People living close to sugar beet fields are at most risk. Allergy ranking for fields of sugar beets is high.

BETEL. See *Piper*.

BETEL NUT PALM. See *Areca*.

BETHLEHEM SAGE. See *Pulmonaria*.

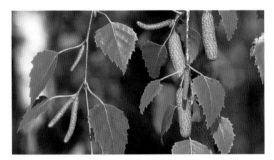

Betula. 9 ◗

BIRCH. (Pictured above.) Many species. Birch trees are probably far too common in landscaping. They shed a great deal of very allergenic pollen, and if they have any saving grace per allergies, it is that their bloom period is fairly short. However, many different species of birch are sold and planted, and each species blooms at a different time. This effectively increases the urban pollen season for birch considerably. Birch are related to alder (see *Alnus*) and their pollens are cross-reactive between the species. An allergy to birch pollen, which is very common in many areas, may often also result in an allergy to numerous foods, including, but not limited to, melons, kiwi, peaches, and strawberries. Until someone comes up with a decent pollen-free birch tree, it would be a very good idea to leave these out of the landscape.

BEVERLY HILLS ARBORVITAE. See *Platycladus orientalis*.

Bidens ferulifolia. 4

YELLOW-FLOWERED DAISY. Mexican annual; easy to grow from seed.

BIG BLUESTEM GRASS. See *Andropogon*.

BIG-CONE SPRUCE. See *Pseudotsuga*.

BIG-LEAF HYDRANGEA. See *Hydrangea macrophylla*.

BIG SAGEBRUSH. See *Artemisia*.

BIG TREE. See *Sequoiadendron giganteum*.

BIGLEAF MAPLE. See *Acer macrophyllum*.

Bignonia.

The old name for many different species of flowering trumpet vines, some hardy and others tender. Most are fast growing and showy, but many trumpet vines can cause contact skin allergies. For allergy rankings, see *Anemopaegma*; *Campsis*; *Clytostoma*; *Distictis*; *Macfadyena*; *Pandorea*; *Pyrostegia*.

Billbergia. 2 ✪

QUEEN'S TEARS, VASE PLANT. A bromeliad.

BILBERRY. See *Vaccinium*.

BIRCH. See *Betula*.

BIRCH BARK CHERRY. See *Prunus serrula*.

BIRD-CATCHER TREE. See *Pisonia*.

BIRD-OF-PARADISE. See *Heliconia*; *Strelitzia*.

BIRD-OF-PARADISE BUSH. See *Caesalpinia*.

BIRD-ON-THE-WING. See *Polygala*.

BIRD'S-EYE BUSH. See *Ochna serrulata*.

BIRD'S EYES. See *Gilia*.

BIRD'S-FOOT FERN. See *Pellaea*.

BIRD'S-FOOT TREFOIL. See *Lotus corniculatus*.

BIRD'S-NEST FERN. See *Asplenium*.

BIRTHWORT. See *Aristolochia*.

Bischofia javanica. MALES 10 ◗, FEMALES 3

A large evergreen tree for zones 10 to 13. Separate-sexed, yet not sold sexed. The sap may cause rash and Bischofia may be especially bad for people with an allergy to latex.

BISCOCHITO. See *Ruprechtia*.

BISHOP'S HAT. See *Epimedium*.

BISHOP'S WEED. See *Aegopodium*.

Bismarckia nobilis. MALES 7, FEMALES 1 ✪

A tropical palm tree occasionally grown in southern Florida and in California. These tall, very handsome fan palms are separate-sexed; the males cause allergy, the females do not. Any that make seeds would be female trees.

BITTERROOT. See *Lewisia*.

BITTERSWEET. See *Celastrus*.

BITTERWOOD. See *Simarouba*.

Bixa orellana. **4**

ANNATTO, LIPSTICK TREE. A small tree with panicles of pink to rose flowers and prickly tan capsules that contain seeds covered with a red coating that is the consistency of lipstick and can be used as a coloring agent. Zones 10 to 12.

BLACK CALLA. See *Arum*.

BLACK-EYED SUSAN. See *Rudbeckia*.

BLACK-EYED SUSAN VINE. See *Thunbergia*.

BLACK LOCUST. See *Robinia*.

BLACK PALM. See *Normanbya*.

BLACK PEPPER. See *Piper*.

BLACK SALLY. See *Eucalyptus*.

BLACK SNAKEROOT. See *Cimicifuga*.

BLACK WALNUT. See *Juglans*.

BLACKBEAD TREE. See *Pithecellobium guadalupensis*.

BLACKBERRY. See *Rubus*.

BLACKBERRY LILY. See *Belamcanda chinensis*.

BLACKBOY. See *Xanthorrhoea*.

BLACKWOOD ACACIA. See *Acacia*.

BLADDER FLOWER. See *Araujia*.

BLADDERNUT. See *Staphylea*.

BLANKET FLOWER. See *Gaillardia*.

BLAZING STAR. See *Chamaelirium luteum*; *Mentzelia*.

Blechnum (Lomaria). **4**

Dwarf tree ferns.

BLEEDING HEART. See *Dicentra*.

Blephilia cilata. **2** ✪

DOWNY WOOD MINT, OHIO HORSEMINT. A wild native mint hardy in zones 4 to 8, with spikes of purple flowers that are very low pollen and full of nectar that attracts large numbers of pollinators, especially bumblebees. See *Mentha* for cautions.

Bletilla striata. **1** ✪

CHINESE GROUND ORCHID. Lavender orchid flowers on a hardy perennial plant (if mulched); does best in shady, moist, rich soil.

Blighia sapida. **MALES 8, FEMALES 1** ✪

AKEE TREE. Four species of evergreen tropical trees, some grown in parts of zones 10 to 12. Fruit on female trees is good to eat, but pollen from male trees may be mildly toxic.

BLISTER CRESS. See *Erysimum*.

BLOOD-LEAF. See *Iresine herbstii*.

BLOOD LILY. See *Hippeastrum*.

BLOOD-RED TRUMPET VINE. See *Distictis*.

BLOODROOT. See *Sanguinaria canadensis*.

BLUE BLOSSOM. See *Ceanothus*.

BLUE BONESET. See *Eupatorium*.

BLUE CROWN PASSION FLOWER. See *Passiflora*.

BLUE CURLS. See *Trichostema lanatum*.

BLUE DAWN FLOWER. See *Ipomoea*.

BLUE DICKS. See *Dichelostemma*.

BLUE DRACAENA. See *Cordyline*.

BLUE-EYED GRASS. See *Sisyrinchium*.

BLUE FESCUE. See *Festuca glauca*.

BLUE GINGER. See *Dichorisandra*.

BLUE GRAMA GRASS. See *Bouteloua gracilis*.

BLUE GUM. See *Eucalyptus*.

BLUE HIBISCUS. See *Alyogyne huegelii*.

BLUE LACE FLOWER. See *Trachymene coerulea*.

BLUE MARGUERITE. See *Felicia amelloides*.

BLUE MIST. See *Caryopteris*.

BLUE PALMETTO. See *Rhapidophyllum hystrix*.

BLUE SPIRAEA. See *Caryopteris*.

BLUE STAR CREEPER. See *Laurentia fluviatilis*.

BLUE STEM, BIG BLUESTEM GRASS. See *Andropogon*.

BLUE THIMBLE FLOWER. See *Gilia*.

BLUE VERVAIN. See *Verbena*.

BLUE YUCCA. See *Yucca*.

BLUEBEARD. See *Caryopteris*.

BLUEBELL. See *Endymion*; *Mertensia*; *Scilla*.

BLUEBELLS, MOUNTAIN. See *Mertensia*.

BLUEBELLS, TEXAS. See *Eustoma grandiflorum*.

BLUEBERRY. See *Vaccinium*.

BLUEBERRY CLIMBER. See *Ampelopsis brevipedunculata*.

BLUEGRASS. See *Poa*.

BLUEWINGS. See *Torenia*.

Boehmeria. MALES 8, FEMALES 1 ✿

A large genus with numerous species of herbs, shrubs, and small trees, all of which can cause allergy from the male plants. *B. nivea*, the Chinese silk plant, is occasionally grown in California. These are nettle relatives and nettle pollen is quite allergenic. The female plants are attractive and useful in the shade, but at the moment no one is yet selling these as selected female plants.

BOG ROSEMARY. See *Andromeda*.

BOKHARA FLEECEFLOWER. See *Polygonum*.

BONESET. See *Eupatorium*.

BORAGE. See *Borago officinalis*.

Borago officinalis. 3

BORAGE. Annual herb for all zones. Sun or shade, easy to grow.

Borassus. MALES 7, FEMALES 1 ✿

DOUB PALM, PALMYRA PALM, TALA PALM, TODDY PALM, WINE PALM. A group of tropical and subtropical separate-sexed fan palms, some used in zone 10, especially in Florida. Some are very large, growing to more than 100 feet. Females of this group produce large seeds, which are used for a popular Asian drink called "toddy." The males of this family cause allergies; the females cause none. Not usually sold sexed. Any Borassus palm with seeds is a female.

Boronia. 3

Small evergreen shrub bearing small, fragrant leaves and pink flowers. Boronia needs light soil and even moisture to thrive.

BOSTON FERN. See *Nephrolepis exalata* 'Bostoniensis'.

BOSTON IVY. See *Parthenocissus*.

BO-TREE. See *Ficus religiosa*.

BOTTLE PALM. See *Beaucarnea recurvata*; *Colpothrinax wrightii*.

BOTTLE PLANT. See *Jatropha*.

BOTTLE TREE. See *Brachychiton populneus*; *Firmiana simplex*.

BOTTLEBRUSH. See *Callistemon*; *Melaleuca*.

Bougainvillea. 1 ✿

Popular flowering evergreen vines and shrubs for zones 9 and 10; used in colder zones as container plants. Most commonly seen with red or purple flowers, but dozens of new colors are available. The plants need warmth, and the roots are especially sensitive to being moved, so transplant carefully. The color in bougainvillea comes mostly from colored leaves, called bracts, not from the actual flowers themselves, which are small and usually yellow. A fine choice for an allergy-free landscape where it will grow, or as a good, sunny window houseplant elsewhere. In Japan, bougainvillea is trained into stunning bonsai plants.

BOUSSINGAULTIA. See *Anredera*.

Bouteloua gracilis. 7

BLUE GRAMA GRASS. Lawn grass for cool areas; best kept mowed at less than 1¾ inches.

Bouvardia. 2 ✿

Evergreen shrub native to desert areas, bearing red, pink, and rose-colored tubular flowers.

BOWDOCK. See *Maclura pomifera*.

BOWER VINE. See *Pandorea*.

BOWSTRING HEMP. See *Sansevieria trifasciata*.

BOWWOOD. See *Maclura pomifera*.

BOX ELDER. See *Acer negundo*.

BOX HOLLY. See *Ruscus*.

BOX, JASMINE. See *Phillyrea decora*.

BOX, SWEET. See *Sarcococca*.

BOXWOOD. See *Buxus*; *Myrsine*; *Paxistima*.

BOYSENBERRY. See *Rubus*.

BRACHYCHITON GENUS

Brachychiton (Sterculia). INDIVIDUALLY RANKED

B. acerifolius. 3

FLAME TREE. Red flowering tree for zones 9 and 10.

B. discolor. 10 ✎

HAT TREE, QUEENSLAND LACEBARK. A very large tree with big leaves and clusters of large trumpet-shaped flowers. The leaves and very large seedpods have tiny stinging hairs that cause severe skin irritation. It should be avoided.

B. populneus. 4

BOTTLE TREE. A large evergreen tree for zones 9 and 10, similar to camphor tree, with 3-inch-long woody seedpods.

Brachycome iberidifolia. 3

SWAN RIVER DAISY. A small annual bearing blue, pink, or rose-colored flowers. Easy to grow.

Brachysema lanceolatum. **3**
SWAN RIVER PEA SHRUB. Drought-tolerant evergreen for full sun; it bears red flowers over an extended bloom period. Brachysema grows well in hot, dry areas.

BRACKEN FERN. See *Pteridium aquilinum.*

BRADFORD PEAR. See *Pyrus.*

BRAHEA GENUS

Brahea (Erythea). **INDIVIDUALLY RANKED**
Perfect-flowered, insect-pollinated attractive fan palms native to Mexico and Central America. Some produce edible fruit. Zones 9 to 13.

B. armata. **2** ✿
MEXICAN BLUE PALM. A palm for warmer areas of zone 10; good blue leaf color.

B. edulis. **2** ✿
GUADALUPE FAN PALM, ROCK PALM. Slow-growing palm for zones 9 or 10. Edible fruit.

B. elegans. **2** ✿
FRANCESCHI PALM. Graceful palm for zone 10.

BRAKE. See *Pteris.*

BRAMBLE. See *Rubus.*

BRASS BUTTONS. See *Cotula squalida.*

Brassaia actinophylla. **MALES 6, FEMALES 1** ✿
QUEENSLAND UMBRELLA TREE, SCHEFFLERA. Popular in Florida, Hawaii, and California.

Brassavola. **2** ✿
Greenhouse orchids with fragrant, spiderlike white or green flowers.

Brassica. **1** ✿ **TO 6 DEPENDING ON SPECIES**
BROCCOLI, BRUSSELS SPROUTS, CABBAGE, CAULIFLOWER, MUSTARD, RAPE, RUTABAGA, TURNIPS, WILD MUSTARD. There are reports of allergy in Sweden to people living near rape fields, although this is not too common. Rape and mustard rank 6, while most vegetable crops such as broccoli, brussels sprouts, cabbage, cauliflower, kale, rutabega, turnip, and wild mustard will only rarely cause pollen allergies and are ranked 1.

BRAZIL NUT. See *Bertholletia excelsa.*

BRAZILIAN FLAME BUSH. See *Calliandra tweedii.*

BRAZILIAN GOLDEN VINE. See *Stigmaphyllon.*

BRAZILIAN PEPPER TREE. See *Schinus terebinthifolius.*

BRAZILIAN PLUME FLOWER. See *Justicia.*

BRAZILIAN SKY FLOWER. See *Duranta.*

BREAD TREE. See *Treculia.*

BREADFRUIT. See *Arctocarpus communis.*

BREATH-OF-HEAVEN. See *Coleonema.*

BRIDAL ROBE. See *Tripleurospermum.*

BRIDAL VEIL. See *Tripogandra multiflora.*

BRIDAL VEIL BROOM. See *Genista.*

BRIDAL WREATH. See *Spiraea.*

Brimeura amethystina. **2** ✿
Bulb hardy in all zones; it bears blue bell-like flowers.

BRISBANE BOX. See *Tristania conferta.*

BRISTLEGRASS. See *Setaria.*

Briza maxima. **4**
RATTLESNAKE GRASS. Annual grass with nodding seeds. Sounds like rattlesnake rattles when shaken.

BROCCOLI. See *Brassica.*

Brodiaea. **1** ✿
Hardy corms for all zones. Easy to grow and may naturalize. (See also *Triteleia.*)

BROME GRASS. See *Bromus.*

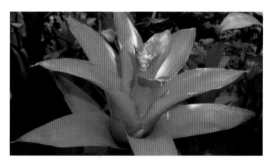

Bromelia (Guzmania; Neoregelia; Nidularium; Tillandsia; Vriesea). **2** ✿
BROMELIAD. (Pictured above.) Perennials of the pineapple family, with strap-shaped leaves and showy, single-flower clusters growing in the center of the plant. Houseplants in most areas except warmer areas of zones 9 and 10. Drought-tolerant plants, easy to grow in pots.

Bromus. **6 TO 9** ◐ **DEPENDING ON SPECIES**
BROME GRASS. An important pasture and hay crop and the cause of many allergies. *B. secalinus,* however, sheds little pollen and causes little allergy. The use of this species should be encouraged.

BRONZE DRACAENA. See *Cordyline*.

BROOKLIME. See *Veronica*.

BROOM. See *Corema*; *Cytisus*; *Genista*.

BROOM PALM. See *Coccothrinax*.

Broussonetia papyrifera. MALES 10 🗲, FEMALES 1 ✪
PAPER MULBERRY. A medium to large fast-growing, deciduous tree or large shrub, hardy to zone 4. It is characterized by its heart-shaped leaves and smooth gray bark. The cause of widespread and severe allergy, males should be removed from the landscape. If planted in your landscape, remove it. Some landscape trees labeled as "fruitless mulberry" may actually be all-male clones of paper mulberry, although many erroneously believe them to be seedless varieties of red or white mulberry. (See also *Morus*.)

Browallia. 2 ✪
Attractive blue flowers on small annual plant. Needs warmth and moisture.

Brugmansia. DOUBLES 2 ✪, SINGLES 4
ANGEL TRUMPET, DATURA. An evergreen subshrub that can be trained as a small tree. For zone 10 or greenhouse; houseplant with good light. It bears large, night-fragrant, trumpet-shaped flowers of white, salmon, pink, or orange. Provide shelter from the wind, which can damage large, soft leaves. Very easy to grow from cuttings. Do not plant angel trumpet under bedroom windows. All parts of these plants are mildly poisonous and contain a powerful, unpleasant hallucinogenic drug.

Brunfelsia pauciflora calycina. 2 ✪
YESTERDAY-TODAY-AND-TOMORROW. An evergreen shrub, slow-growing, for warm areas of zone 9 and all of zone 10. Related to nightshade, it does best in acid soil with plenty of iron and moisture. When in full bloom three colors of flowers—blue, purple, and white—are on the bush at the same time. The small, round seedpods are poisonous if eaten.

Brunnera macrophylla. 2 ✪
BRUNNERA. Hardy, very attractive perennial for all zones. Brunnera grows well in the shade beneath deciduous trees.

BRUNSVIGIA ROSEA. See *Amaryllis belladonna*.

BRUSSELS SPROUTS. See *Brassica*.

Buchloe dactyloides. MALES 9 🗲, FEMALES 1 ✪
BUFFALO GRASS. Drought-tolerant lawn grass native to Rocky Mountain areas. If a mixed-sex lawn, keep this lawn mowed short to prevent allergies. New all-female cultivars, grown from sod or plugs, are low-growing and drought-tolerant, need little mowing, and produce no pollen. They are excellent choices for the allergy-free lawn. At the moment there is no type of buffalo grass that can be grown from seed that will be all-female. The cultivars '609', 'Prairie', 'Legacy', 'Buffalo Girl', and 'UC Verde' (selected especially for California and southern Arizona) are all useful female buffalo grass clones. 'Prestige' is another newer all-female cultivar that is drought-tolerant, attractive, and winter hardy and has wide applications. Wayne Thorson from Todd Valley Farms tells me that he's grown it for fifteen years and has never seen a single male flower on it. Buffalo grass goes fully dormant in winter and then greens back up again in spring. Plant buffalo grass from plugs, or as sod. Do not plant buffalo grass from seed, as this will result in a large number of allergenic male plants.

BUCKEYE. See *Aesculus*; *Ungnadia*.

BUCKTHORN. See *Hippophae*; *Rhamnus*.

BUCKWHEAT. See *Eriogonum*.

BUCKWHEAT TREE. See *Cliftonia monophylla*.

BUCKWHEAT, WILD. See *Eriogonum*.

Buddleia. 3
BUTTERFLY BUSH. Tall fast-growing perennial, shrub, or small tree, hardy in all zones. These do attract butterflies; plants should be pruned back hard at least once a year or else they get woody and look ragged. Considerable nectar in the flowers and very little pollen. Some species are poisonous.

BUFFALO BERRY. See *Shepherdia*.

BUFFALO GRASS. See *Buchloe dactyloides*.

BUGBANE. See *Cimicifuga*.

BUGLE LILY. See *Watsonia*.

BUGLOSS. See *Anchusa*.

Bulbine. 3
BULBINE LILY, CAT'S TAIL, SNAKE FLOWER. Easy to grow perennials with orange flowers for zones 9 to 11.

Bulbinella floribunda. 4
Perennial tuberous flowers for zones 9 and 10. Easy to grow.

BULL BAY. See *Magnolia grandiflora*.

BULRUSH, LOW. See *Scirpus*.

Bumelia lanuginose. **SPECIES 6, MALES 7, FEMALES 1** ⊗
CHITTAMWOOD. A tall tree native to the U.S., very heat- and drought-tolerant but little used in landscaping. Zones 5 to 11. Some of this species will be separate-sexed but not all of them. Any Bumelia that never makes any of the small cherry-size fruits is probably a male and considerably more allergenic than the fruiting ones. Birds like the fruit. A female selection of this tree could be very useful.

BUNCHBERRY. See *Cornus.*

BUNNY EARS CACTUS. See *Cactus.*

BUNYA-BUNYA. See *Araucaria.*

Buphthalmum speciosum. **5**
Quite tall yellow daisy, grown as an annual from seed.

Bupleurum rotundifolium. **5**
Grown as an annual from seed for its large leaves and little yellow flowers.

BURDEKIN PLUM. See *Pleiogynium.*

BURMESE PLUMBAGO. See *Ceratostigma.*

BURNING BUSH. See *Euonymus; Kochia.*

BURRO TAIL. See *Sedum.*

Bursera. **MALES 7, FEMALES 1** ⊗
ELEPHANT TREE, GUMBO-LIMBO TREE. Subtropical trees occasionally grown in zone 10. Many of these are separate-sexed, and males are potentially allergenic. If the tree fruits (small red fruit), then it is female and safe.

Burseraceae. **MALES 7, FEMALES 1** ⊗
TORCHWOOD. Many species of tropical and sub-tropical trees and shrubs; most are separate-sexed and only female, fruiting plants would be desired. Zones 10 to 13.

BUSH ANEMONE. See *Carpenteria californica.*

BUSH CHERRY. See *Syzygium paniculatum.*

BUSH MORNING GLORY. See *Convolvulus.*

BUSH PALM. See *Sabal.*

BUSH POPPY. See *Dendromecon rigida.*

BUSHMAN'S POISON. See *Acokanthera.*

BUSY LIZZY. See *Impatiens.*

BUTCHER'S BROOM. See *Ruscus.*

BUTCHER'S VINE, CLIMBING. See *Semele androgyna.*

Butia capitata (Cocos australis). **4**
JELLY PALM, PINDO PALM. A tall (to 20 feet), hardy palm with a thick trunk, grows slowly and is hardier than most. It produces edible, sweet, apricot-flavored yellow fruit.

BUTTER DAISY. See *Verbesina.*

BUTTERCUPS. See *Eranthis hyemalis; Ranunculus; Thalictrum.*

BUTTERFLY BUSH. See *Buddleia.*

BUTTERFLY FLOWER. See *Schizanthus.*

BUTTERFLY ORCHID. See *Orchids.*

BUTTERFLY PALM. See *Chrysalidocarpus.*

BUTTERFLY PEA. See *Clitoria.*

BUTTERFLY VINE. See *Stigmaphyllon.*

BUTTERFLY WEED. See *Asclepias.*

BUTTERNUT. See *Juglans.*

BUTTONBALL TREE. See *Platanus.*

BUTTONWOOD. See *Platanus.*

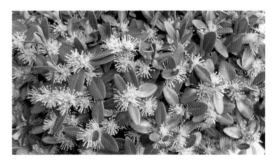

Buxus. **7**
BOX, BOXWOOD. (Pictured above.) Numerous species of evergreen shrubs and small trees, often used for low hedges. The very small, rounded leaves and dense growth habit make boxwood a good hedge plant. Boxwood flowers are small, greenish, and inconspicuous; however, they do cause allergies. Boxwood flowers on old wood, so if hedges are kept closely sheared, the plants will not flower. All parts of the plant are highly poisonous if eaten.

CABBAGE. See *Brassica*.

CABBAGE, FLOWERING. See *Brassica*.

CABBAGE PALMETTO. See *Sabal*.

CABBAGE TREE. See *Cordyline*; *Cussonia spicata*.

CACAO TREE. See *Theobroma cacao*.

Cactus. 1 ☼

A large group of spiny, succulent plants, some very
cold-hardy and others frost-tender. Almost all cactus
need fast-draining, light soil, warmth, full sun, and
little water in the summer. Because they are pollinated
at night by moths, cactus flowers, though often rare,
are usually showy and highly attractive. Some members
of the Euphorbia genus look like cactus, but are not
similar either botanically or in allergen potential. True
cactus, although often covered with sharp spines, some
often tiny, is a very fine choice for allergy-free landscaping. Cactus should not be confused with the many species of Euphorbia, a great many of which do look quite
a bit like a true cactus; all Euphorbia have potential for
allergy, especially from their sap.

Caesalpinia. 4

BIRD-OF-PARADISE BUSH, POINCIANA. Deciduous or
evergreen small tree or shrub. Leguminous plants that
grow well in hot, low-desert areas. All parts of these
plants, especially the seeds, are poisonous if eaten.

CAJEPUT TREE. See *Melaleuca*.

Caladium bicolor. 4

Big, fancy-leafed tuberous perennial for mild winter
areas. Houseplants elsewhere. The flowers may cause
allergies, yet flowers are seldom seen on these plants,
which are grown only for their leaves.

CALAMINT. See *Satureja*.

CALAMONDIN. See *Citrus*.

Calamus. MALES 9 ◗, FEMALES 1 ☼

Large group of tropical palms. Separate-sexed trees;
use only those that make fruit.

Calathea. 1 ☼

ZEBRA PLANT. Houseplants. Many species, most with
large, unusual leaves.

Calceolaria. 2 ☼

Perennials; some hardy in all zones. Small, pouchlike
yellow-orange flowers.

Calendula officinalis. DOUBLES 3, SINGLES 4

CALENDULA, POT MARIGOLD. Cool-season annual
grown in all zones. Edible yellow or orange flowers.
Easy to grow. Best not to use as cut flowers indoors,

as they may shed more pollen if brought inside. Double-flowered Calendulas have less pollen than singles.

CALICO BUSH. See *Kalmia*.

CALICO FLOWER. See *Aristolochia*.

CALIFORNIA BAY. See *Umbellularia californica*.

CALIFORNIA CHRISTMAS TREE. See *Cedrus deodara*.

CALIFORNIA FAN PALM. See *Washingtonia filifera*.

CALIFORNIA FUCHSIA. See *Zauschneria*.

CALIFORNIA GERANIUM. See *Senecio*.

CALIFORNIA HOLLY. See *Heteromeles arbutifolia*.

CALIFORNIA HOLLY GRAPE. See *Mahonia aquifolium*.

CALIFORNIA LAUREL. See *Umbellularia californica*.

CALIFORNIA NUTMEG. See *Torreya*.

CALIFORNIA POPPY. See *Eschscholzia californica*.

CALIFORNIA WAX MYRTLE. See *Myrica*.

CALLA LILY. See *Zantedeschia*.

Calliandra. 6
A large genus of evergreen, flowering shrubs. *C. tweedii*, the Trinidad flame bush, is a graceful, evergreen shrub with bright red powderpuff flowers. Hardy in zones 9 and 10. An attractive shrub, but keep this one away from the house.

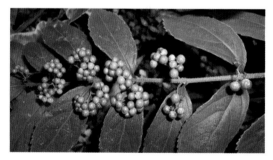

Callicarpa bodinieri giraldii. 3
BEAUTYBERRY. (Pictured above.) Hardy, deciduous shrub for zones 5 to 8. Small lilac-colored flowers followed by purple fruit, which persist into winter.

Callicoma serratifolia. 8
An Australian evergreen shrub or small tree, hardy in zones 9 to 10. Leaves toothed, glossy above, and hairy below. Sneezy-looking flowers are white with many exposed stamens.

CALLIOPSIS. See *Coreopsis*.

Callirhoe involucrata. 2 ✪
A poppylike trailing mallow, grown from seed. Good in hot sunny areas. Purple-red flowers.

Callisia. 4
Houseplants related to wandering Jew. May cause allergies in dogs, especially red, watery eyes.

Callistemon. 9 ✦
BOTTLEBRUSH. Evergreen trees or shrubs. Many species. Some species hardy into warmer areas of zone 8. Most have bright red clusters of flowers that look like baby-bottle brushes. Some confusion in the trade with the genus Melaleuca, to which they are related. Native to Australia, bottlebrush has heavy, triangular-shaped pollen that does not travel far in the air; however, up close it can be a very potent allergen. People with allergies should never attempt to smell or sniff one of these flower clusters or the result may often be fast and severe. Do not bring these flowers inside as cut flowers.

Never plant a bottlebrush tree next to a driveway where the pollen will fall on your car, as exposure can result from this. Watch pets, especially dogs, around bottlebrush shrubs, as not only can they become allergic to the pollen, but they can also easily bring it inside the house on their coats.

Bottlebrush is attractive and the flowers are good for many pollinators. In addition, it is visited by many wild birds, especially tanagers and orioles, who like to eat the flowers.

If bottlebrush is kept in the back of the landscape or planted far from doors, windows, patios, or swimming pools, it is much less of a problem.

Callistephus chinensis. 5
CHINA ASTER. Annual in all zones. Do not use these for cut flowers, as they may shed more pollen if brought indoors.

Callitris. 9 ✦
CYPRESS PINE. Group of species from Australia, occasionally grown in zones 9 and 10. Not a true pine.

Calluna. DOUBLES 2 ✪, SINGLES 4
HEATHER, SCOTCH HEATHER. A species of flowering shrub native to Europe and Asia Minor, grown in zones 5 to 10 in the United States. To thrive, heathers need acid soil (peat or sand is best) and a good supply of water. They are low-growing plants with tiny leaves and masses of small pink, white, or purple flowers. Heather grows best in full sun or partial shade in hot summer areas. There are several cultivars with double flowers.

'County Wicklow' has double pink flowers, 'Else Frye' has double white flowers, and 'Tib' has double rosy purple flowers.

Calocedrus decurrens (Libocedrus). 7
INCENSE CEDAR. Large evergreen tree, not a true cedar. This tree is often used when small as a pyramidal arbor-vitae, but it quickly outgrows the ordinary yard and is far too large for most gardens. Its smell is pungent and will affect some with perfume or pine-type sensitivities. Pollen can be a problem.

Calochortus tolmiei. 2 ✪
CAT'S EARS, MARIPOSA LILY, PUSSY EARS. Lilylike native corms, hardy in all zones.

Calodendrum capense. 4
CAPE CHESTNUT. Profuse blooming lilac-colored flowers in late spring. Grown in California and Florida. A slow-growing beautiful tree to 40 or more feet. Citrus relative, despite its disparate appearance. On occasion people who have a Cape chestnut in their yard may develop an allergy to its pollen, but for most yards this tree gets far too big. Zones 9 to 13.

CALONYCTION. See *Ipomoea*.

Calothamnus. 8
NET BUSH. Evergreen Australian shrub similar to bottlebrush but smaller, with gray leaves.

Caltha palustris. 1 ✪
MARSH MARIGOLD. Perennial; hardy in all zones. Grows well next to streams, ponds, and moist areas.

Calycanthus floridus. 3
CAROLINA ALLSPICE. Deciduous shrub hardy to zone 4. Purple fragrant flowers. *C. occidentalis*, the spice bush, is hardy to zone 5. A West Coast native, it can be trained into a small tree.

Calylophus. 3
SUNDROPS. Drought-tolerant native perennial with bright yellow flowers for full sun in zones 5 to 10.

Calypso bulbosa. 1 ✪
Pink-flowered orchid that grows best in the shade of trees. This hardy little plant needs humus-rich soil with good moisture.

Calyptrogyne. 5
Small group of Mexican palms.

CAMAS. See *Camassia*; *Zigadenus*.

Camassia. 3
CAMAS. Perennial bulb, hardy in all zones. Grows best in heavy soil with abundant moisture. Blue or white lilylike flowers.

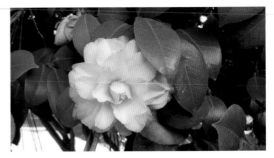

Camellia. DOUBLES 1 ✪, SINGLES 3
(*Camellia japonica*, double, pictured above.) Of the many species, the most common and popular is *C. japonica*, an evergreen shrub or small tree. Camellia flowers are white, red, pink, or mixed and resemble tuberous begonias. Hardy to zone 6, Camellias are grown in cool greenhouses worldwide. Culture is exacting; they need acid soil, rich in humus; perfect drainage, but also constant moisture; and lots of iron. Keep a deep mulch of leaf litter around the base.

Camellia flowers may be singles, semi-doubles, or full doubles. In some fully double varieties, the flowers have no stamens (the male parts) and so have no potential to release pollen. Camellias belong to the tea family and, although sometimes difficult to grow, they're worth the effort. The full doubles, known as formal doubles, are excellent choices for the allergy-free landscape; the single-flowered varieties only slightly less so.

CAMOMILE. See *Chamaemelum nobile*.

Campanula. 1 ✪
BELLFLOWER, CANTERBURY BELL, STAR OF BETH-LEHEM. Annuals and perennials for all zones. Many species, generally with blue or lavender flowers. Grow best in filtered shade inland and full sun near the coast. Keep well watered in summer.

CAMPHOR TREE. See *Brachychiton acerifolius*; *Cinnamomum camphora*.

CAMPION. See *Lychnis*; *Silene*.

Campsis. 5
COW ITCH VINE, TRUMPET CREEPER, TRUMPET VINE. Hardy vine to zone 3, where it may die back to the ground and regrow in spring. Several species; most have

large orange flowers. Vigorous climbers cling to brick, wood, and stucco surfaces. Contact with the leaves can cause skin rash, inflammation, and blistering in some individuals. Use care when pruning.

Camptotheca acuminata. MALES 7, FEMALES 1 ✪
Deciduous tree, native to China. Sometimes grown in California. Zones 8 to 10.

Canarium ovatum. MALES 7, FEMALES 1 ✪
PILI NUT. A big (to 65 feet) evergreen tree grown mostly in the Philippines at low elevations for the hard-shelled, fat-filled nuts. Pili nut trees are separate-sexed; the males produce airborne pollen. The female trees (which bear nuts) cause no allergies.

CANARY BIRD BUSH. See *Crotalaria.*

CANARY BIRD FLOWER. See *Tropaeolum.*

CANARY GRASS, CANARY REED GRASS. See *Phalaris.*

CANDLE BUSH. See *Cassia.*

CANDLE PLANT. See *Senecio.*

CANDLEBERRY. See *Myrica.*

CANDOLLEA CUNEIFORMIS. See *Hibbertia.*

CANDYTUFT. See *Iberis.*

CANDYWEED. See *Polygala.*

CANE PALM. See *Chrysalidocarpus.*

Canella. 4
WILD CINNAMON. Evergreen tree occasionally grown in warmer areas of Florida and California. Zones 10 to 13.

Canna. 3
Hardy in all zones, but in the coldest climates the tuberous roots should be lifted and stored. Tall, broad-leafed plants with terminal flower clusters of many colors. Easy to grow, but does best with full sun and good moisture.

Cannabis sativa. MALES 7, FEMALES 1 ✪
MARIJUANA. A very popular tall annual plant, occasionally grown (often illegally) in gardens. Separate-sexed; male plants shed airborne pollen profusely and cause limited local allergy.

CANTERBURY BELL. See *Campanula.*

Cantua buxifolia. 3
FLOWER-OF-THE-INCAS, MAGIC FLOWER. Tender perennial shrub that does best in light shade. Drought-tolerant. Long, pendulous, tubular flowers; plants should be staked for support. Grown in cool greenhouses outside of zone 10.

CAPE CHESTNUT. See *Calodendrum capense.*

CAPE COWSLIP. See *Lachenalia.*

CAPE DAISY. See *Venidium.*

CAPE FORGET-ME-NOT. See *Anchusa.*

CAPE FUCHSIA. See *Phygelius capensis.*

CAPE HONEYSUCKLE. See *Tecomaria capensis.*

CAPE MARIGOLD. See *Dimorphotheca; Osteospermum.*

CAPE MYRTLE. See *Myrsine.*

CAPE PITTOSPORUM. See *Pittosporum.*

CAPE PLUMBAGO. See *Plumbago auriculata.*

CAPE PONDWEED. See *Aponogeton distachyus.*

CAPE PRIMROSE. See *Streptocarpus.*

CAPE WEED. See *Arctotheca calendula.*

Capsicum. 1 ✪
PEPPERS. Vegetable garden plants; bell peppers and hot chile peppers. Members of the potato family. Flowers, usually white but sometimes purple, do not release pollen into the air. Peppers are nutritious and the plants can be ornamental if grown well. All peppers do best with full sun, rich, well-drained soil, plenty of fertilizer, and water. Bell pepper fruits will often sunburn if the leaf canopy is not thick enough—to grow enough and large enough leaves, use a fertilizer with plenty of nitrogen.

Caragana arborescens. 4
SIBERIAN PEASHRUB. Large, deciduous, yellow-flowered shrub hardy into coldest zones.

CARAWAY. See *Carum carvi.*

CARDINAL CLIMBER. See *Ipomoea.*

CARDINAL FLOWER. See *Lobelia.*

CARDOON. See *Cynara.*

Carex. MONOECIOUS 6, MALES 8, FEMALES 1 ✪
SEDGE. Large group of grasslike plants, all of which cause allergies. Some are separate-sexed.

Carica papaya. MALES 6, FEMALES 1 ✪
PAPAYA. Tropical evergreen fruit tree. Separate-sexed trees with limited airborne pollen. Females are excellent, pollen-free trees. Best in zones 10 to 13.

Carissa. 2 ✪
NATAL PLUM. Evergreen shrub for zones 9 and 10. White flowers; red, edible but tasteless, fruit. Sap may cause skin rash. A very good, low-pollen shrub.

Carlina. 4
ANNUAL DAISY. Large flowers, one to a plant. Used as dried flowers.

CARMEL CREEPER. See *Ceanothus*.

CARNATION. See *Dianthus*.

CARNAUBA WAX PALM. See *Copernicia*.

Carnegiea gigantea. 1 ✪
SAGUARO CACTUS. Giant cactus, native to Southwest. White flowers bloom at night.

CAROB. See *Ceratonia siliqua*.

CAROLINA ALLSPICE. See *Calycanthus floridus*.

CAROLINA BUCKTHORN. See *Rhamnus*.

CAROLINA JESSAMINE. See *Gelsemium sempervirens*.

CAROLINA LAUREL CHERRY. See *Prunus caroliniana*.

Carpentaria. 6
A palm from Australia, to 40 feet.

Carpenteria californica. 1 ✪
BUSH ANEMONE. Evergreen shrub native to the West Coast and hardy to zone 6. Does best in dry areas. Handsome shrub with fragrant white flowers.

CARPET BUGLE. See *Ajuga*.

CARPET PLANT. See *Episcia*.

Carpinus. 7
HORNBEAM. Common, deciduous hardy trees with leaves similar to an elm. All can cause some limited allergies.

Carpobrotus. 2 ✪
HOTTENTOT FIG, ICE PLANT, SEA FIG. Coarse, fast-growing perennial common along coastal areas. Flowers yellow- or rose-colored.

CARRION FLOWER. See *Smilax*; *Stapelia*.

CARROT. See *Daucus*.

CARROTWOOD TREE. See *Cupaniopsis anacardioides*.

Carthamus tinctorius. 4
FALSE SAFFRON, SAFFLOWER. Annual grown for safflower oil and also used as garden annual for its blue flowers. Full sun. Drought-tolerant.

Carum carvi. 2 ✪
CARAWAY. Hardy herb for all zones. Used to flavor pickles and rye bread.

Carya. 8 TO 10 ◐
HICKORY, PECAN. *C. illinoensis*, the pecan, is hardy to zone 7 but produces its best crops of nuts in zone 9.

It causes severe allergy. *C. ovata*, the shagbark hickory, causes the most severe allergies of any hickory species. Hickory is related to walnut, and cross-allergic responses between the two are common.

Caryopteris. 5
BLUE MIST, BLUE SPIRAEA, BLUEBEARD. Hardy deciduous shrub with blue flowers. Full sun. Drought-tolerant. In the garden these are excellent plants, but direct skin contact with the leaves or flowers has caused itch, rash, and even some asthmalike symptoms. Use extreme care when handling or pruning plants; avoid the sap. Not recommended as cut flowers, as they may shed more pollen if brought indoors. Use care when pruning or deadheading old flowers.

Caryota. 9 ◐
FISHTAIL PALM, WINE PALM. Handsome palm tree for zone 10. The cause of widespread allergy in the tropics.

CASCARA SAGRADA. See *Rhamnus*.

CASHEW. See *Anacardium occidentale*.

Casimiroa edulis. 2 ✪
SAPOTE. Evergreen fruit tree that grows anywhere lemons thrive. Large, round, edible fruit ripens in late summer. Large seeds. Trees grow fast and are easy to start from seed, although quality of the fruit is variable. The best fruit is from budded trees. Leaves and sap are poisonous.

Cassia. 5 TO 7 DEPENDING ON SIZE OF SPECIES
CANDLE BUSH, GOLD MEDALLION TREE, SENNA. Many species of evergreen or deciduous shrubs and trees. Most Cassias have abundant bright yellow flowers. Mimosa-like plants. Zones 8 to 13. Oil of Cassia has been known to cause skin rash. Seeds are poisonous. *Cassia leptophylla* (ranked 7) is a popular street tree in a number of cities, including San Diego, and its large, bright yellow flowers produce considerable pollen and are the cause of allergies.

Castanea. MONOECIOUS 6, FEMALE-ONLY OR MALE-STERILE 1 ✪
CHESTNUT. Large, hardy deciduous nut-bearing trees. Because of a widespread fungal disease, the American chestnut is almost extinct, but there are Chinese and Spanish chestnuts that are immune to the blight. The pollen, although abundant, is mixed with nectar, sticky, mostly insect-pollinated, and does not travel far. It is only a problem when contacted directly. There are some newer hybrids that are male-sterile, all-female, and these produce no pollen.

Castanopsis. 6
CHINQUAPIN. Many species of evergreen trees and shrubs. Hardy in zones 8 to 10.

Castanospermum australe. 3
MORTON BAY CHESTNUT. Large evergreen tree for zones 10 to 12. Bright red and yellow flowers. Seeds are edible.

CAST-IRON PLANT. See *Aspidistra elatior.*

CASTOR BEAN. See *Ricinus communis.*

CASTOR-OIL PLANT. See *Ricinus communis.*

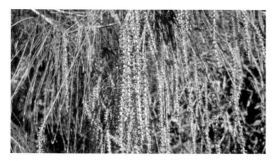

Casuarina. MALES 10 ◔, FEMALES 1 ✪
AUSTRALIAN PINE, BEEFWOOD, HORSETAIL TREE, SHE-OAK. (*Casuarina equisetifolia*, male, pictured above.) Australian evergreen tree much planted in zones 9 and 10. Cause of increasing allergy. Trees may naturalize (become invasive) in some areas and force out native species. Female trees make many small cones that persist on the branches for years. Male trees produce prodigious amounts of pollen over a long period of time. Existing males of this species should be removed as health hazards.

CAT GUT. See *Tephrosia.*

CATALINA CHERRY. See *Prunus lyonii.*

CATALINA IRONWOOD. See *Lyonothamnus floribundus.*

CATALINA PERFUME. See *Ribes viburnifolium.*

Catalpa. 6
Large deciduous trees hardy in all zones. Many large white flowers followed by long, beanlike seedpods. Although perfect-flowered, Catalpa trees are fairly well known in allergy studies. The hybrid between the Catalpa and the Desert Willow, Chitalpa, looks a good bit like a Catalpa, but sheds no pollen.

Catananche caerulea. 5
CUPID'S DART. Hardy perennial for all zones. Corn-flower-blue flowers are often used as dried flowers, but these may (occasionally) cause allergy.

CATBERRY. See *Nemopanthus.*

CATCHFLY. See *Lychnis*; *Silene.*

Catha edulis. 2 ✪
ARABIAN TEA, CHAT, KHAT. Big evergreen shrubs for zones 9 to 13. Shiny green leaves with red stems and reddish bark. Small white flowers. Drought-tolerant; tolerant of poor soil and wind. In Ethiopia and some other countries the fresh leaves are chewed for their stimulant properties, and the cured leaves are used for tea.

Catharanthus roseus. 1 ✪
ANNUAL VINCA, MADAGASCAR PERIWINKLE. Frost-tender perennial, usually grown as a heat-loving annual. These plants have been greatly improved in the past twenty years, largely due to the efforts of plant breeder Ronald Parker, a professor of horticulture at the University of Connecticut. Low-growing, spreading garden plants for hot, sunny areas. Many hybrid colors, including white with red eyes and red with white eyes. Beautiful, easy to grow, fairly drought-tolerant. (See also *Vinca rosea.*)

CATMINT. See *Nepeta.*

CATNIP. See *Nepeta.*

CAT'S CLAW. See *Macfadyena unguis-cati.*

CAT'S EARS. See *Calochortus tolmiei.*

CATTAIL. See *Typha.*

Cattleya. 2 ✪
An epiphytic orchid. Greenhouse plant, grown in bark mixture. Cattleyas are among the showiest of the orchids. Need warm nights, filtered light, and high humidity.

CAUCASIAN MAPLE. See *Acer cappadocicum.*

CAULIFLOWER. See *Brassica.*

Caulophyllum thalictoides. 5
BLUE COHOSH, PAPOOSE ROOT. Hardy native perennial with large leaves, yellow flowers, and small interesting blue fruit; best in shady areas with moist soils in zones 3 to 7; native to the eastern U.S. and Canada. Fruits not edible but seeds sometimes used as a coffee substitute.

Ceanothus. GROUND COVERS 3, SHRUBS 4, TREES 5
BLUE BLOSSOM, WILD LILAC. Mostly evergreen shrubs, ground covers, and small trees for zones 6 to 10. Native to Pacific coastal mountains. Many clusters of blue and occasionally white flowers. Drought-tolerant. Needs good drainage. Beautiful flowers but the plants are not very long-lived in the landscape.

CEDAR. See *Cedrus*.

CEDAR, ALASKA YELLOW. See *Chamaecyparis*.

CEDAR, ARIZONA. See *Cupressus arizonica*.

CEDAR, BATTLE AX. See *Thujopsis dolabrata*.

CEDAR, CIGAR BOX. See *Cedrela odorata*.

CEDAR, CLANWILLIAM. See *Widdringtonia*.

CEDAR, COLORADO RED. See *Juniperus scopulorum*.

CEDAR, DEERHORN. See *Thujopsis dolabrata*.

CEDAR ELM. See *Ulmus crassifolia*.

CEDAR, GIANT. See *Thuja*.

CEDAR, GROUND. See *Lycopodium*.

CEDAR, HIBA. See *Thujopsis dolabrata*.

CEDAR, INCENSE. See *Calocedrus decurrens*.

CEDAR, JAPANESE. See *Cryptomeria japonica*.

CEDAR, JAPANESE RED. See *Cryptomeria japonica*.

CEDAR, MEXICAN. See *Cupressus*.

CEDAR, MLANJE. See *Widdringtonia*.

CEDAR OF GOA. See *Cupressus*.

CEDAR OF LEBANON. See *Cedrus libani*.

CEDAR, PINK. See *Acrocarpus fraxinifolius*.

CEDAR, PLUME. See *Cryptomeria japonica*.

CEDAR, PORT ORFORD. See *Chamaecyparis*.

CEDAR, PORTUGUESE. See *Cupressus*.

CEDAR, RED. See *Juniperus virginiana*.

CEDAR, SALT. See *Tamarix*.

CEDAR, SOUTHERN RED. See *Juniperus silicicola*.

CEDAR, SPANISH. See *Cedrela odorata*.

CEDAR, STINKING. See *Torreya*.

CEDAR, TAIWAN. See *Taiwania cryptomeriodes*.

CEDAR, TECATE. See *Cupressus forbesii*.

CEDAR, WEST INDIAN. See *Cedrela odorata*.

CEDAR, WESTERN RED. See *Thuja*.

CEDAR, WHITE. See *Chamaecyparis*; *Juniperus*; *Thuja*.

CEDAR, WILLOWMORE. See *Widdringtonia*.

Cedrela. 2 ⊙
BARBADOS CEDAR, CIGAR BOX CEDAR, SPANISH
CEDAR, TOONA TREE, WEST INDIAN CEDAR. An
interesting group of about twenty species of subtropical timber trees, of the mahogany family, deciduous
and evergreen, some planted in California and Florida.

Certain species of Cedrela, especially *C. odorata*, are
called cedars although they are not related. *C. odorata* is
hardy to zone 6 and the wood is used for making cigar
boxes because it has a pungent smell that repels insects.
Another, *C. toona*, commonly called the toona tree, is
an evergreen tree for zone 10 that has lightly fragrant
loose clusters of white flowers.

Cedronella. 3
BALM-OF-GILEAD. Perennial subshrub from the Canary
Islands, occasionally grown in California.

CEDRUS GENUS

Cedrus. INDIVIDUALLY RANKED
CEDAR, TRUE CEDARS. Four species of evergreen trees
native to Africa and Asia. All four are pine relatives, and
like the pines, although they shed abundant pollen, they
are not responsible for much allergy. Cedar pollen is large
and often has a waxy coating. Nonetheless, if a female
cedar tree can be used, it will be far superior in any
allergy-fighting garden. There is an occasional allergic
response to the lumber, which is aromatic and used in
making cedar chests and similar forms of furniture.

C. atlantica. 2 ⊙
ATLAS CEDAR. Hardy to zone 7. Grows to 100 feet.

C. brevifolia. 2 ⊙
CYPRESS CEDAR. Hardy to zone 7. It is similar to cedar
of Lebanon but with shorter leaves.

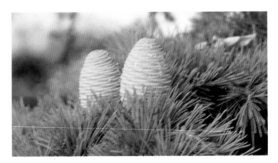

C. deodara. MONOECIOUS 4, MALES 6, FEMALES 1 ⊙
CALIFORNIA CHRISTMAS TREE, DEODAR CEDAR.
(*Cedrus deodara*, female, pictured above.) Hardy to zone
7. A tall, long-lived evergreen tree common in California cities, but native to the Himalayas. The trees have
grayish needles and drooping, curved tops. Many were
once sold as living Christmas trees in the Los Angeles
area. Many named varieties are sold. Most deodar
cedars are separate-sexed, but none are sold sexed. At
least one of them, *C. deodara* 'Repandens', also sold as

C. deodara 'Pendula', is a weeping, all-male form ranked at 5. In the near future it may well be possible to buy sexed cedars. It will be easy then to pick females, which would be near-perfect allergy-free trees.

C. libani. 2 ✪

CEDAR OF LEBANON. A tall, evergreen tree hardy in zones 6 to 10. Many varieties are sold. In biblical times, there were vast forests of these lofty trees growing on the slopes of Lebanon. The prophet Ezekiel said they were so beautiful that they were the envy of all the trees in the garden of Eden. King Solomon used the wood of *C. libani* for the beams and panels in the Temple in Jerusalem and in his grand royal palace.

Celastrus. MALES 6, FEMALES 1 ✪

BITTERSWEET. Hardy, deciduous vines for all zones. Does best in cold winter areas. Red seeds stay on plants for much of winter and are not especially prized by birds. These are separate-sexed plants, and only the females produce the berries. Female plants are pollen-less and excellent choices for the allergy-free landscape. Seeds and leaves are highly poisonous if eaten.

CELERY. See *Apium graveolens*.

Celosia. 4 TO 5

COCKSCOMB. Heat-loving annual for all zones. Red or yellow flowers in plumelike clusters, some tall and others short like combs of a rooster. Full sun. For best results, set out transplants that are not yet in bloom. Best not to use the tall varieties as cut flowers indoors, as they may shed more pollen if brought inside.

Celtis. 7

HACKBERRY, SUGARBERRY. Deciduous trees related to elm. Hardy in all zones. More work needs to be done to determine which species produce the most airborne pollen, because some are much better (or worse) than others. All Celtis, however, can contribute to allergy. In the United States, allergy to Celtis is common. In other countries—Argentina, for example—Celtis is considered a major allergy tree.

Centaurea. 3

BACHELOR'S BUTTON, DUSTY MILLER, SWEET SULTAN. Hardy annuals and perennials for all zones. There are more than 500 species of Centaurea, but only a few are popular garden plants. Although relatives of the Helianthus family of daisies and sunflowers, Centaurea flowers do not pose much of an allergy risk. Avoid use as a cut flower in the house, as they may shed more pollen if brought indoors.

CENTIPEDE GRASS. See *Eremochloa*.

CENTIPEDE PLANT. See *Homalocladium platycladum*.

Centranthus ruber. 2 ✪

JUPITER'S BEARD, RED VALERIAN. An easy-to-grow perennial for zones 8 to 10. A European native, Centranthus has naturalized in many California locations. Drought-tolerant and long-lived. Reddish flowers most common, but there are also white, which are more attractive than the red. The rather malodorous flowers shed little pollen.

CENTURY PLANT. See *Agave americana*.

Cephalanthus occidentalis. 5

BUTTONBUSH. Native flowering shrub used in zones 4 to 8.

Cephalocereus senilis. 1 ✪

OLD MAN CACTUS. Mexican native for zone 10. Tall (eventually to 40 feet), with long, gray hairs. Old plants have rose-colored flowers in April or May.

Cephalophyllum 'Red Spike' (*Cylindrophyllum*). 2 ✪

Perennial ice plant with bright red flowers. Zones 9 and 10.

Cephalotaxus. MALES 9 🍃, FEMALES 1 ✪

CHINESE PLUM YEW, PLUM YEW. Asian evergreen trees or shrubs hardy to zones 4 and 5. Plumlike edible fruit. Most species are separate-sexed plants, and only the females bear fruit. Common landscape shrubs in the southeastern United States, plum yews grow best in moist, shady spots. Some named cultivars to avoid are all-males: *C.* 'Harringtonia', *C.* 'Pedunculata', *C. harringtonia* 'Fastigiata', *C. koraiana*, and two others mistakenly sold as Podocarpus, *P. coraianus* and *P. koraiana*. Because they are pollen-free, female plants are excellent in the allergy-free landscape, but they are (as of this writing) still very hard to find in nurseries.

Cerastium tomentosum. 3

SNOW-IN-SUMMER. Low-growing perennial hardy in all zones. Short-lived ground cover with masses of white flowers.

Ceratiola ericoides. MALES 6, FEMALES 1 ✪

FLORIDA ROSEMARY, SANDHILL ROSEMARY. Not to be confused with *Rosmarinus officinalis*, the true culinary rosemary, Ceratiola is a low, evergreen, spreading, separate-sexed shrub native to the southern coastal plain, occasionally used in landscaping. Pollen-free female plants are good choices for the allergy-free garden.

Ceratonia siliqua. **MALES 7, FEMALES 1 ⊘**
CAROB TREE, ST. JOHN'S BREAD. Carob may be an all-male tree, an all-female tree, or both, which explains why some bear so many long seedpods while others (the males) have none. Carob sheds abundant pollen, and the trees are messy. In some neighborhoods in zone 9 and 10 these trees are very common street trees, and in these locations allergy to carob is not rare.

Ceratopetalum. **5**
Five species of trees or shrubs from New Zealand occasionally grown in California.

Ceratostigma. **3**
One of several plants sold as Plumbago. Several species of evergreen shrubs or perennials for zones 5 to 10, these have bright blue flowers that are darker than the sky-blue of the Cape plumbago, *Plumbago auriculata*.

Ceratozamia mexicana. **3**
A cycad grown in zones 10 to 13. Slow-growing, short, palmlike plant.

Cercidiphyllum japonicum. **MALES 6, FEMALES 1 ⊘**
KATSURA TREE. Slow-growing, deciduous tree hardy to zone 3; native to Japan, good fruit.

Cercidium. **5**
PALO VERDE. Deciduous tree native to desert areas of the Southwest. These trees will grow in areas where no other tree will grow. Small yellow flowers and green bark, thorns.

Cercis. **4**
REDBUD. Some species hardy to zone 5. Deciduous flowering tree with reddish flowers. The bark is occasionally used to relieve diarrhea, usually as a tea.

Cercocarpus. **4**
MOUNTAIN MAHOGANY, SWEET BRUSH. Evergreen or deciduous tall shrub or small tree native to the West Coast. Hardy in all zones and quite drought-tolerant. Good plants for cold, dry areas. Member of the rose family. Leaves are poisonous.

Cereus. **1 ⊘**
NIGHT-BLOOMING CACTUS. With long, white, beautiful fragrant flowers. Zones 9 and 10. (See also *Selenicereus*.)

Cerinthe. **2 ⊘**
BLUE SHRIMP PLANT. Erect perennial hardy to zone 7; strong blue flower colors.

Ceropegia woodii. **1 ⊘**
ROSARY VINE. Outdoors in warmest parts of zone 10 and houseplant elsewhere. Small evergreen vine with tiny leaves. Needs shade and abundant water.

Ceroxylon. **MALES 8, FEMALES 1 ⊘**
WAX PALM. A group of about fifteen species that includes some of the world's tallest palms, some to over 185 feet. Native to Columbia and Peru, they are all separate-sexed. Not sold in the United States, the males are potent allergy trees; the females cause none.

Cestrum nocturnum. **4**
Tall evergreen for zone 10, or easy-to-grow greenhouse plant in colder climates. Tends to get leggy in shade. Small white flowers have powerful fragrance that could bother those with sensitivities to perfumes and odors. Do not plant Cestrum next to any bedroom windows as the fragrance may also be slightly hallucinogenic and could trigger bad dreams. Seeds are poisonous.

CEYLON GOOSEBERRY. See *Dovyalis hebecarpa*.

Chaenomeles. **2 ⊘**
FLOWERING QUINCE, QUINCE. Deciduous shrub hardy in all zones. Quince is one of the first shrubs to bloom in early spring, with showy, bright pink, white, or red blossoms. Most have thorns but a few varieties are thornless. (Fruiting quince is Cydonia.)

Chaenorrhinum. **1 ⊘**
FALSE SNAPDRAGON. Annual or tender perennial from seed. Fine blue flowers.

CHAIN FERN, GIANT. See *Woodwardia fimbriata*.

CHAIN PLANT. See *Tradescantia*.

Chamaecrista fasciculata. **3**
PARTRIDGE PEA. Wildflower annual for any zone, with lacy leaves and bright yellow pealike flowers that are highly attractive to pollinators. Seeds are mildly poisonous.

Chamaecyparis (Retinispora). **8**
ALASKA YELLOW CEDAR, FALSE CYPRESS, LAWSON CYPRESS, PORT ORFORD CEDAR, WHITE CEDAR. A large group of many species of hardy, evergreen trees and shrubs. Often commonly called cedars, these are actually closely related to cypress instead. Several are from Japan, and some are native to the northwest coastal areas. All Chamaecyparis may cause allergy. Good substitutes are pines, true cedars, and selected female juniper cultivars.

Chamaedorea. **MALES 7, FEMALES 1 ⊘**
A large group of about 100 species of Mexican and tropical palms, all separate-sexed. Males cause allergy; females do not. One species is a common houseplant,

C. elegans, the parlor palm or good-luck palm. Your luck will be better if your parlor palm is female. Occasionally sold under the invalid name of *Neanthe bella*.

Chamaelirium luteum. MALES 6, FEMALES 1 ✪
BLAZING STAR. A tuberous perennial lily, native to the south-central United States and occasionally planted in shady spots in the garden. Separate-sexed. Do not bring in any flower spikes of a male and use them in the house as a cut flower.

Chamaemelum nobile. 5
CAMOMILE, CHAMOMILE. Hardy, low-growing ever-green perennial. Used for tea and occasionally grown as a substitute for lawns. Skin rash occasionally reported from using chamomile flowers as a hair wash or tonic, as are allergic reactions to drinking the tea. See also *Matricaria recutita*.

Chamaerops humilis. MALES 8, FEMALES 1 ✪
MEDITERRANEAN FAN PALM. The only palm tree native to Europe, this is among the hardiest of all palms. Short, with a very thick trunk, this tree grows as far north as Seattle, Washington. Propagated from clumps that develop at the base. As a rule, almost all fan palms are insect-pollinated and do not pose allergy problems. The Mediterranean fan palm is, however, an exception: it is a separate-sexed, wind-pollinated tree that, when mature, may cause allergy. Female trees bear no pollen and are good choices in the allergy-free landscape. When buying, look for plants that already have the small, grape-size fruits on them, as they'll be the females.

Chamelaucium. 2 ✪
WAX PLANT, WAXFLOWER. Native to Australia, shrubs for zones 9 to 10, drought-tolerant with cute little wax-like flowers, full sun.

Chamelaucium uncinatum. 4
GERALDTON WAXFLOWER. Evergreen shrub native to Australia and grown in zones 9 and 10. Needlelike leaves and small pink flowers often used in flower arrangements. Needs fast-draining soil in full sun.

CHAMOMILE. See *Chamaemelum nobile*.

Chamveyronia. 7
Tropical and subtropical palms.

CHASTE TREE. See *Vitex*.

CHAT. See *Catha edulis*.

CHECKERBERRY. See *Gaultheria*.

Cheiranthus cheiri. 3
WALLFLOWER. Perennial, hardy to zone 6. Easy to grow in full sun. Prune to shape.

Chelone obliqua. 4
Tall, attractive pink-flowering native perennial for rich, moist soils in full sun or partial shade in zones 4 to 9. Native to the Midwest and southeastern parts of the U.S. Attractive to bumblebees and hummingbirds.

CHENILLE PLANT. See *Acalypha*.

Chenopodium. GENUS 9 TO 10 ◙
GOOSEFOOT FAMILY. Many weeds, but some Cheno-podiums are grown as herbs, vegetables, or ornamentals. Some common names are mercury, Mexican tea, quinoa, Spanish tea, wild spinach, and wormseed. The crushed leaves of many Chenopodiums give off volatile organic compounds (VOCs), which can cause dizziness if inhaled. Contact with the leaves often results in allergic skin reactions. All species of Chenopodium can cause pollen-related allergies. Nonetheless, there are some separate-sexed species in this group (especially Atriplex and also Grayia), and with these there are now some useful female clones available. (See each in this chapter.) Many species are poisonous.

CHERIMOYA. See *Annona cherimola*.

CHERRY. See *Prunus*.

CHERRY PALM. See *Pseudophoenix*.

CHERRY, WEST INDIAN. See *Malpighia glabra*.

CHERVIL. See *Anthriscus*.

CHESTNUT. See *Castanea*.

Chiastophyllum oppositifolium. 3
Hardy, spreading succulent with bright yellow flowers, easy to grow in zones 6 to 10.

CHILEAN BELLFLOWER. See *Lapageria rosea*.

CHILEAN GUAVA. See *Ugni molinae*.

CHILEAN INCENSE CEDAR. See *Austrocedrus*.

CHILEAN JASMINE. See *Mandevilla laxa*.

CHILEAN WINE PALM. See *Jubaea*.

Chilopsis linearis. 4
DESERT WILLOW. Small, flowering, deciduous tree native to western deserts. Easy to grow from seed or hardwood cuttings, this tree grows best in hot, dry desert climates. Many small Catalpa-like flowers, which are used in Mexico to make a cough medicine. The flowers are also occasionally used as a heart stimulant

medicine. Desert willow is a very attractive small tree that's quite drought-tolerant and should be used more.

CHIMING BELLS. See *Mertensia*.

Chimonanthus praecox. 3

MERATIA, WINTERSWEET. Deciduous shrub from China, hardy to zone 6; needs winter cold to thrive. Fragrant yellow flowers bloom very early in the spring. Needs plenty of water.

CHINA ASTER. See *Callistephus chinensis*.

CHINA BERRY. See *Melia*.

CHINA FIR. See *Cunninghamia*.

CHINA TREE. See *Saponaria*.

CHINCHERINCHEE. See *Ornithogalum*.

CHINESE BOTTLE TREE. See *Firmiana simplex*.

CHINESE DATE. See *Ziziphus*.

CHINESE ELM. See *Ulmus parvifolia*.

CHINESE EVERGREEN. See *Aglaonema*.

CHINESE FIR. See *Cunninghamia*.

CHINESE FORGET-ME-NOT. See *Cynoglossum*.

CHINESE FOUNTAIN PALM. See *Livistona*.

CHINESE GROUND ORCHID. See *Bletilla striata*.

CHINESE HOUSES. See *Collinsia heterophylla*.

CHINESE JUJUBE. See *Ziziphus*.

CHINESE LANTERN. See *Abutilon*; *Physalis*.

CHINESE LAUREL. See *Antidesma*.

CHINESE MAIDENHAIR TREE. See *Ginkgo biloba*.

CHINESE PARASOL TREE. See *Firmiana simplex*.

CHINESE PISTACHE TREE. See *Pistache*.

CHINESE PLUM YEW. See *Cephalotaxus*.

CHINESE RICE PAPER PLANT. See *Tetrapanax papyriferus*.

CHINESE RUKKIS TREE. See *Eucommia ulmoides*.

CHINESE SCHOLAR TREE. See *Sophora japonica*.

CHINESE SOAPBERRY. See *Sapindus*.

CHINESE SWAMP CYPRESS. See *Glyptostrobus lineatus*.

CHINESE TALLOW TREE. See *Sapium sebiferum*.

CHINESE THREAD TREE. See *Eucommia ulmoides*.

CHINESE VARNISH TREE. See *Rhus*.

CHINESE WATER PINE. See *Glyptostrobus lineatus*.

CHINQUAPIN. See *Castanopsis*.

Chionanthus. MALES 8, FEMALES 1 ✪

FRINGE TREE. Two deciduous tree species, one native and one Chinese. Both are hardy in zones 5 to 10. Fringe trees are separate-sexed trees and both sexes flower profusely, similar to white lilacs. Members of the olive family, these (male) trees can cause severe allergy. The male trees have slightly larger flowers and only the female trees produce clusters of the small olivelike fruits; females are pollen-free and good selections for the allergy-free landscape.

Chionodoxa. 2 ✪

GLORY-OF-THE-SNOW. Hardy bulb in all zones. Bright blue flowers on small plants bloom very early in spring and occasionally naturalize.

Chiranthodendron pentadactylon. 5

MONKEY-HAND TREE. Fast-growing, large evergreen tree for zone 10. Small, red, tuliplike flowers resemble small hands. Large green leaves.

Chitalpa. 1 ✪

Chitalpa is an intergeneric hybrid cross between Catalpa and Chilopsis (desert willow). This hybrid is male sterile and makes no viable pollen. Zones 9 and 10.

CHIVES. See *Allium*.

Chloris. 8

FINGER GRASS, RHODES GRASS. An imported grass that causes allergy, especially in the western United States. This species is spreading quickly and is taking over much native habitat along parts of the Pacific Coast. Invasive and allergenic.

Chlorophora (Milicia excelsa). MALES 10 ✎, FEMALES 3

AFRICAN TEAK, IROKO. Several species of large evergreen tropical trees, occasionally used in zones 10 to 13. Pollen from these males is exceptionally allergenic; the sawdust from the wood of the trees is also a potent allergen. The smaller branches hang down in female trees and curve upward in male trees. The latex sap of the trees is also allergenic and will cause skin problems.

Chlorophytum comosum. MALES 6, FEMALES 1 ✪

SPIDER PLANT. Easy-to-grow houseplant. Sensitive to chlorine in water, which causes tip burn on the long, strap-shaped leaves. Can be used as a ground cover in shady areas of zone 10. Spider plant was found by the National Aeronautic and Space Administration (NASA) to be the best houseplant for "scrubbing" indoor air pollution. Plants are separate-sexed and only the female plants make any of the small seeds. Both the all-green and the variegated types can be of either sex. In the near future it is hoped that there will be some female-only plants available to buy.

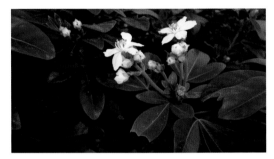

Choisya ternata. 3
MEXICAN ORANGE. (Pictured above.) Evergreen shrub for zones 9 and 10. Fragrant white flowers.

CHOKEBERRY, RED. See *Aronia arbutifolia*.

CHOKECHERRY. See *Prunus virginiana*.

Chorisia. 6
FLOSS SILK TREE, KAPOK. Evergreen or briefly deciduous trees with stout, heavily thorned trunks. Hardy in zones 8 to 10. Showy large white or pink flowers. Sheds lots of silky down called kapok, which was used to stuff pillows and as insulation for vests, especially used during World War II. Close contact with kapok is known to cause allergies, including hay fever, asthma, and contact skin rash. In the garden it is relatively safe and the flowers are not big producers of pollen, but keep the large fruits cleaned up and disposed of.

CHRISTMAS BERRY. See *Heteromeles arbutifolia*.

CHRISTMAS CACTUS. See *Schlumbergera*.

CHRISTMAS PALM. See *Veitchia*.

CHRISTMAS ROSE. See *Helleborus*.

CHRISTMAS TREES. See *Abies*; *Cedrus*; *Pinus*.

Chrysalidocarpus. MALES 8, FEMALES 1 ✿
Twenty species of palms from the tropics. *C. lutescens*, the butterfly palm, cane palm, or yellow palm, is frequently used in Florida landscaping. Trees are separate-sexed and only the males cause allergy.

Chrysanthemum. DOUBLES 4, SINGLES 6
COSTMARY, DUSTY MILLER, FEVERFEW, FLORIST'S CHRYSANTHEMUM, GARDEN CHRYSANTHEMUMS, MARGUERITES, OX-EYE DAISY, PAINTED DAISY, SHASTA DAISY. A large group of more than 200 species of annuals and perennials, including some of our most common garden flowers. Allergy to Chrysanthemum is common. Allergy to the insecticide pyrethrum, made from a type of Chrysanthemum, is also common. A few people are very sensitive to the leaves of Chrysanthemums and may get skin rashes from handling the plants. Some people may also be allergic to their fragrance.

Chrysanthemums are short-day plants and bloom best in autumn, when day length is less than twelve hours. Pollen may cause allergy, especially in those already sensitive to ragweed. The double-flowered varieties shed far less pollen than single-flowered types. Mums brought inside as cut flowers may well shed pollen, especially single-flowered cultivars. These are often used as potted flowering plants that are brought to people in the hospital; this is not the best idea. There may be a few very doubled forms that are pollen-free.

Chrysogonum virginianum. 3
GOLDENSTAR. Native creeping perennial ground cover for moist, acid, shady soils in zones 5 to 9. Forms a mat 3 to 4 inches tall; each plant may spread 18 inches or so wide. Little bright yellow flowers are highly attractive.

CHRYSOLARIX. See *Pseudolarix*.

Chrysophyllum cainito. 2 ✿
STAR APPLE. A tall evergreen tree of the American tropics, grown for its star-shaped sweet green or purple fruits.

Chrysophyllum oliviforme. 6
A frost-tender tree with attractive leaves, hardy only in the warmest parts of zone 10.

CHUPAROSA. See *Justicia*.

Cibotium. 6
Several species of tree ferns, some of which may reach over 12 feet. Popular landscape plants in Florida and California. These large ferns shed spores, which drop directly under the tree. Do not place them next to patios or directly over where people sit. Also do not position them next to windows, because the spores are minute enough to easily pass through most screens. Planted in just the right spot, these may present little problem.

Cichorium intybus. 3
CHICORY. A hardy, blue-flowered perennial, native of Europe, with thick, tuberous roots that are used to flavor coffee. Very easy to grow and often naturalizes.

CIDER GUM. See *Eucalyptus*.

CIGAR BOX CEDAR. See *Cedrela*.

CIGAR PLANT. See *Cuphea*.

CILANTRO. See *Coriandrum*.

Cimicifuga. 3
BUGBANE, COHOSH, SNAKEROOT. Hardy perennials for all zones. Used in shady gardens with moist soil; some species are native to the eastern United States.

Cineraria. 5
Short-lived perennials. Many hybrids with vivid colors, developed for shady, moist areas. Popular potted flowering plants. (See also *Senecio*.)

Cinnamomum camphora. 8
CAMPHOR TREE. Large evergreen tree of zones 9 and 10, the source of camphor. Leaves have a pleasing smell when crushed. Camphor trees are very popular street trees in much of California and Florida. During spring, these trees bear thousands of persistent, tiny yellowish flowers, which shed copious amounts of pollen that rarely drifts far from the tree. On city blocks that are lined with camphor trees on both sides of the street (as is fairly common in Southern California), residents with severe allergies or asthma may need to leave the area for several weeks or longer at the peak of bloom.

CINNAMON FERN. See *Osmunda*.

CINNAMON, WILD. See *Canella*.

CINQUEFOIL. See *Potentilla*.

Cirsium. 9 ◐
Various thistles; many cause allergies.

Cissus. 4
Evergreen vine for zones 8 to 10. Vigorous growth and handsome leaves. Easy to grow. Some, especially *C. rhombifolia*, the grape ivy, are used as houseplants. Some Cissus are separate-sexed, but there are no female selections available to buy at the moment.

Cistanthe grandiflora. 2 ✿
ROCK PURSLANE. A tough, easy-to-grow, spreading, drought-tolerant gray-leafed succulent with very attractive rose-colored flowers on long stems. Full sunlight in zones 9 to 13.

Cistus. 3
ROCKROSE. Evergreen shrub, hardy in zones 8 to 10. Good in full sun. Drought-tolerant. Large, showy white or purple flowers on easy-to-grow, 3- to 6-foot bushes.

Citharexylum fruticosum; C. spinosum.
MALES 9 ◐, FEMALES 3
FIDDLEWOOD, FLORIDA FUDDLEWOOD. Small tree for zones 10 to 13, with small, lightly fragrant flowers. Male plants of these species are allergenic and all the plants have a very high potential to become very invasive.

Citrus. 1 TO 5 ✿
CALAMONDIN, CITRON, GRAPEFRUIT, KUMQUAT, LEMON, LIME, ORANGE, TANGERINE. Long-lived, handsome evergreen trees for zones 9 and 10 in favored locations with good frost drainage. Citrus needs good soil drainage and summer irrigation to thrive. Most also need high summer heat to produce sweet fruit, especially grapefruit. Mature trees bear fragrant, white blossoms during most of the year and most allergy to citrus is in response to the heavy fragrance. Allergy to the pollen is less common. People living in or next to citrus groves are more likely to develop sensitivity. The flowers of most tangerines and kumquats are smaller and much less fragrant, making them better choices for individuals with fragrance sensitivities.

Allergy to citrus is neither particularly common nor severe. On rare occasions, however, some people develop photodermatitis from contact with citrus plants or fruit. Photodermatitis is a rash caused by exposure to sunlight after contact with an allergen. Many of the seedless cultivars of citrus have pollen-free flowers.

Cladrastis lutea. 5
YELLOWWOOD. Deciduous native trees hardy in all zones. Long clusters of very fragrant white flowers late in spring. Young trees are slow to mature and may not bloom for many years.

Clarkia. 2 ✿
FAREWELL-TO-SPRING, GODETIA. Native annual for all zones. Full sun. Good cut flowers in red, white, pink, rose, and purple, both single- and double-flowered varieties. Fast-growing from direct seeding.

Claytonia. 1 ✿
MAYFLOWER, SPRING BEAUTY. Small perennial with early spring bloom for moist, shady areas.

Clematis. FORMAL DOUBLES 1, BISEXUAL 5, MALES 8, FEMALES 1 ✪

Several hundred species of evergreen or deciduous hardy flowering vines. Clematis are among the most beautiful vines for winding up the trunks of trees, climbing on a trellis, or growing up and through climbing roses. Clematis does best when the roots are kept cool (mulch) and the tops have warmth and sunlight. They should have fast-draining soil and do well in large pots. Acid soil should be limed before planting. There are some well-documented cases of skin rashes caused by contact with Clematis foliage. Slow-growing at first and hard to establish, Clematis is often worth the effort. Poisonous if eaten.

Cleome spinosa. 3

SPIDER FLOWER. Tall, easy-to-grow summer annual.

Clerodendrum. 3

GLORYBOWER. More than 400 species of evergreen trees, shrubs, and vines, some hardy to zone 6. Unusual red, white, or red-and-white flowers, some resembling bleeding hearts (Dicentra).

Clethra alnifolia. 4

Deciduous shrub native to the eastern United States. Culture is similar to that of rhododendron: shade, mulch, acid soil, good moisture, fast drainage. Small white flowers are richly fragrant. May pose problems for the odor-sensitive individual.

Clethra arborea. 4

LILY-OF-THE-VALLEY TREE. Evergreen tree for zones 9 and 10. White flowers closely resemble lily-of-the-valley, and the fragrance is also similar. Not a tree for the odor-sensitive individual.

Cleyera japonica. 4

Handsome evergreen shrub, for zones 8 to 11, with small, white, fragrant flowers followed by clusters of dark red berries, which persist through winter. Culture similar to Camellia, to which it is related.

Clianthus puniceus. 2 ✪

PARROT BEAK. A shrubby evergreen vine or shrub from New Zealand, grown in zones 9 to 10. Small leaflets edge long leaves. Flowers are red, pink, or white, shaped like a parrot's beak. Full or part shade.

CLIFF-BRAKE. See *Pellaea*.

CLIFF ROSE. See *Cowania mexicana*.

Cliftonia monophylla. 2 ✪

BUCKWHEAT TREE. Small native evergreen tree for zones 7 to 10. Flowers are small, pink or white, and attractive to bees.

CLIMBING BUTCHER'S VINE. See *Semele androgyna*.

CLIMBING FERN. See *Lygodium japonicum*.

CLIMBING LILY. See *Gloriosa rothschildiana*.

Clintonia. 2 ✪

BEAR-TONGUE LILY, COW-TONGUE LILY. Small tuberous, native lilies hardy to zone 4. Grows best in shady, moist situations.

Clitoria. 2 ✪

BUTTERFLY PEA. A large genus of perennial flowering vines, some of which can be grown in most zones. The double-flowering variety is hardy only in zones 8 to 10. Showy, pealike flowers.

Clivia. 2 ✪

KAFFIR LILY. Popular greenhouse plant, also used in well-protected, deep-shade landscapes in zones 9 and 10. Easy to grow under the right conditions. Flowers are bright orange, rarely yellow, on irislike plants with broad, strap-shaped leaves. Container plants flower best when root bound.

CLOVE. See *Syzygium aromaticum*.

CLOVE PINK. See *Dianthus*.

CLOVER. See *Melilotus*; *Trifolium*.

CLUB MOSS. See *Lycopodium*.

Clytostoma callistegioides. 2 ✪

VIOLET TRUMPET VINE. For zones 7 to 12, this vine dies back to the ground outside of zone 10. Grown from cuttings of old wood.

Cnidoscolus. 10 ✦

SPURGE NETTLE. Large group of perennial herbs, shrubs, or small trees native to North and South America. All have dangerous sap and can cause skin rash and inhalant allergy. Many of these are separate-sexed but neither sex would be recommended, as the potential for contact allergy is too high.

COCA PLANT. See *Erythroxylum coca*.

Coccoloba. MALES 8, FEMALES 1 ✪

PIGEON PLUM, SEA GRAPE, SNAILSEED. Large group of tropical and subtropical evergreen trees, vines, and shrubs, some with edible fruit. A few species are grown in southern Florida. The female plants make fruit and are not difficult to identify; they can be grown from softwood cuttings taken in spring. Zones 10 to 13.

Coccothrinax. 1 ✿
BROOM PALM, SILVER PALM. Slow-growing palms for sunny areas in zone 10. Good allergy choices.

Cocculus laurifolius. MALES 9 🍃, FEMALES 1 ✿
CORAL BEADS, MOONSEED, SNAILSEED. Evergreen small tree, shrub, or vinelike plant, hardy in zones 7 to 10. Bears many small white flowers in early summer on plant covered with 3-inch-long, deeply veined leaves. Separate-sexed plants; only females produce the red or black fruits. The female plants produce no pollen, but males produce a great deal of potentially allergenic (and poisonous) pollen. Unfortunately, Cocculus is rarely sold sexed and so gets a poor ranking. There are a great many of these trees and shrubs at the arboretum in Los Angeles, and every single one of them is a male.

The bark of Cocculus contains a powerful alkaloid poison, coclaurina, which has the same properties as the poison curare. It would make good sense to be especially careful not to get fresh sap in your eyes or in a cut or scratch on your hands. Take care when pruning.

COCKLE. See *Silene*.

COCKSCOMB. See *Celosia*.

COCKSPUR CORAL TREE. See *Erythrina crista-galli*.

COCOS AUSTRALIS. See *Butia capitata*.

Cocos nucifera. 7
COCONUT PALM. Many palms are sold as Cocos species, but only *C. nucifera* is a true coconut palm. These are the tall, coconut-bearing palms of the tropics. Monoecious, they do cause some allergy in areas where very common.

COCOS PLUMOSA. See *Arecastrum romanzoffianum*.

COCOS PALM. See *Syagrus*.

Codiaeum. 4
CROTON. Several species of evergreen trees or shrubs from the tropics, grown in the United States as houseplants. Large variegated, colorful leaves. Needs good heat and light to thrive in the house. As houseplants these are rarely seen in bloom, yet the flowers may cause allergy. Remove blooms as soon as they appear. On large-leafed houseplants such as croton, the foliage should be wiped down with a moist cloth every week to cut down on allergenic house dust. Poisonous.

CODONOPSIS CLEMATIDEA. See *Campanula*.

Coelogyne. 2 ✿
Greenhouse orchid with showy white flowers, for partial shade. Grow these pseudobulbs in containers of orchid bark and feed them regularly.

Coffea arabica. 2 ✿
COFFEE. Grown commercially for coffee beans. Can be grown outside in frost-free areas of zone 10, where it needs partial shade to thrive. An attractive small tree for greenhouse or houseplant use. In zone 9 these can often be grown outside if planted directly underneath an evergreen tree, such as a large citrus. Self-fruiting, only one plant is needed to make coffee berries.

COFFEE FERN. See *Pellaea*.

COFFEE TREE, WILD. See *Colubrina arborescens*.

COFFEEBERRY. See *Rhamnus californica*.

COHOSH. See *Cimicifuga*.

COHUNE PALM. See *Orbignya*.

Coix lacryma-jobi. 6
JOB'S TEARS. Perennial grasslike plant grown as an annual in cold climates. Grows to 6 feet, with shiny white seedpods with beadlike seeds often used for bracelets and rosaries. Sun or part shade.

Colchicum autumnale. 3
AUTUMN CROCUS, MEADOW SAFFRON. Perennial corm, often used as a blooming houseplant; the plant will flower from a corm simply watered and set in a dish. As a garden plant, Colchicum does not pose much potential for allergy. Because the corms contain the powerful drug colchicine, which is used in genetic experiments, it is wise for pregnant women not to handle them, and for them to be kept away from small children.

Coleonema (Diosma). 4
BREATH-OF-HEAVEN. Evergreen shrub for zones 9 and 10, with tiny leaves and many small fragrant white or pink flowers. Needs full sun and good drainage. Greenhouse plant in cooler regions. Popular landscape shrub in California.

Coleus hybridus. 1 ✿
Perennials used as annuals in all zones. Good foliage plant for shady spots. Large colored leaves in a wide variety of colors available. Houseplant for sunny rooms. Easy to root from cuttings. A member of the mint family.

Collinsia heterophylla. 1 ✿
CHINESE HOUSES. California native annual, grown from seed. White or rose-colored snapdragon-like flowers.

Colocasia esculenta. 2 ✿

ELEPHANT'S EARS, TARO. Zone 10 to 13 perennials with big tuberous roots and huge green leaves. Give them shade, plenty of moisture, and protection from the wind because the big leaves tear easily. Plants seldom flower. Poisonous.

Colpothrinax wrightii. 1 ✿

BARREL PALM, BELLY PALM, BOTTLE PALM, CUBAN BELLY PALM. Central American and Cuban palms with trunks swollen in middle at maturity.

COLTSFOOT. See *Galax urceolata*; *Tussilago*.

Colubrina arborescens. MALES 8, FEMALES 1 ✿

WILD COFFEE TREE. Shrub or small evergreen tree for zone 10 and tropics. Not normally sold sexed, but look for plants with fruit on them.

COLUMBINE. See *Aquilegia*.

Columnea. 2 ✿

NORSE FIRE PLANT. Many species. Trailing houseplants with orange, red, or yellow flowers. Related to African violets and have similar culture requirements.

Comarostaphylis diversifolia. 5

SUMMER HOLLY. Small evergreen tree native to California. Needs fast drainage and partial shade to thrive. Dark green leaves, small white flowers; red berries persist into winter.

COMFREY. See *Symphytum officinale*.

Commiphora mollis. 3

CORKWOOD TREE, VELVET-LEAF. East African native, hardy only in frost-free areas, zones 11 to 13; sap is used as medicine. Wildlife eats the fruit.

COMPASS PLANT. See *Silphium*.

COMPTIE. See *Zamia*.

Comptonia peregrina. MALES 7, FEMALES 1 ✿

SWEET FERN. Hardy perennial native to the eastern United States. Not a true fern. Female plants make excellent ground covers and are good for covering large slopes. (See also *Myrica*.)

Condalia obovata. 6

A Central American native tree, hardy only in warmest areas of zone 10.

CONEFLOWER, PURPLE. See *Echinacea purpurea*.

CONFEDERATE JASMINE. See *Trachelospermum*.

Consolida ambigua. 3

LARKSPUR. Hardy annual for all zones. Many double-flowering varieties in white, blue, or purple. Grows to 2 feet, depending on variety.

Convallaria majalis. 4

LILY-OF-THE-VALLEY. Hardy perennial grown from pips. Grown as ground cover underneath taller, shade-loving plants. Very fragrant white flowers may cause allergy in fragrance-sensitive individuals. Plants, especially the roots, are highly poisonous if eaten.

Convolvulus. 2 ✿

Several species of shrublike morning glory. Grows well in dry, sunny locations of zones 7 to 10.

COONTIE. See *Zamia*.

Copernicia. 1 ✿

CARNAUBA WAX PALM, PETTICOAT PALM. A group of tall, handsome subtropical palms, some used in zones 9 and 10, especially in Florida.

COPPER LEAF. See *Acalypha*.

Coprosma. MALES 9 🍃, FEMALES 1 ✿

MIRROR PLANT. A large group of very attractive evergreen shrubs and small trees with shiny leaves, native to Australia, New Zealand, and the Pacific Islands. *C. repens*, the mirror plant, is often used in landscaping in zones 7 to 10. Male and female flowers are borne on separate plants. The female plants, which can be identified by their small red or yellow berries, cause no allergy. Generally not yet sold sexed, so whole group is often suspect; however, there will be some new female cultivars released in the next few years. Look for ones with an OPALS #1 ranked tag on them.

COQUITO PALM. See *Jubaea*.

CORAL BEADS. See *Cocculus laurifolius*.

CORAL BELLS. See *Heuchera*.

CORAL PLANT. See *Jatropha*.

CORAL TREE. See *Erythrina*.

CORAL VINE. See *Antigonon*.

CORALBERRY. See *Symphoricarpos*.

CORDGRASS. See *Spartina*.

Cordia. 5

Large group of mostly tropical evergreen or deciduous trees or shrubs occasionally used as greenhouse plants, houseplants, or landscape material in zone 10. *C. myxa*, the Assyrian plum, is a small deciduous tree found in California.

Cordyline. 3
CABBAGE TREE, DRACAENA, DRAGON TREE, GRASS PALM, TI. Twenty species of large evergreen shrubs or small trees. Those grown outdoors in zones 9 and 10 are tall and resemble yucca, to which they are related. Small, fragrant white flowers.

Corema. MALES 8, FEMALES 1 ☻
BROOM, CROWBERRY, POVERTY GRASS. Hardy evergreen separate-sexed shrubs used as ground cover.

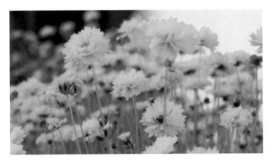

Coreopsis (Calliopsis). DOUBLES 3, SINGLES 5
PERENNIAL DAISY, TICKSEED. (Pictured above.) Yellow flowers on easy-to-grow, sun-loving plants. Double- and single-flowered varieties are available; doubles shed far less pollen.

Coriandrum. 3
CILANTRO, CORIANDER. Aromatic herbs grown and used for seasoning. Small white flowers.

Coriaria japonica. 9 ◗
TANNER'S TREE. Group of shrubs and small trees, some hardy to zone 4. They bear many small greenish flowers. They produce very poisonous fruit.

CORK FIR. See *Abies*.

CORK OAK. See *Quercus*.

CORK TREE. See *Phellodendron*.

CORKWOOD. See *Leitneria floridana*.

CORN. See *Zea mays*.

CORN COCKLE. See *Agrostemma githago*.

CORN LILY. See *Ixia*; *Veratrum*.

CORN PLANT. See *Dracaena*.

CORNELIAN CHERRY. See *Cornus*.

Cornus. 5
BUNCHBERRY, CORNELIAN CHERRY, CRACKERBERRY, DOGWOOD, FLOWERING DOGWOOD, OSIER, RED OSIER. Large group of hardy deciduous shrubs and trees, many

native to the United States. On rare occasions implicated in allergy. Avoid direct contact with flowers.

Corokia cotoneaster. 3
Small evergreen shrub native to New Zealand, hardy to zone 6. Oddly shaped branches with tiny leaves and small yellow flowers followed by orange berries. Needs little water and fast drainage.

Coronilla varia. 3
CROWN VETCH. Hardy perennial legume used as hay crop or for ground cover in large, sunny areas. Pealike flowers are usually purple. Dried flowers, as found in hay, can cause allergy, but fresh flowers rarely do so.

Corozo. 7
OIL PALM. Tropical palm tree.

Correa. 2 ☻
AUSTRALIAN FUCHSIA. Low-growing evergreen shrubs hardy to zone 8. Plants bear pink or red fuchsialike flowers. Often used as ground covers, they need fast drainage and should not be overwatered.

Cortaderia selloana. MALES 8, FEMALES 1 ☻
PAMPAS GRASS. Tall, clump-forming perennial grass with tall erect white or pink flower spikes. Hardy to zone 6, these occasionally naturalize in zones 8 to 10. Pampas grass is unusual in that, although it is a separate-sexed species, most individual plants are female and are able to set viable seed without pollination by a male plant. Female Cortaderia plants are excellent additions to the landscape but care must be taken not to use them in exposures where they may become invasive and spread into nearby wild areas. The cultivar 'Pumilia' is smaller and said to be more winter hardy.

Corylopsis. 7
WINTER HAZEL. Deciduous shrubs and small trees, hardy to zone 4. Very early flowering, the yellow flowers appear on bare branches early in the spring. Branches of Corylopsis are often brought into the house to bloom in late winter, where they may cause allergy.

Corylus. 7
FILBERT, HAZELNUT. Deciduous, hardy, nut trees or shrubs, these are known to cause allergy, especially among individuals living close to filbert orchards.

Corynocarpus laevigata. 4
NEW ZEALAND LAUREL. Evergreen shrub or small tree, for zones 9 to 10, with dark green, glossy leaves and small, orange, 1-inch-long ovoid fruits. Fruit is very poisonous.

Cosmos. 5
Tall flowering annuals of many colors. Easy and fast growing from seed.

COSTA RICAN HOLLY. See *Olmediella betschlerana.*

Cotinus. MALES 8, FEMALES 2 ✪
SMOKE BUSH, SMOKE TREE. Two species of unusual but attractive deciduous shrubs or small trees, hardy in all zones. Relatives of poison ivy, the pollen of Cotinus is highly allergenic but, because the smoky-colored flowers are borne on old wood, the pollen can be avoided by hard yearly pruning. In the future there may well be some selected female clones of this sold with OPALS tags. Contact with the sap of this plant is known to cause skin rashes.

Cotoneaster. GROUND COVERS 3, SHRUBS 5
A large group of evergreen and deciduous shrubs, trees, and ground covers, with small grayish leaves, small white flowers, and clusters of orange-red berries that are attractive to birds. The low-growing ground cover Cotoneaster cultivars shed less pollen than do the taller, shrubby plants. Berries and leaves are poisonous.

COTTON. See *Gossypium hirsutum.*

COTTONWOOD. See *Populus.*

Cotula squalida. 4
NEW ZEALAND BRASS BUTTONS. Low-growing evergreen perennial for zones 6 to 10. Yellow, buttonlike flowers and soft, gray-green feathery leaves. Ground cover in full sun or part shade with plenty of water.

Cotyledon. 2 ✪
Succulent for zones 9 and 10; houseplant elsewhere. Full sun or partial shade, easy to grow.

COW ITCH TREE. See *Lagunaria patersonii.*

COW ITCH VINE. See *Campsis.*

COW-TONGUE LILY. See *Clintonia.*

Cowania mexicana. 2 ✪
CLIFF ROSE. Hardy to zone 3. Native to western deserts and drought-tolerant, this shrubby perennial can grow to 6 feet. Attractive little white or yellow flowers.

COWBERRY. See *Viburnum; Vaccinium.*

COWSLIP. See *Primula.*

COWSLIP, CAPE. See *Lachenalia.*

COYOTE BRUSH, COYOTE BUSH. See *Baccharis pilularis.*

CRAB CACTUS. See *Schlumbergera.*

CRABAPPLE. See *Malus.*

CRABGRASS. See *Digitaria sanguinalis.*

CRACKERBERRY. See *Cornus.*

Crambe cordifolia. 4
Very large perennial plant with huge leaves and masses of tiny white flowers on spikes that may be almost 6 feet tall; good garden accent plant for moist soils in zones 6 to 9, native to Europe and related to kale and cabbage. Flowers very attractive to bees and small butterflies.

CRANBERRY. See *Vaccinium; Viburnum.*

CRANESBILL. See *Erodium; Geranium.*

CRAPE MYRTLE. See *Lagerstroemia indica.*

Craspedia globosa. 5
Tall, round, yellow-flowering plants grown from seed as annuals and used for dried flowers.

Crassula. 2 ✪
JADE PLANT. Succulent perennial, hardy in zones 9 and 10 and common as sun-loving houseplants. Very easy to grow and drought-tolerant.

Crataegus. 3
HAWTHORN, WASHINGTON THORN. Many species of thorny, deciduous, flowering trees, some hardy to zone 3. White, pink, or red flowers are followed by small red berries, which are attractive to birds. Double-flowered varieties shed less pollen than single-flowered ones do. Allergy to hawthorn pollen is not common, and when it occurs, is rarely severe. Hawthorn needs a period of winter chill to thrive; in warm zone 10 in particular, they will grow, but not well, and often are infested with aphids. Best grown in zones 3 to 9.

CRAZYWEED. See *Oxytropis.*

CREAM BUSH. See *Holodiscus.*

CREAM NUT. See *Bertholletia excelsa.*

CREEPING CHARLIE. See *Pilea.*

CREEPING SAGE. See *Salvia.*

CREEPING ZINNIA. See *Sanvitalia procumbens.*

CREOSOTE BUSH. See *Larrea tridentata.*

Crescentia. 5
Group of small fruiting trees native to Mexico. Not hardy except in warmest areas of zone 10.

CRIMEAN LINDEN. See *Tilia.*

Crinodendron (Tricuspidaria). 2 ✪

FLOWERING OAK, LILY-OF-THE-VALLEY TREE. Evergreen trees native to Chile and grown in zones 9 and 10. Grows well in shade with moist, acid soil. Lots of attractive bell-shaped white flowers in summer, followed by many seedpods.

Crinum. 3

SPIDER LILY. Large lilylike flowers on bulb-grown plant. Perennial in zones 9 and 10, in partial shade or full sun. Fragrant flowers are borne atop long stems.

Crocosmia (Montbretia). 3

Hardy corm grows to zone 6, if mulched in winter. Will naturalize in mild areas. Orange, red, or yellow blooms make long-lasting cut flowers.

Crocus. 2 ✪

Low-growing, early-blooming spring flowers grown from corms. Many colors. Will naturalize where conditions are perfect. One species, *C. sativus*, is grown for the pollen, which is collected and sold as the spice saffron. Poisonous. (See also *Colchicum autumnale*.)

Crossandra infundibuliformis. 2 ✪

A houseplant with dark green leaves and showy orange or scarlet flowers. Needs a warm room and filtered sunlight.

Crotalaria. 4

CANARY BIRD BUSH, RATTLEBOX. Large group of evergreen perennials and shrubs for zone 10. Large, fast-growing plants must be pruned back often. Numerous small yellow-green flowers and gray-green leaves. Very poisonous.

CROTON. See *Codiaeum*.

CROTON JAPONICUM. See *Mallotus japonica*.

Croton megalobotrys. 9 🍃

Large, tropical evergreen tree. *C. monanthogynus*, known as prairie tea, is an annual native of the southern United States and Mexico. Sap of all species is quite allergenic.

CROWBERRY. See *Corema*; *Vaccinium*.

CROWFOOT. See *Ranunculus*.

CROWN-BEARD. See *Verbesina*.

CROWN-OF-THORNS. See *Euphorbia*.

CROWN VETCH. See *Coronilla varia*.

Cryosophila. 1 ✪

Several species of small palm trees grown in zones 9 and 10; occasionally sold as the genus Acanthorrhiza.

Cryptanthus. 1 ✪

EARTH-STAR. Fancy-leafed perennials in tropical zones and houseplants elsewhere, earth-stars are members of the pineapple family.

Cryptocarya rubra. 2 ✪

Evergreen tree native to Chile and hardy in zones 9 and 10. Copper-red new leaves and glossy green older leaves on an attractive tree, slow-growing to 60 feet.

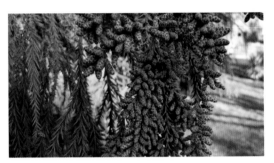

Cryptomeria japonica. 10 🍃

JAPANESE CEDAR. (Pictured above.) Hardy to zone 5, this is not a true cedar but more closely related to cypress. A tall evergreen Asian tree, it is native to Japan, where it is now considered the primary source of allergenic airborne pollen and, in Tokyo, the most common cause of both asthma and hay fever. Most of the recent severe Cryptomeria allergy in Japan is from a mass planting of these trees initiated by the Japanese Department of Agriculture.

Several kinds of Cryptomeria are sold in the United States, including a dwarf variety and one called 'Plume Cedar'. The dwarf cultivars are not very allergenic. In Japan they have developed a female, pollen-free Cryptomeria, but these are not yet available for sale in the U.S.

Cryptotaenia. 4

Tall foliage plant, grown as an annual in all zones. Small yellow flowers.

Ctenanthe. 3

BAMBURANTA. Grown in light shade in the warmest parts of zone 10, or as a houseplant elsewhere. Prized for its unusual, leathery leaves.

CUBAN BELLY PALM. See *Colpothrinax wrightii*.

CUBAN ROYAL PALM. See *Roystonea regia*.

CUCUMBER TREE. See *Magnolia*.

Cudrania. MALES 6, FEMALES 1 ✿
Five species of deciduous spiny trees, vines, or shrubs from China and Australia, related to mulberry. Some are hardy to zone 5. *C. tricuspidata* is a small thorny tree occasionally used as a hedge plant. Separate-sexed, but not sold sexed. The pollen-less females plants are a good choice for the allergy-free garden. The fruit is quite good.

Cunninghamia. 9 🍂
CHINESE FIR. Three species of large, Asian, evergreen coniferous trees, none of which is an actual fir. They are closely related to *Cryptomeria japonica* and, like Crypto-meria, can cause allergy. Hardy in zones 8 to 10.

Cunonia capensis. MALES 9 🍂, FEMALES 1 ✿
AFRICAN RED ALDER. A large group of trees and shrubs mostly native to South America, some of which are seen in California. Almost all of the Cunonia pose allergy potential. Separate-sexed plants, not yet sold sexed. Females do not produce pollen and are good choices for the allergy-free landscape.

CUP FLOWER. See *Nierembergia*.

CUP-OF-GOLD VINE. See *Solandra maxima*.

Cupaniopsis anacardioides. 6
CARROTWOOD, TUCKEROO. Australian native evergreen tree much used as street tree in Florida and California. Wood just under the bark is carrot colored. Carrotwood trees look similar in many ways to carob trees and, like carob, they also cause allergy. Some of these trees may be separate-sexed but none is sold sexed.

Cuphea. 2 ✿
CIGAR PLANT. Large group of Mexican native herbs and shrubs useful in the warmer zones. Small, tubular red flowers like little cigars. Sun or part shade. Easy to grow from cuttings.

CUPID'S DART. See *Catananche caerulea*.

Cupressocyparis leylandii. 8
LEYLAND CYPRESS. Evergreen hybrid tree, fast growing and often used for tall screens. In many areas this tree is dying off due to canker infection. These are often sold as being pollen-free trees, but that is not correct.

CUPRESSUS GENUS

Cupressus. 10 🍂
CYPRESS. A large group of evergreen trees with short, needlelike leaves, often grayish-green colored, similar to junipers, with which they are sometimes confused. Seeds form in round, golf-ball-size brown pods. Cypress are used in landscaping in warm, Mediterranean regions, but are not hardy enough for use in either northern Europe or the colder parts of the United States. They are drought-tolerant and very common on the West Coast. All shed profuse amounts of allergenic pollen, and may do so throughout as much as six or seven months of the year in warm climates. Reactions to cypress pollen are often severe. No cypress are recommended.

C. forbesii. 10 🍂
TECATE CYPRESS. Large evergreen bush native to Southern California.

C. glabra, C. arizonica. 10 🍂
ARIZONA CYPRESS. A large, gray-leafed shrub, to 40 feet tall and wide. Does well in the desert. In many areas of the Middle East, especially in Israel, this is the most allergenic species planted and the cause of considerable allergy and asthma. No cypress are good for those with allergies or asthma, but *C. glabra* and *C. arizonica* may well be the most allergenic of them all. At schools in particular, these should be removed and replaced with allergy-friendly shrubs.

C. macrocarpa. 10 🍂
MONTEREY CYPRESS. Tall, native tree growing along the central coast of California. This species may be somewhat less allergenic than the others. Livestock have been poisoned by eating Monterey cypress.

C. sempervirens. 10 🍂
ITALIAN CYPRESS. Tall, common, narrow landscape shrub, much overused in landscaping. Although this is not a separate-sexed (dioecious) species, nonetheless, modern horticulture has figured out a way to produce all-male Italian cypress trees, and most now sold are males. Very allergenic.

CURRANT. See *Ribes*.

CUSHION PINK. See *Silene*.

Cussonia spicata. 3
CABBAGE TREE. Small evergreen tree for zone 10, grown mostly for its large, fancy leaves. Small yellow flowers on 6-inch-long spikes.

Cyanotis. 3
PUSSY EARS, TEDDY BEARS. Evergreen houseplants. Needs good light indoors.

Cycas. MALES 6, FEMALES 1 ✿
SAGO PALM. Dwarf palms for zones 9 and 10. Often grown as container plants in greenhouses in colder

climates. Cycas are separate-sexed trees and both sexes bear cones. Female trees can be distinguished by their much larger cones. Males cause limited allergy; females none. Plants are expensive, so when buying mature trees, insist on females, which cause no allergy.

Cyclamen. 1 ✪
Tuberous perennials, some hardy to zone 4. Good flowering potted plants for the house but move them outside in the shade after they bloom. Red, pink, white, and salmon-colored flowers. *C. hederifolium* is the hardiest. Outside all need shade, moisture, and yearly fertilizer.

CYCLOPHORUS. See *Pyrrosia lingua*.

CYLINDROPHYLLUM. See *Cephalophyllum*.

Cymbalaria. 1 ✪
Small, creeping perennials for zones 5 to 10. Little leaves and small purple flowers on this ground cover for shady, moist areas.

Cymbidium. 1 ✪
Greenhouse orchids, grown in containers of bark, with regular water, feeding, and filtered shade. Good cut flowers.

Cynara. 3
ARTICHOKE, CARDOON. Perennial vegetables of the thistle family. Artichokes are hardy in zones 9 and 10. Cardoon is grown for its edible leaf stalks; hardy in zones 8 to 10.

Cynodon dactylon. COMMON 10 ◆, HYBRIDS INDIVIDUALLY RANKED
BERMUDA GRASS. A tough lawn grass for southern states that flowers even when quite short. The flowers produce plenty of pollen of the worst sort. To reduce flowering and pollen production, keep Bermuda grass lawns well fertilized, watered, and mowed often and low.

Hybrid Bermuda grasses are better choices because they grow more slowly and flower less often, if at all. Some of the lowest, tightest-growing Bermuda grass hybrids are pollen-free. Bermuda grass can also be a very difficult weed to eradicate when it spreads into perennial beds, because it spreads by underground rhizomes. Eradicate Bermuda grass by applying a nonselective, systemic herbicide. Bermuda grass that has spread to vacant lots has great potential to produce pollen; insist that owners of empty lots keep them mowed frequently.

Mow Bermuda grass lawns late in the afternoon, because the pollen is most active early in the morning. In general, lawn grasses that do not flower unless they are tall are the best choices. 'Princess 77' is a hybrid Bermuda grass that can be grown from seed, and it is pollen-free and OPALS ranked 1.

Cynoglossum. 2 ✪
CHINESE FORGET-ME-NOT. Annual or short-lived blue-flowered perennial. Grows best in full sun, with abundant water.

Cyperus. 7
NUT GRASS, PAPYRUS, PERENNIAL SEDGE. Bog and pond plants often regarded as weeds.

CYPRESS. See *Cupressus*.

CYPRESS CEDAR. See *Cedrus brevifolia*.

CYPRESS, FALSE. See *Chamaecyparis*.

CYPRESS PINE. See *Callitris*.

CYPRESS, SWAMP. See *Cyrilla racemosa*; *Glyptostrobus lineatus*.

Cypripedium. 4
LADY SLIPPER ORCHID, LADY SLIPPER, MOCCASIN FLOWER. Native orchid bearing pink, white, or yellow flowers. Moisture- and shade-loving hardy perennials, they look good planted with ferns and other shade lovers. Contact with the leaves and flowers of pink lady slipper occasionally causes severe skin rash.

Cyrilla racemosa. 2 ✪
HE HUCKLEBERRY, IRONWOOD, MYRTLE, SWAMP CYPRESS, TITI. Neither a true cypress nor an allergy plant, Cyrilla is hardy in zones 8 to 10. Small flowers are attractive to bees.

Cyrtanthus mackenii. 2 ✪
FIRE LILY. Bulb, hardy in zones 9 and 10. Small, irislike plants with white, red, or yellow flowers for moist shady areas. Contact with lily bulbs of all species can on occasion trigger lily rash.

Cyrtomium. 4
HOLLY FERN. Tall leathery-leafed fern for zones 8 to 10, grows to 3 feet in shady, moist locations.

Cytisus. 5
ATLAS BROOM, BROOM, SCOTCH BROOM. Lots of bright yellow flowers on these lacy-leafed subshrubs. Protect from snails near the coast. Allergy to broom is uncommon, except in areas where there is a great deal of it growing. All parts of these plants—seeds, leaves, flowers—are poisonous if eaten. Often becomes invasive and naturalizes in mild winter areas. Do not plant if there is wild land close by.

Allergy Index Scale: 1 is Best, 10 is Worst.

✪ for 1 and 2   🍂 for 9 and 10

No matter what the ranking, always read the full plant description carefully and take note of any warnings.

Daboecia. 2 ✪

HEATH, HEATHER. Small evergreen flowering shrub of the heather family, hardy in zones 6 to 10. Needs acid soil, good drainage, and ample water. Thrives in partial shade inland; full sun near the coast. Small, drooping pink-, white-, red-, or rose-colored egg-shaped flowers.

Dactylis. 10 🍂

ORCHARD GRASS. A common forage grass in the southern and eastern United States, orchard grass is one of the worst allergy grasses. If used, it should be pastured or cut early in the season as a hay crop to avoid flowering.

DAFFODIL. See *Narcissus.*

DAGGER PLANT. See *Yucca.*

DAHLBERG DAISY. See *Dyssodia tenuiloba.*

Dahlia. FORMAL DOUBLES 2 ✪, SINGLES 5

Perennial flowers from seed and tubers. Hardy to zone 7; dahlias must be lifted and overwintered indoors in colder areas. They thrive in full sun. Dahlias come in a wide variety of sizes and colors and are popular as cut flowers. Dahlias are related to ragweed and cross-allergic reactions occur. Full doubles do not shed much

pollen, although some single-flowered varieties produce pollen copiously. Some formal dahlias produce no pollen and are good allergy-free plants.

Dais cotinifolia. 3

POMPOM TREE. South African native shrub or small tree, grown in full sun in zones 9 and 10. Resembles crape myrtle, with clusters of puffy pink flowers.

DAISY. See *Anthemis; Bellis perennis; Bidens ferulifolia; Carlina; Coreopsis; Euryops; Heliopsis; Tripleurospermum; Venidium; Verbesina.*

DAISY TREE. See *Montanoa.*

DAISYBUSH. See *Olearia.*

DALEA SPINOSA GENUS

Dalea spinosa. 2 ✪

SMOKE TREE. A thorny native of the western deserts, zones 8 to 10, Dalea bears fragrant violet flowers. Summer deciduous, it drops its leaves in summer when the soil gets dry, then grows new leaves in autumn. Can be propagated from seed.

D. greggii. 2 ✪

A drought-tolerant, spreading perennial. Zones 9 to 10.

D. purpurea. 2 ✪

PURPLE PRAIRIE CLOVER. A fine wildflower for sunny areas. Zones 3 to 8.

DALLIS GRASS. See *Paspalum.*

DAME'S ROCKET. See *Hesperis matronalis*.

DAMMAR PINE. See *Agathis robusta*.

DANDELION. See *Taraxacum officinale*.

DANEWORT. See *Sambucus*.

Daphne odorata. **5**
SPURGE LAUREL, WINTER DAPHNE. Sweet-smelling, white-flowered small evergreen shrubs for shady areas with fast drainage, acid soil, and constant moisture. The sap and juice from the berries may cause dermatitis, and the fragrance may bother odor-sensitive individuals. Small fruits are highly poisonous if eaten.

Daphniphyllum. **MALES 8, FEMALES 1** ✪
Group of evergreen shrubs and trees native to Japan, Korea, and Australia, occasionally used in the United States. Hardy to zone 7, all cause allergy. Dioecious, but not sold sexed.

DARNEL. See *Lolium*.

Dasylirion. **MALES 8, FEMALES 1** ✪
SPOON FLOWER. Desert natives related to Agave, these are separate-sexed and the males can cause allergy.

DATE PALM. See *Phoenix dactylifera*.

Datisca cannabina. **9** ✎
A tall perennial herb that closely resembles *Cannabis sativa*, or marijuana.

Datura. **2** ✪
ANGEL TRUMPET, DEVIL WEED, JIMSON WEED, LOCOWEED, THORN APPLE. Perennial natives of dry areas. Big, white, trumpet-shaped flowers shed little pollen. Plants contain narcotic that produces dramatic, unpleasant reactions. (See also *Brugmansia*.)

Daucus. **10** ✎
CARROT, QUEEN ANNE'S LACE, WILD CARROT. A tall weed of waste areas, occasionally allowed to grow in the back of perennial borders; a common allergen.

Davidia involucrata. **5**
DOVE TREE. A medium-size, beautiful deciduous shade tree from China, hardy in zones 5 to 10.

DAVID'S MAPLE. See *Acer davidii*.

DAWN REDWOOD. See *Metasequoia glyptostroboides*.

DAYLILY. See *Hemerocallis*.

DEAD NETTLE. See *Lamium maculatum*.

DEADLY NIGHTSHADE. See *Solanum*.

DEATH CAMAS. See *Zigadenus*.

DEERHORN CEDAR. See *Thujopsis dolabrata*.

DEERWOOD. See *Ostrya*.

Delosperma. **3**
SUCCULENT ICEPLANT. Trailing, white-flowered perennial for zones 9 and 10.

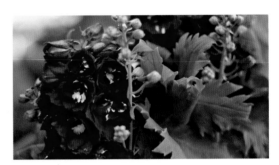

Delphinium. **3**
LARKSPUR. (Pictured above.) Tall flowering perennials, some hardy to zone 2. Many species and colors, especially blues, purples, and whites; some western native species have red flower spikes. They thrive in full sun, rich, acidic soil, and ample moisture. Delphinium leaves and seeds are very poisonous. The annual Delphinium is called larkspur, and it is also poisonous, occasionally fatal, especially if eaten by cattle, sheep, or horses.

Dendrobium. **2** ✪
A group of tropical orchids that are popular as greenhouse plants. They are grown under cool, dry, and lean conditions until flower buds form, then watered and fed. One plant may produce hundreds of flowers.

Dendromecon rigida. **3**
BUSH POPPY. West Coast native shrub with large yellow flowers. Does best in full sun; drought-tolerant.

Dentaria lacinita. **3**
TOOTHWORT. A hardy spring-blooming perennial with white-to-pink flowers for shady gardens with moist soils in zones 3 to 8. Plants will spread in right areas.

DEODAR CEDAR. See *Cedrus deodara*.

Derris. **5**
FLAME TREE, JEWEL VINE. A group of evergreen leguminous trees and vines; one source of the insecticide rotenone.

DESERT BROOM. See *Baccharis pilularis*.

DESERT CANDLE. See *Eremurus*.

DESERT HOLLY. See *Atriplex*.

DESERT HONEYSUCKLE. See *Anisacanthus*.

DESERT IRONWOOD. See *Olneya tesota*.

DESERT OLIVE. See *Forestiera*.

DESERT PALM. See *Washingtonia*.

DESERT WILLOW. See *Chilopsis linearis*.

Desmanthus. 6

A group of about twenty species of trees, shrubs, and herbs native to the Western Hemisphere and Madagascar, all of them suspect in allergy studies. One species, *D. illinoensis*, prickleweed or prairie mimosa, is a perennial with dense clusters of white flowers, native from Ohio to Florida and also in New Mexico. Occasionally used as a flowering perennial, it may naturalize.

Desmoncus. 7

A large group of tropical and subtropical palm trees, occasionally planted in Florida.

Deutzia. 3

Hardy deciduous flowering bushes with many small white, pink, or purple flowers.

DEVIL WEED. See *Datura*.

DEVIL'S BACKBONE. See *Pedilanthus tithymaloides*.

DEVIL'S IVY. See *Epipremnum aureum*.

DEVIL'S WOOD. See *Sambucus*.

Dianella tasmanica. 3

TASMANIA FLAX LILY. Dianella is a small perennial from Australia and Tasmania with long, strap-shaped leaves. Hardy in zones 9 to 10, it can be used as a houseplant in other areas. Easy to grow, drought-tolerant, blue flowers followed by small, edible blue fruits, plants are best grown in shade. There are variegated forms with extra-attractive foliage.

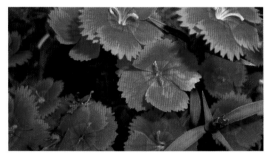

Dianthus. 1 ✪ TO 3 DEPENDING ON CULTIVAR

CARNATION, PINK, SWEET WILLIAM. (Pictured above.) Many hardy species of annual and perennial herbs and flowers, popular as garden and cut flowers. Low

pollen producers, but highly fragrant, Dianthus may affect people with odor sensitivities. Grown from seed or cuttings, Dianthus thrives in full sun with regular watering, especially during cool weather. Pinch off old flowers or cut plants back after bloom. A few cultivars of Dianthus and carnation are pollen-free female plants.

Diascia. 2 ✪

TWINSPUR. Annuals and perennials.

Dicentra. 4

BLEEDING HEART, DUTCHMAN'S BREECHES, GOLDEN EAR-DROPS, SQUIRREL CORN, STEER'S HEAD, TURKEY CORN. Hardy perennials for shady, moist spots. About twenty species in the genus, most are grown from corms or tubers. The unusual flowers, occasionally shaped like small red or pink hearts, produce little exposed pollen. Dicentra would be almost perfect allergy-free plants except that handling the leaves, flowers, or roots can cause skin rash in some people. All parts of Dicentra are poisonous if eaten.

Dichelostemma. 3

BLUE DICKS, FIRECRACKER LILY, SNAKE LILY, WILD HYACINTH. Several species of perennials native to the West Coast.

Dichondra. 2 ✪

Nine species of small, creeping, or prostrate perennials. *D. micrantha* is occasionally used as a good, allergy-free lawn substitute (for small areas) in warm winter areas, mostly Florida and California. It grows best in full sun, but will tolerate some shade. Dichondra can be planted from seed, plugs, or flats; it spreads by surface root runners. If heavily fertilized and watered, Dichondra can grow to 6 inches and require mowing. Soil is prepared as for planting a lawn, and seeded with 2 to 3 pounds of seed for every 1,000 square feet.

Dichorisandra. 4

BLUE GINGER. Perennial houseplants, related to wandering Jew. Small blue flowers.

Dicksonia. 5

TASMANIAN TREE FERN. Hardiest of the tree ferns, to about 20°F. May attain a height of 15 feet. Do not plant right next to doors or underneath windows.

Dictamnus albus. 6

FRAXINELLA, GAS PLANT. Hardy perennial for all zones. Volatile oils in the plant will ignite in the air if a match is held close to a flower on a warm, still night. With this in mind, odor-sensitive individuals might want to be careful with this plant. Contact with this plant can cause photodermatitis.

Dictyosperma. 6
PRINCESS PALM, YELLOW PALM. Two species of palms, occasionally grown in zone 10.

DIDISCUS. See *Trachymene coerulea*.

Dieffenbachia seguine. MALES 7, FEMALES 1 ☺
DUMB CANE. Large evergreen houseplants with big, often variegated leaves. Needs fairly good light and should not be overwatered. Dumb cane gets its name because tiny, needle-sharp crystals of calcium oxalate in the sap, if ingested, immediately irritate the tongue, mouth, and throat, causing pain and making speech difficult. The effect can last for up to twenty hours. The sap or juice can also cause skin rash. When grown as houseplants, these plants seldom bloom, but if they are males, the flowers have a good capacity for allergy. In a greenhouse they are more likely to flower and present allergy problems.

Diervilla lonicera. 4
Northern bush honeysuckle. Native to the eastern U.S., winter hardy into much of Canada. Easy-to-grow small subshrub.

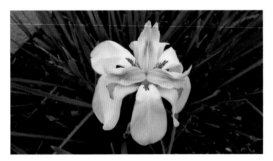

Dietes (Moraea). 2 ☺
FORTNIGHT LILY, MORAEA. (Pictured above.) Easy-to-grow, long-lived, clumping perennials with long, strap-shaped leaves and flat, bright white flowers. Popular and common in zones 9 and 10.

Digitalis. 2 ☺
FOXGLOVE. Tall, hardy, flowering perennials or bienni-als that produce spikes of bell-shaped flowers in pastel colors. Easy to grow in full sun or partial shade. An annual variety is available. When used as cut flowers, they may shed pollen; foxgloves are best kept in the garden. Source of the drug digitalis. All parts of this plant are highly poisonous.

Digitaria sanguinalis. 6
CRABGRASS. This weed grass blooms when still low and, although it does cause allergy, the plants do not produce much pollen.

DILL. See *Anethum*.

Dillenia. 3
Large seguine group of mostly Asian evergreen shrubs and trees, some grown in zone 10.

Dimorphotheca. 4
AFRICAN DAISY, CAPE MARIGOLD. Sun-loving, low-growing, spreading annuals for all zones.

Dioon. MALES 5, FEMALES 1 ☺
A cycad. The flowers of the male plants are taller and thinner than those on the female plants. Each plant only has one large flower cone at a time. Pollen from male plants can be avoided by removing the male cone before it matures and sheds pollen. All cycad pollen is poisonous.

Dioscorea. 2 ☺
SWEET POTATO.

DIOSMA. See *Coleonema*.

Diospyros. MALES 6, FEMALES 1 ☺
PERSIMMON. Many species of deciduous and evergreen trees in the ebony family. Two species of deciduous fruit trees are used in the United States. Beautiful landscape trees, *Diospyros* is Latin for "two fires," refer-ring to the bright fiery color of the ripe fruits and also to the unusually good scarlet–fiery orange fall color of the leaves. *D. virginiana*, the American persimmon, is a tall fruiting tree, native to the southeastern United States and hardy in zones 3 to 10. In zones 6 or 7, with good soil and regular water, this persimmon may reach 100 feet, although 50 feet is average.

D. kaki, the Japanese persimmon, is a shorter, rounder tree. The cultivar 'Fuyu' has orange fruits, flattened rather than round, that can be eaten any time after they turn orange. The fruits of the American persimmon must be dead ripe before eating; otherwise, they are inedible and astringent. 'Fuyu', a female tree, grows slowly but matures to a very handsome, spread-ing small tree with netted bark and excellent fall color. Ornamental in all seasons. Any persimmon tree that makes fruit is a female tree.

DIPLACUS. See *Mimulus*.

DIPLADENIA. See *Mandevilla*.

DIPLOPAPPUS. See *Felicia amelloides*.

Dirca palustris. 3
LEATHERWOOD, MOOSEWOOD. Eastern and western species of shrubs native to the U.S. and southern Canada, hardy to zone 5; best in deep soil with abundant moisture. A fine plant, but very slow-growing.

Disanthus. 2 ✪
Deciduous shrub from Japan, grown for its good fall color in zones 8 to 10.

Distichlis. MALES 9 🗲, FEMALES 1 ✪
SALTGRASS. Several species of low-growing, spreading grasses used to control erosion, especially in alkaline soils. Saltgrass is separate-sexed and can be grown asexually from rhizomes; hence, an all-female cultivar may be developed. Look for an OPALS #1 ranked female selection in the near future. Saltgrass grows in the wild in the hottest parts of Death Valley, and it also grows coast to coast all across the U.S. This grass has great potential because it can be selected as a pollen-free female, and because it is so tough and adaptable.

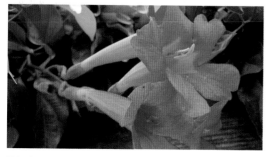

Distictis. 5
TRUMPET VINE. (Pictured above.) Evergreen vines for zones 8 to 10. Several related species, all producing large flowers on fast-growing vines. All species may cause contact skin allergies, so use caution when pruning.

Dizygotheca (Schefflera elegantissima). 4
FALSE ARALIA. Houseplant or zone 10 outdoors in shade.

DOCK, DOCK SORREL. See *Rumex*.

Dodecatheon. 1 ✪
SHOOTING STAR. Hardy perennials for all zones. Resembles Cyclamen.

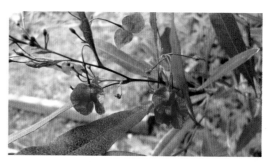

Dodonaea viscosa. MONOECIOUS 7, MALES 9 🗲, FEMALES 1 ✪
HOP BUSH, PURPLE HOPSEED. (*Dodonaea viscosa*, female, pictured above.) Australian native evergreen shrub or small tree for zones 8 to 10. This is a very useful, fast-growing, drought-tolerant hedge plant, but only female plants should be used. I recently saw close to a hundred of them for sale at a large home improvement store, and all were clonal male plants. Male plants do not make any of the attractive, hoplike seedpods. See the hedges section in chapter 4 for more suggestions on female hopseed plants. *D. microzyga*, brilliant hopbush, zones 9 to 10, is an evergreen shrub 4 feet tall and as wide. Female plants are pollen-free and very attractive; males are allergenic. Look for OPALS-tagged female plants.

DOG FENNEL. See *Anthemis*.

DOG TOOTH VIOLET. See *Erythronium*.

DOGBANE. See *Apocynum*.

DOGWOOD. See *Cornus*.

Dolichos. 4
HYACINTH BEAN. Fast-growing flowering pea vines, easy to grow from seed. Perennial in mild areas.

Dombeya. 3
PINK BALL DOMBEYA. Tender, winter-blooming evergreen shrubs, with large leaves and round clusters of pink or red flowers. Dombeya needs sun, warmth, and ample water to thrive.

DONKEY TAIL. See *Sedum*.

Doronicum. 8
LEOPARD'S BANE. Hardy perennials with yellow daisy flowers borne on erect stems.

Dorotheanthus bellidiformis. 3
LIVINGSTONE DAISY. Profusely flowering, low and spreading annual iceplant for all zones.

Doryanthes palmeri. 2 ✪
SPEAR LILY. Giant succulent resembling Agave. Flower spike may reach 10 feet.

DOUB PALM. See *Borassus*.

DOUBLE COCONUT PALM. See *Lodoicea*.

DOUGLAS FIR. See *Pseudotsuga*.

DOUM PALM. See *Hyphaene*.

DOVE TREE. See *Davidia involucrata*.

Dovyalis hebecarpa. MALES 6, FEMALES 1 ✪
CEYLON GOOSEBERRY, KEI APPLE, UMKOKOLO. Small group of subtropical spiny evergreen fruit trees, occasionally grown in zone 10. Trees are usually separate-sexed; male trees may cause allergy, females do not, and a few bisexual trees are less likely to produce severe allergy. The trees produce enormous yields of fruit the size of large marbles, with apricot-colored flesh and very sweet, intensely red juice, which is used for jelly and beverages.

DOXANTHA. See *Macfadyena unguis-cati*.

Dracaena. 4 TO 6 DEPENDING ON SPECIES
CORDYLINE, CORN PLANT, DRAGON TREE. Outside in zone 10; houseplants elsewhere. Palmlike trees and strap-leafed, erect houseplants. The large dragon tree, *D. draco*, is the most allergenic of the numerous species; avoid direct contact with the flowers.

DRAGON TREE. See *Cordyline*; *Dracaena*.

DRAGONHEAD, FALSE. See *Physostegia virginiana*.

Drimys winteri. 5
PEPPER TREE, WINTER'S BARK. Small evergreen trees for zones 8 to 10. Winter's bark has fragrant leaves and clusters of jasmine-scented small white flowers. It thrives in sunny coastal areas, or in partial shade elsewhere.

Drosanthemum. 3
ICEPLANT. Perennial for zones 9 and 10. Drought-tolerant, it grows best in coastal regions.

Dryas. 2 ✪
Hardy, white- or yellow-flowered perennial used in sunny rock gardens or as a ground cover.

Drymophloeus. 7
A group of small palms, some grown in Florida.

Dryopteris. 4
WOOD FERN. Hardy in most regions.

Duchesnea indica. 1 ✪
INDIAN MOCK STRAWBERRY. Ground cover for small areas, Duchesnea bears yellow flowers and fruits that resemble strawberries but are bland and tasteless. Attractive to birds.

Dudleya. 1 ✪
LIVE FOREVER. Small perennial succulent for full sun and dry conditions in zones 9 and 10.

DUMB CANE. See *Dieffenbachia seguine*.

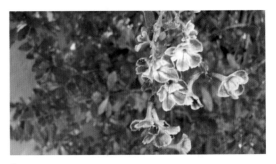

Duranta. 3
PIGEON BERRY, SKY FLOWER. (Pictured above.) Spiny, blue-flowered evergreen shrubs for zones 9 and 10. Small tubular violet flowers are followed by long, trailing clusters of small yellow fruit. Fruit is poisonous.

DUSTY MILLER. See *Artemisia*; *Centaurea*; *Chrysanthemum*; *Senecio*.

DUTCHMAN'S BREECHES. See *Dicentra*.

DUTCHMAN'S PIPE VINE. See *Aristolochia*.

DWARF PALM. See *Sabal*.

Dypsis decaryi. 6
TRIANGLE PALM. Zone 10 palm with interesting trunk.

Dyssodia tenuiloba (Thymophylla). 4
DAHLBERG DAISY, GOLDEN FLEECE. Annual native of the Southwest, with yellow flowers and small needlelike leaves. It thrives in sandy soil and full sun.

Allergy Index Scale: 1 is Best, 10 is Worst.
✪ for 1 and 2 ❧ for 9 and 10
No matter what the ranking, always read the full plant description carefully and take note of any warnings.

EARTH-STAR. See *Cryptanthus.*

EASTER LILY CACTUS. See *Echinopsis.*

EASTER LILY VINE. See *Beaumontia grandiflora.*

Ebenopsis ebano. 5
TEXAS EBONY TREE. Southern Texas native tree or shrub. Thorny, evergreen, and very drought-tolerant. Zones 7 to 11.

Echeveria. 1 ✪
HENS-AND-CHICKS. Easy-to-grow, drought-tolerant succulent for zones 8 to 10. Good in pots.

Echinacea purpurea. 5
PURPLE CONEFLOWER. Hardy perennials for all zones. Grows bigger in cold winter areas and has naturalized in the Midwest. It is a popular medicinal plant.

Echinocactus. 1 ✪
BARREL CACTUS. Big, round, slow-growing cactus for desert areas in zones 9 to 10.

Echinops exaltatus. 5
GLOBE THISTLE. Tall perennial for all zones; used for dry flowers.

Echinopsis. 2 ✪
EASTER LILY CACTUS. Small cactus to 10 inches. White or red flowers rise above plants.

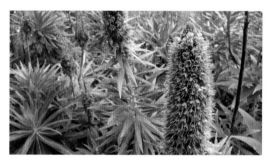

Echium fastuosum. 5
PRIDE OF MADEIRA. (Pictured above.) Big, shrubby perennials for zones 9 to 10. Large spikes of purple or blue flowers are impressive and attractive to bees. The large gray leaves are covered with tiny prickles that may cause contact skin rash, common in those working around these plants.

EDELWEISS. See *Leontopodium alpinum.*

EDRAIANTHUS GRAMINIFOLIUS. See *Campanula.*

EEL GRASS. See *Vallisneria.*

EGGPLANT. See *Solanum.*

EGLANTINE. See *Rosa.*

Ehretia anacua. 5
A small flowering Texas native tree, hardy only in zone 10.

Eichhornia crassipes. 2 ✪
WATER HYACINTH. Pond plant with lilac blooms and floating leaves. Needs warmth to grow well.

ELAEAGNUS GENUS

Elaeagnus. INDIVIDUALLY RANKED
Group of hardy, deciduous and evergreen shrubs or small trees. Variegated species of Elaeagnus, with green leaves marked with yellow or white, are sold as *E. marginata* or *E. variegata* and all can cause allergies.

E. angustifolia. 9 ◗
RUSSIAN OLIVE. Medium-size deciduous tree commonly planted in the Midwest as a windbreak. Not a true olive. Small yellow flowers in early summer are the cause of much local allergy in some areas.

E. commutata. 6
SILVERBERRY, WOLFBERRY. Deciduous shrub, hardy in all zones. Birds relish the small fruits.

E. ebbingei. 6
Thornless evergreen shrub bearing edible red berries.

E. pungens. 7
EVERGREEN SILVERBERRY. A large, hardy, thorny shrub often used as hedge plant.

Elaeis. 7
Tropical palms.

ELDERBERRY. See *Sambucus*.

ELEPHANT TREE. See *Bursera*.

ELEPHANT'S EAR. See *Alocasia*; *Colocasia*.

ELEPHANT'S EAR TREE. See *Enterolobium cyclocarpum*.

ELEPHANT'S FOOD. See *Portulacaria afra*.

ELM. See *Ulmus*.

ELM, WATER. See *Planera aquatica*.

Elymus canadensis. 5
WILD RYE. A forage grass widely used across the United States. This useful grass is neither highly allergenic nor a high pollen producer.

Emblica officinalis (Phyllanthus emblica).
MONOECIOUS 5, MALES 9 ◗, FEMALES 1 ✪
INDIAN GOOSEBERRY. An important medicinal plant in Ayurveda natural medicine; semitropical, medium-size deciduous tree, hardy in zones 9 to 10. Fruits have many medicinal properties.

EMERALD LEAF. See *Peperomia*.

Empetrum. 2 ✪
ROCKBERRY.

EMPRESS TREE. See *Paulownia tomentosa*.

Encelia farinosa. 4
BRITTLEBUSH, INCIENSO. Native to southwestern deserts of the U.S. and Mexico, perennial, full sun, very drought-tolerant, many yellow flowers that are pollinated by bees, butterflies, wasps, and beetles. Zones 8 to 10.

Endymion. 2 ✪
ENGLISH OR SPANISH BLUEBELLS, SCILLA. Hardy bulbs for sun or partial shade. Plant bulbs deeper in colder climates. Many colors, but blue is most common.

ENGLISH DAISY. See *Bellis perennis*.

ENGLISH IVY. See *Hedera helix*.

ENGLISH PEA. See *Pisum sativum*.

ENGLISH WALNUT. See *Juglans*.

Enkianthus. 3
Deciduous shrubs hardy to zone 4. Attractive upright trunk with spreading horizontal branches bearing small bell-shaped white or red flowers in spring.

Ensete. 2 ✪
ABYSSINIAN BANANA. A native of Ethiopia, where the flowers and seeds are eaten, these large palmlike perennials for zones 9 to 10 have enormous leaves up to 20 feet long. Plants die after flowering.

Entelea arborescens. 6
An evergreen shrub or small tree from New Zealand, used in zones 9 to 10. Relative of the lindens.

Enterolobium cyclocarpum. 6
ELEPHANT'S EAR TREE. Large-leafed ornamental for the tropics and the warmest parts of zone 10.

EPAULETTE TREE. See *Pterostyrax*.

Ephedra. MALES 7, FEMALES 1 ✪
JOINT FIR, MORMON TEA. Planted in dry locations as ground cover for its green stems. Source of drug ephedra. All female Ephedra plants will form some kind of small fruits. In the U.S. the fruits are usually white or almost clear; those I saw recently in Israel were a bright red. Female plants will make large numbers of these fruits, making them fairly easy to identify. Males shed

considerable pollen and are allergenic. Once established, all species of Ephedra are very tough, drought-resistant, and long-lived. Native Ephedra in the U.S. seldom get more than 4 feet tall, but in some countries plants get to 10 feet tall and almost as wide.

EPIDENDRUM. See *Orchid*.

Epigaea repens. 3
TRAILING ARBUTUS. Very hardy, low-growing, pink-flowered subshrub or ground cover for shady areas. Needs well-drained, peaty, acid soil and constant moisture to grow well.

Epilobium. 6
FIREWEED. A tall red or pink flowering annual, known to cause occasional allergy. (See also *Zauschneria*.)

Epimedium. 1 ✪
BISHOP'S HAT. Low-growing perennial for shady, moist, acid-soil areas to zone 7. Good under trees or below camellias and azaleas. Tiny white or rose-colored blooms resemble larkspur.

Epipactis gigantea. 2 ✪
STREAM ORCHID. Hardy terrestrial orchid native to the western United States. Purple, bird-shaped flowers are borne on 10-inch stalks. It needs moist soil in partial shade to thrive.

Epiphyllum. 2 ✪
ORCHID CACTUS. Shade-house cactus for zones 8 to 10 or houseplant elsewhere. These are jungle, not desert, cactus, and their culture reflects this. Spring-blooming with large showy flowers in many colors.

Epipremnum aureum (Rhapidophora). 2 ✪
DEVIL'S IVY, POTHOS. Formerly called *Pothos aureus* or *Scindapsus aureus*. Easy-to-grow houseplants, propagated from cuttings. The sap of these plants may cause skin rash in nursery workers making many cuttings. Pothos is one of the better plants at cleaning up indoor air pollution; however, the broad leaves collect dust and may harbor dust mites. Give plants an occasional lukewarm rinse in a shower.

Episcia. 2 ✪
CARPET PLANT, FLAME VIOLET, LOVEJOY. Houseplants for hanging baskets; easy to grow in good light and with ample water. Small flowers resemble African violets. They spread by runners.

Equisetum hyemale. 5
HORSETAIL RUSH. Spore-bearing fern relative for garden wet spots. Hardy in all zones.

Eranthemum pulchellum. 2 ✪
Evergreen shrub for shady, moist areas of zone 10 or greenhouse plant elsewhere. Tubular blue flowers in late winter to early spring.

Eranthis hyemalis. 3
BUTTERCUPS, WINTER ACONITE. Early spring-blooming tuberous perennials, hardy in all zones. Thrives in partial shade and moist soil. Plant tubers deeper in coldest climates. All parts are very poisonous if eaten.

Eremocarpus setigerus. 6
TURKEY MULLEIN. Not a true mullein (*Verbascum*). Turkey mullein is a common low-growing, very strongly scented California native, rarely used in landscapes. The smell of the crushed leaves affects some. The sap is poisonous and may cause rash.

Eremochloa. 7
CENTIPEDE GRASS. A lawn grass for southern areas, often escaped to vacant lots, where it grows rampantly and produces copious amounts of pollen.

Eremophila. 4
FUCHSIA BUSH, POVERTY BUSH. Drought-tolerant subshrubs for zones 9 to 10, native to Australia.

Eremurus. 5
DESERT CANDLE, FOXTAIL LILY. Hardy perennial with tall spires of flowers to 6 feet.

Erica. 4
HEATH, HEATHER. A very large group of evergreen shrubs or small trees, with small, needlelike leaves, mostly from Europe and South Africa. No species of Erica are hardy below 28°F. Used as greenhouse flowering plants in all zones. Needs good light, acid soil, fast drainage, and good soil moisture to grow well. Heather blooms profusely with many small, often fragrant, flowers in many colors. Poisonous.

Erigeron. 4
BEACH ASTER, FLEABANE. Low-growing perennials for full sun in zones 5 to 10. Small daisylike flowers on spreading, occasionally invasive plants. Easy to grow.

Erinus alpinus. 3
ALPINE BALSAM. Low-growing, spreading, small perennial for zones 3 to 7, best in shade or semi-shade. A rock garden plant with attractive white or pink flowers. Short-lived but may reseed itself.

Eriobotrya. 3
LOQUAT. Tall (to about 30 feet) evergreen trees for zones 7 to 10. Big, handsome leaves and small,

yellow, slightly fragrant flowers followed by round, sweet yellow fruits with large brown shiny seeds. These trees are easy, but slow, to grow from seed; budded varieties produce larger fruit, but are hard to find. *E. deflexa* is a bronze-leafed ornamental tree. Leaves and seeds are mildly poisonous.

Eriogonum. BISEXUAL 5, MALES 7, FEMALES 1 ✿
WILD BUCKWHEAT. Annuals and perennials native to the West. Very drought-tolerant; full sun.

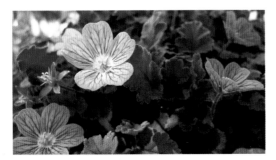

Erodium chamaedryoides. 2 ✿
CRANESBILL. (Pictured above.) Low-growing evergreen perennials hardy in zones 8 to 10. Small pink or white flowers for full sun or partial shade. Member of the Geranium family.

Eryngium. 4
SEA HOLLY. Hardy perennial for all zones. Erect plants resemble flowering thistle.

Erysimum. 3
BLISTER CRESS. Hardy, drought-tolerant perennials with orange or yellow flowers, which thrive in full sun. Related to wallflowers.

ERYTHEA. See *Brahea*.

Erythrina. 5 TO 6 DEPENDING ON SPECIES
CORAL TREE. Evergreen or deciduous flowering trees for zones 9 to 10. The cockspur coral tree, *E. crista-galli*, is the hardiest of the group. Some species are thorny. All have large leaves and heavy blooms of bright coral-red or orange flowers followed by long beanlike seedpods. *E. herbacea* is a U.S. native shrub that attracts birds and supplies food for native butterflies. Pollen from all Erythrina species is considered mildly allergenic. Seeds, flowers, and leaves of most species are poisonous.

Erythronium. 2 ✿
DOG TOOTH VIOLET, FAWN LILY. Perennial corms native to the West. Plant in moist, shady areas.

Erythroxylum coca. 4
COCA PLANT. Evergreen shrubs or small trees from tropical America. Plant from which the drug cocaine is derived. The plants, which make attractive small red fruits, are not the source of any known allergy, but they are illegal in most countries around the world.

Escallonia. 3
RED ESCALLONIA. Dense, evergreen shrubs much used for landscaping in zones 8 to 10. They grow largest and flower best near the coast. Small white flowers (when present) and shiny leaves; fairly good foundation shrubs. Certain cultivars have flowers that are much redder than the norm, but they seem difficult to find. Attracts bees.

Eschscholzia californica. 3
CALIFORNIA POPPY. Perennial often grown as annual for full sun, in all zones. Fast from seed. Bright orange to yellow flowers. State flower of California.

Esenbeckia runyonii. 3
Small tree native to Mexico, used as a shade tree or for hedges. Attractive leaves and flowers, drought-tolerant and very easy to start from cuttings. Zone 10.

Espostoa lanata. 1 ✿
OLD MAN CACTUS. Erect cactus to 9 feet with small hairlike spines and tubular pink flowers.

Eucalyptus. 2 ✿ TO 8 DEPENDING ON SPECIES
GUM TREE, IRONBARK, MALLEE, MARLOCK, SALLY, YATE. A very large group of evergreen shrubs and trees native to Australia and widely planted throughout mild areas of the world. Almost all Eucalyptus cause some allergy, but some species cause far more problems than others. The odor of fresh or dried Eucalyptus leaves and flowers is offensive to some individuals and may cause an allergic odor response.

There are more than 500 species of Eucalyptus in Australia, and well over 100 species are grown in the United States. Very overplanted in California, Arizona, and Florida; most Eucalyptus shed profuse amounts of pollen. Eucalyptus flowers are pollinated by insects but imperfectly so, and each flower has an unusually high number of pollen-producing stamens. Most species will only be hardy in zones 9 to 13, but a few will live in zone 8.

Several species, such as the fuchsia gum, the square-fruited mallee, and the coral gum, pose a constant problem because they flower throughout the year. In areas directly below large blue gum trees, the fall of pollen goes on for months and covers everything with a persistent dust. Some of the Eucalyptus, such as *E. ficifolia*, the red-flowered gum, have sticky pollen mixed with nectar, and these do not cause nearly as much allergy. (Some claim that they have gained a measure of allergy protection by eating Eucalyptus honey, and this does make considerable sense.) Eucalyptus pollen is large, triangular in shape, and usually sheds in clumps. Crawling around on these clumps of pollen, I have often observed many tiny insects, probably some form of thrip. These insects and their dander are allergenic. In Australia there appear to be a few cultivars with bright red flowers that are rich in nectar but lack any pollen. In the U.S. the safest species would be *E. ficifolia*.

Eucomis. 3
PINEAPPLE FLOWER. Bulb for zones 7 to 10. A lily family member that produces a central flower that resembles a pineapple, Eucomis is easily grown from seed.

Eucommia ulmoides. MALES 8, FEMALES 1 ⊕
CHINESE RUKKIS TREE, CHINESE THREAD TREE, GUTTA PERCHA TREE, HARDY RUBBER TREE, STONE COTTON TREE. Large deciduous trees from China, hardy in zones 5 to 12. Leaves resemble elm. Sap is a rubber-forming latex that might cause contact allergies. Separate-sexed trees, they are not usually sold sexed. The females are a good choice for the allergy-free garden. Usually flowering in mid-spring, the winged seeds resemble those of the ash. The bark of the Eucommia tree is purported to be a natural androgenic substance, and some weight-lifters drink tea made from this bark. Most bark sold comes from China.

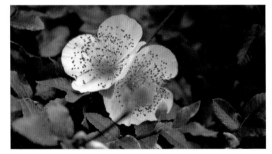

Eucryphia. 4
(Pictured above.) Evergreen shrub or tree for zones 7 to 10. Not commonly used, the shiny-leafed, white-flowered Eucryphia thrive in full sun to partial shade and moist, acidic soil.

Eugenia (Pitanga). 5
SURINAM CHERRY. Very common landscape evergreen shrub, tree, or hedge plant in zones 9 to 11. Small edible fruit ripens from yellow to orange to dark red. In many areas of California, where Eugenia trees and hedges are quite common, all of them are now infected with some sort of leaf thrip, and this makes the plants a source of insect dander. (See also *Syzygium paniculatum*.)

Euonymus. 1 ⊕ TO 7 DEPENDING ON SPECIES AND SOMETIMES SEX
SPINDLE TREE, WINTER CREEPER. Large group of deciduous and evergreen shrubs and vines. Deciduous Euonymus is hardy to zone 3. Although all members of this species have a potential for allergy, as a group they pose little threat if sheared hard annually to prevent flowering. *E. alata*, the burning bush or winged euonymus, is one of the hardiest deciduous varieties, prized for its intense red autumn color, although in some areas it has become an invasive plant.

E. fortunei is the hardiest of the evergreen Euonymus and is occasionally used as a ground cover. *E. japonica*, the Japanese evergreen Euonymus, has many variegated forms, some of which never bloom. Some of the native Euonymus species in Europe are dioecious, and only female plants will make the small fruits. All-male plants would be allergenic. All parts of the plant are poisonous if eaten.

Eupatorium. 6
BLUE BONESET, BONESET, JOE-PYE WEED, MIST FLOWER. Upright flowering perennials for sun or partial shade, hardy in all zones. The tubular flowers are pink, purple, rose, or white. One species, *E. rugosum*, called white snakeroot, grows wild in much of the southeastern United States and causes an illness called "the trembles" in milk cows. The toxicity of the leaves passes into the milk and, when consumed by humans, causes "milk sickness," which is characterized by vomiting, delirium, and death. Milk sickness was the cause of death of Abraham Lincoln's mother when he was seven years old. It was not until 1928 that the relationship between snakeroot and milk sickness was understood.

Euphorbia. VARIES BY SPECIES, ALL WITH POTENTIAL FOR ALLERGY
BASEBALL PLANT, CROWN-OF-THORNS, GOPHER PLANT, MILK BARREL, MILKBUSH, MEXICAN FIRE PLANT, MOLE PLANT, PENCIL TREE, POINSETTIA, SNOW-ON-THE-MOUNTAIN, SPURGE. Very large group of evergreen shrubs, perennials, biennials,

vines,succulents, and annuals. With well over 1,000 different species, Euphorbia is a complex genus, all members of which have potential for allergy. The milky sap or latex from many is often poisonous and usually has potential to cause skin rash. The white sap of the annual ground cover, snow-on-the-mountain (*E. marginata*), can cause severe skin burns even on people who are not allergic. This same highly caustic sap was once used to brand cattle.

Some of the succulent, leafless Euphorbias release a potent gas (VOCs) when cut that may be carcinogenic. Take care when making cuttings; a worker at the University of California, Davis, became violently ill and passed out while making Euphorbia cuttings in a small enclosed greenhouse.

Pollen from various Euphorbias is suspect because none has complete flowers, and all may bear separate male (pollen-producing) flowers. Many Euphorbias are "short day" plants and only bloom in the autumn when the days are short.

The most famous and popular of all Euphorbias is the poinsettia. Native to Mexico, poinsettias may reach 10 feet when planted outdoors. The red "flowers," which often appear around the Christmas holiday season, are composed not of petals but of colored leaflike structures called bracts. The actual flowers are inconspicuous yellow structures near the center of the rosette of bracts. These flowers are unisexual and shed pollen, especially at midday, although it is not normally airborne. Given their many noxious relatives, it would not be wise to inhale this pollen. Those with an allergy to rubber would be advised not to get the white latex milky sap of poinsettia on their skin.

It would be wise to consider all species of Euphorbia as poisonous. There are a great many very scary stories about contact with the sap of the common garden plant, *E. cooperi*. The very common pencil tree has caused blindness, permanent scarring, and death.

The males of the many Euphorbias that are completely separate-sexed plants can be counted on to contribute to possible dangerous inhalant allergy. (See also *Hevea brasiliensis*.)

EUROPEAN CRANBERRY BUSH. See *Viburnum opulus*.

EUROPEAN MOUNTAIN ASH. See *Sorbus*.

EUROPEAN SPINDLE TREE. See *Euonymus*.

EUROPEAN WHITE HELLEBORE. See *Veratrum*.

Eurya emarginata. MALES 8, FEMALES 3
Ferny-leafed evergreen shrub from Japan, hardy to zone 6, in partial shade and moist, acid soil. These are separate-sexed plants; males produce a malodorous scent that may cause allergy. Not sold unsexed, so best to avoid use.

Euryops. 4
GREENLEAF DAISY. Shrubby evergreen perennials, very common in zones 9 and 10. Fast growing and easy to maintain, Euryops produces its yellow flowers almost year-round.

Eustoma grandiflorum. 3
GENTIAN, LISIANTHUS, TEXAS BLUEBELL. Short-lived perennial for sunny areas in all zones. The colorful blooms make long-lasting cut flowers.

Euterpe. 7
A group of tropical and subtropical palm trees.

EVENING LYCHNIS. See *Silene*.

EVENING PRIMROSE. See *Oenothera*.

EVENING STAR. See *Mentzelia*.

EVERGLADES PALM. See *Acoelorrhaphe wrightii*.

EVERGREEN GRAPE. See *Rhoicissus capensis*.

EVERGREEN MAPLE. See *Acer oblongum*.

EVERGREEN PEAR. See *Pyrus*.

EVERGREEN SILVERBERRY. See *Elaeagnus pungens*.

EVERLASTING. See *Helichrysum*.

Evodia tretradium. 5
BEE BEE TREE. Native to China, zones 4 to 8, best in moist, acid soils. Large deciduous trees with ashlike leaves and small white flowers. Citrus relatives.

Exacum. 2 ✪
GERMAN VIOLET, PERSIAN VIOLET. Houseplants requiring good light and warmth. Plants are sensitive to touch and don't do well if handled often.

Exbucklandia. 6
Evergreen trees from the Himalayas, related to *Liquidambar*.

Exochorda. 3
PEARLBUSH. Deciduous shrubs, native to China and hardy to zone 5. Pearl-like buds open to white flowers. Thrives in full sun.

F

Allergy Index Scale: 1 is Best, 10 is Worst.
✪ for 1 and 2   ◐ for 9 and 10
No matter what the ranking, always read the full plant description carefully and take note of any warnings.

Fabaceae.

PEA FAMILY. A huge group of plants with over 20,000 species. All are legumes with flowers that have wings and a keel. Some are important food crops and others are very poisonous. Most species are not highly allergenic, but there are numerous exceptions to this. Allergy-ranked by genus-species.

Fagus. 6

BEECH. Large, hardy, deciduous trees; several species are native to the eastern United States. Fast growing with attractive foliage, some varieties have purple or bronze leaves. The trees produce small edible nuts. Beech trees are related to oaks, and like the oaks, they cause allergies, although beech pollen is rarely as potent an allergen as oak. Leaves and bark are poisonous but the beechnuts are eaten.

FAIRY LILY. See *Zephyranthes.*

FALSE ACACIA. See *Robinia.*

FALSE ARALIA. See *Dizygotheca.*

FALSE ARBORVITAE. See *Thujopsis dolabrata.*

FALSE BIRD-OF-PARADISE. See *Heliconia.*

FALSE BUCKEYE. See *Ungnadia.*

FALSE CYPRESS. See *Chamaecyparis.*

FALSE HELLEBORE. See *Veratrum.*

FALSE SAFFRON. See *Carthamus tinctorius.*

FALSE SNAPDRAGON. See *Chaenorrhinum.*

FALSE SOLOMON'S SEAL. See *Smilacina.*

FALSE SPIRAEA. See *Sorbaria sorbifolia.*

FALSE SYCAMORE. See *Melia.*

FAN PALM. See *Washingtonia.*

FAREWELL-TO-SPRING. See *Clarkia.*

FARFUGIUM. See *Ligularia.*

Fatshedera lizei. 2 ✪

FATSHEDERA. Evergreen subshrub, vine, or ground cover, hardy in zones 9 to 10. A naturally occurring hybrid between *Fatsia japonica* and *Hedera helix*. All Fatshedera are mules, or sterile hybrids, that bear flowers and produce some limited nonviable pollen but set no viable seeds. The plants are propagated by cuttings.

Fatsia japonica. 4

JAPANESE ARALIA. Evergreen subshrubs for zones 7 to 10, in partial shade.

FAWN LILY. See *Erythronium.*

FEATHER BUSH. See *Lysiloma thornberi.*

FEATHER-DUSTER PALM. See *Rhopalostylis.*

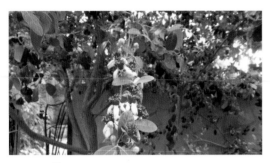

Feijoa sellowiana. 3

PINEAPPLE GUAVA. (Pictured above.) Attractive evergreen shrub or small (to 18 feet), multi-trunked tree native to Brazil. Hardy to 15°F, in full sun or partial shade. Flowers are large, red and white, and followed by egg-size, oblong green fruit. Reputed to have very high vitamin C content, Feijoa fruit has a pleasantly sweet citrus taste. The trees drop a large quantity of fruit, so placement near sidewalks should be avoided.

Most Feijoa are seedling grown, and the fruit may vary greatly in size and quantity; grafted varieties are available but are difficult to find. In California, Feijoa are often pollinated by mockingbirds or orioles, which pull off the sweet, edible white petals and, in doing so, distribute the sticky pollen. Irrigation will increase the size of the fruit.

Felicia amelloides (Diplopappus). 3

BLUE MARGUERITE. Small evergreen perennial for zones 7 to 10 that grows best in full sun with average care. Covered with small, blue daisylike flowers with yellow centers.

FELT FERN, JAPANESE. See *Pyrrosia lingua*.

FEMALE LINDEN. See *Tilia*.

FENNEL. See *Foeniculum*.

FENUGREEK. See *Trigonella*.

Fern. 3 TO 6 DEPENDING ON SPECIES AND SIZE

A very large group of spore-bearing plants. Most grow best in moist, shady situations, and they vary greatly by species in ability to withstand cold and frost. All ferns produce airborne spores on the undersides of the leaves, which can cause allergy. People who are already allergic to molds (or more precisely, to the spores of molds) may well find themselves allergic to ferns. Club moss (Lycopodium) is a related species that also bears spores; allergy to club moss spores is common and often severe, and cross-allergic reactions between ferns and club moss is common.

In the garden, and if not overused, most small ferns do not present a great allergy problem. Hanging ferns and large tree ferns, however, may drop spores on tables, chairs, pets, and people below them and should be used with care. Tree ferns should not be planted right next to bedroom windows or doorways. Tree ferns also shed tiny plant hairs that can trigger rash.

FERN PINE. See *Podocarpus*.

Ferocactus. 1 ✪

BARREL CACTUS. Native to deserts from Texas to New Mexico, Arizona, and Mexico and hardy to 0°F. It thrives with full sun and little water.

FESTUCA GENUS

Festuca. INDIVIDUALLY RANKED

FESCUE. Many species of fescue are used for pasture, ornamental, or lawn grass.

F. elatior. 3

TALL FESCUE. A common sod grass for lawns. It is a good choice because it does not flower if mowed regularly. *F. rubra*, red fescue, is also a good choice for the well-kept lawn.

F. glauca. 6

BLUE FESCUE. An ornamental variety that blooms for an extended period and produces abundant pollen. If one wishes to have a few blue fescue plants, it is easy enough to cut off the flower stalks before any pollen is shed.

FETTERBUSH. See *Pieris*; *Leucothoe*.

FEVERFEW. See *Chrysanthemum*.

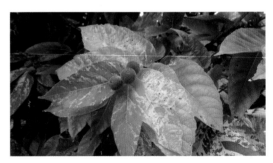

Ficus. 2 ✪ TO 3

FIG. (*Ficus aspera*, pictured above.) Evergreen or deciduous vines, shrubs, houseplants, or trees, hardy to zone 6. Although related to mulberry, a known allergen producer, most Ficus are relatively benign. All Ficus are capable of provoking skin rash from their milky sap.

F. benjamina is a common indoor tree that normally never flowers and so presents few problems. A few people report contact rash from F. benjamina. The edible fig, F. carica, has its flowers inside the fruits and presents little problem, except that the fuzzy, slightly hairy leaves of edible fig can cause a contact rash in people with sensitive skin. The milky sap from fresh domestic figs also can cause contact skin rash.

The huge evergreen tree, the Morton Bay fig, with great spreading heavy branches and large, leathery leaves, also makes tiny figs, and does not pose an allergy problem. A Morton Bay fig, one of the largest fig trees in the United States, grows beside the freeway on the west side of U.S. 101 in the heart of Santa Barbara, California, near the train station. Local lore has it that a sailor gave the seedling to a Santa Barbara girl and she planted it in 1876.

F. microcarpa, the Indian laurel fig, is a common street tree in California and Florida. It presents a low allergy risk, but its roots are famous for breaking up sidewalks. The rubber plant, F. elastica decora, also makes tiny figs and as a houseplant almost never blooms. The same can be said for the huge-leafed F. lyrata, the fiddleleaf fig.

Although once used for rubber production, F. elastica, the common rubber tree, is no longer commercially grown. Rubber is commercially produced from Hevea brasiliensis, a Euphorbia relative. Ficus trees are not recommended as houseplants because all Ficus are heavy VOC producers, and they will not improve the indoor air quality.

F. religiosa. 3
THE BODHI TREE, BO-TREE, TREE OF BUDDHA. Native to India, not hardy, houseplant.

FIDDLEWOOD. See Citharexylum fruticosum.

FILBERT. See Corylus.

Filipendula. 4
MEADOWSWEET. Hardy perennial herbs and flowers, some native to the United States.

FINGER GRASS. See Chloris.

FINOCCHIO. See Foeniculum.

FIR. See Abies.

FIRE LILY. See Cyrtanthus mackenii.

FIREBUSH. See Streptosolen jamesonii.

FIRECRACKER LILY. See Dichelostemma.

FIRETHORN. See Pyracantha.

FIREWEED. See Epilobium; Zauschneria.

FIREWHEEL TREE. See Stenocarpus sinuatus.

Firmiana simplex. 7
CHINESE BOTTLE TREE, CHINESE PARASOL TREE, JAPANESE VARNISH TREE, PHOENIX TREE. Small evergreen or deciduous tree native to Japan and China, for zones 8 to 12. Large three-lobed tropical-looking leaves and greenish white flower clusters. This species has become highly invasive in many areas of the U.S.

FISH POISON PEA. See Tephrosia.

FISHTAIL PALM. See Caryota.

Fittonia. 1 ✪
NERVE PLANT. Houseplant for warm, moist conditions and filtered light.

FIVE-FINGERS. See Neopanax.

FIVE-LEAF AKEBIA. See Akebia quinata.

Flacourtia. 7
MADAGASCAR PLUM, RAMONTCHI. Frost-tender small evergreen trees grown in mildest parts of zone 10; best in zones 11 to 13. One-inch round fruits are edible. There are many species of Flacourtia, and most are dioecious; hence, males would pose an allergy concern. In Florida these have become a serious invasive plant.

FLAME FREESIA. See Tritonia.

FLAME TREE. See Brachychiton acerifolius; Derris.

FLAME VINE. See Pyrostegia venusta; Senecio.

FLAME VIOLET. See Episcia.

FLANNEL BUSH. See Fremontodendron.

FLANNEL PLANT. See Verbascum.

FLAX. See Linum.

FLAX, YELLOW. See Reinwardtia indica.

FLEABANE. See Erigeron.

FLEECEFLOWER. See Polygonum.

FLORIDA ARROWWOOD. See Zamia.

FLORIDA FUDDLEWOOD. See Citharexylum fruticosum.

FLORIDA THATCH PALM. See Thrinax.

FLORIDA TORREYA. See Torreya.

FLOSS SILK TREE. See Chorisia.

FLOWER-OF-THE-INCAS. See Cantua buxifolia.

FLOWERING DOGWOOD. See *Cornus.*

FLOWERING GARLIC. See *Allium.*

FLOWERING MAPLE. See *Abutilon.*

FLOWERING OAK. See *Crinodendron.*

FLOWERING ONION. See *Allium.*

FLOWERING QUINCE. See *Chaenomeles.*

FLOWERING SNEEZEWEED. See *Helenium autumnale.*

FLOWERING STONES. See *Lithops.*

FLOWERING TOBACCO. See *Nicotiana.*

Foeniculum. 5
ANISE, FENNEL. Perennial herbs grown as annuals. Odor can bother a few people. Anise oil occasionally causes skin rashes, so it is reasonable to suspect that the leaves may also.

Fontanesia. 8
Two species of deciduous shrubs, from China, resembling privet. Olive relatives, hardy to zone 5. Some of the plants may be separate-sexed and with these the males will be especially allergenic. At any rate, the whole group has large potential for allergy, especially for anyone who already has an existing olive-pollen allergy.

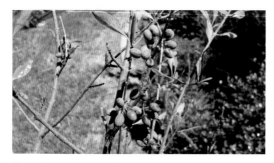

Forestiera. MALES 9 🌑, FEMALES 1 ⊙
DESERT OLIVE, SWAMP PRIVET. (*Forestiera neomexicana*, pictured above.) Olive relatives. Twenty species of shrubs and small deciduous or evergreen trees for zones 5 to 10. Separate-sexed. Some species can grow to 15 feet tall and can be used in desert areas as single-trunked trees. In the western U.S. the native species is *F. pubescens*, also called *F. neomexicana*. This species grows from the Mexican border north into Montana. Very tough, drought-resistant, easy and fast growing; female selections of all species of Forestiera have great potential as landscape plants. Male plants have large

potential for allergy and can be expected to cross-react with existing olive allergies. A female cultivar of desert olive is called 'Desert Girl' and is useful for large wild-looking hedges. Not suitable for acid soils, although *F. acuminata*, the swamp privet, will tolerate wet, acid conditions.

FORGET-ME-NOT. See *Cynoglossum; Mertensia.*

FORMOSAN REDWOOD. See *Taiwania cryptomerioides.*

Forsythia. 6
GOLDEN BELLS. Several species of deciduous, hardy shrubs grown for their early, bright yellow flowers. Related to olives.

FORTNIGHT LILY. See *Dietes.*

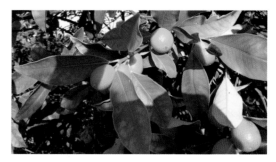

Fortunella. 2 ⊙
KUMQUAT. (Pictured above.) Kumquats have smaller flowers than oranges or lemons, are less fragrant, and are somewhat hardier. They need high summer heat to bear their small fruit, which resemble oranges. These sharp and sweet-tasting fruits are often eaten whole, rind and all. Kumquat trees are usually much smaller than most other citrus.

Fortuneria. 7
Deciduous shrub from China occasionally grown in the United States in zones 6 to 9.

Fothergilla. 5
Native deciduous shrubs hardy in zones 5 to 10. Good fall color and easy to grow in wet soil.

FOUNTAIN GRASS. See *Pennisetum setaceum.*

Fouquieria splendens. 1 ⊙
OCOTILLO. Tall (to 10 feet), thorny, mostly leafless deciduous shrubs native to hot, dry desert areas of the Southwest. Very drought-tolerant; needs light soil and full sun. Bright red flowers. Easily propagated by cuttings.

FOUR O'CLOCK. See *Mirabilis jalapa*.

FOXBERRY. See *Vaccinium*.

FOXGLOVE. See *Digitalis*.

FOXTAIL GRASS. See *Alopecurus*.

FOXTAIL LILY. See *Eremurus*.

FOXTAIL MILLET. See *Setaria*.

Fragaria. 1 ✪

STRAWBERRY. Hardy perennial fruiting plants. *F. chiloensis* is a good ground cover for small areas, sun or shade. Strawberries grow best on sandy loam soils.

FRAGRANT SNOWBALL. See *Viburnum*.

FRAGRANT SNOWBELL. See *Styrax*.

FRAGRANT SUMAC. See *Rhus*.

FRANCESCHI PALM. See *Brahea elegans*.

Francoa ramosa. 2 ✪

MAIDEN'S WREATH. Evergreen, spreading perennial, native to Chile, bearing spikes of small pink or white flowers. It grows well in filtered shade.

FRANGIPANI. See *Plumeria*.

Franklinia alatamaha (Gordonia). 3

Deciduous tree, once native to the eastern United States but now only known in cultivation. Small to medium-size; has large, unusual white flowers and smooth, tan, very attractive bark. Large leaves turn orange-red in fall. They do best in well-drained, moist acid soil under conditions similar to the Camellia, to which they are related.

FRAXINELLA. See *Dictamnus albus*.

FRAXINUS GENUS

Fraxinus. INDIVIDUALLY RANKED

ASH, BLACK ASH, FLOWERING ASH, WHITE ASH. Related to the olives, ash are large, native, deciduous trees that produce copious amounts of potent pollen. In some countries, ash is a primary allergy plant. Various ash species are hardy in almost any zone.

Luckily, most ash are separate-sexed trees; females are easy to identify by their drooping clusters of winged seeds. Commercial budded or grafted varieties sold as seedless ash are male trees that produce pollen. The inconspicuous flowers appear early in the year, often before the leaves. Ash are handsome, large, fast-growing shade trees, and their strong wood makes good firewood and fine lumber. White ash is used to make professional baseball bats.

F. americana. MALES 7, FEMALES 1 ✪

WHITE ASH. Common named male varieties are 'Autumn Applause', 'Autumn Purple', 'Blue Mountain', 'Cimmaron', 'Rosehill' or 'Rose Hill', and 'Skyline'.

F. angustifolia. 1 ✪

NARROWLEAF ASH. Common named female varieties are 'Flame', 'Moraine', and 'Raywood'.

F. anomala. 6

SINGLELEAF ASH.

F. bungeana. 2 ✪

CHINESE DWARF ASH.

F. dipetala. 4

CALIFORNIA SHRUB ASH.

F. excelsior. MALES 7, FEMALES 1 ✪

ENGLISH ASH. Common named male varieties are 'Gold Cloud', 'Hessei', 'Juglandifolia', and 'Kimberly'. The weeping ash, *F. excelsior* 'Pendula', is an excellent tree for the allergy-free landscape.

F. nigra. MALES 9 ✦, FEMALES 1 ✪

BLACK ASH. 'Fallgold' is a common named male variety.

F. ornus. MALES 6, FEMALES 1 ✪

FLOWERING ASH, MANNA ASH. 'Emerald Elegance' and 'Victoria' are pollen-producing trees that may cause some allergy. 'Aire Peters', however, is an excellent choice for allergy-free landscapes.

F. pensylvanica. MALES 7, FEMALES 1 ✪

GREEN ASH. Common named male varieties of this heavy pollen producer are 'Aerial', 'Bergeson', 'Cardan', 'Dakota Centennial', 'Emerald', 'Honeyshade', 'King Richard', 'Mahle', 'Marshall Seedless', 'Newport', 'Patmore', 'Prairie Dome' or 'Prairie Spire', 'Robinhood', and 'Select'.

Several named varieties, 'Jewel', 'Niobara', 'Summit' or 'Summit Ash', and 'Tornado', are excellent female pollen-free trees for the allergy-free landscape.

F. uhdei. MALES 7, FEMALES 1 ✪

EVERGREEN ASH, FRESNO ASH, MEXICAN ASH, SHAMEL ASH. 'Majestic Beauty' is a male cultivar. 'Tomlinson' is a good female.

F. uhdei 'Majestic Beauty'. 7

F. uhdei 'Tomlinson'. 1 ✪

F. velutina. 7

ARIZONA ASH, DESERT ASH, VELVET ASH. Some common named male varieties are 'Fan West', 'Modesto', 'Stribling', 'Sunbelt', and 'Von Ormy'.

In the north and eastern U.S., a nonnative insect pest, the emerald ash borer (EAB), is spreading very fast and killing all ash trees in a great many areas. Millions of ash trees have been killed in the past few years. Some of the spread of EAB is from people transporting firewood from dead ash trees. As a result of EAB, ash trees in general are suddenly not a popular choice for many to consider using. It is important to note here that almost all of the ash trees planted in U.S. and Canadian cities in the past forty years were male clones. These were allergenic trees and as EAB kills them off, it represents a great once-in-a-lifetime opportunity to replace these trees with female, allergy-friendly trees.

Freesia. 3
Low-growing flowers with wispy stems and grasslike leaves. The corms are fully hardy only in zones 7 to 10; elsewhere, they must be lifted and overwintered indoors. Many colors, all strongly fragrant. The fragrance may cause allergy in odor-sensitive individuals.

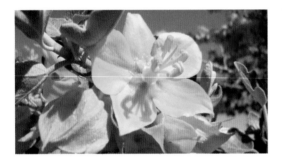

Fremontodendron. 6
FLANNEL BUSH. (Pictured above.) Very large evergreen shrubs with gray hairy leaves and large, bright yellow flowers, for zones 8 to 11. This plant was named for John Frémont, the first governor of California. Very drought-tolerant, it grows well on sunny, dry hillsides. Leaves and seedpods have sharp hairs that cause skin rash. Handle and prune with care.

FRENCH TARRAGON. See *Artemisia*.

FRINGE BELLS. See *Shortia*.

FRINGE CUP. See *Tellima grandiflora*.

FRINGE HYACINTH. See *Muscari*.

FRINGE TREE. See *Chionanthus*.

FRINGED GALAX. See *Shortia*.

FRINGED WORMWOOD. See *Artemisia*.

Fritillaria. 2 ✪
FRITILLARY. Hardy bulbs for zones 3 to 10. Tall plants with bell-shaped red, yellow, or orange flowers grow well in partial shade with good moisture. The flowers and plants are attractive but malodorous.

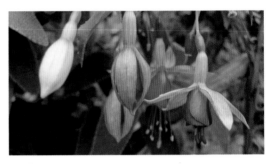

Fuchsia. 3
(Pictured above.) Evergreen in zones 9 to 13, and houseplants or summer annuals elsewhere. Hanging, tubular flowers with brightly colored petals and sepals. Easily grown from cuttings, Fuchsia flowers attract hummingbirds. They grow best in filtered sunlight with good soil, plenty of moisture, and regular feeding. Plants are occasionally bothered by aphids or whiteflies; these can be controlled with a soap spray. In New Zealand there are native species of Fuchsia that grow to be 40-foot-tall trees.

In California, a tiny insect called the fuchsia gall mite has infested many Fuchsia, causing distorted leaves and branches. Cut off diseased portions well below the affected parts and dispose of them.

F. magellanica is hardier than other species and can be grown outside into zones 4 or 5 if the roots are heavily mulched. Tops die back in autumn and resprout from crowns in spring. (See also *Correa*.)

FUCHSIA GUM. See *Eucalyptus*.

FUDDLEWOOD. See *Citharexylum fruticosum*.

FUNKIA. See *Hosta*.

Furcraea. 4
Very large perennial plants related to Agave, for zones 9 to 10, as large accent plants. Drought-tolerant. Monocarpic. Possible danger from contact rash.

Allergy Index Scale: 1 is Best, 10 is Worst.
✿ for 1 and 2   ✿ for 9 and 10
No matter what the ranking, always read the full plant description carefully and take note of any warnings.

Gaillardia. 6
BLANKET FLOWER. Annuals and perennials for full sun in all zones. Easy and fast to grow from seed; many varieties and different species.

Galanthus. 2 ✿
SNOWDROPS. Hardy bulbs for all zones but grow best in cool climates. Needs moist, rich soil. White flowers bloom very early in spring. Bulbs are very poisonous.

Galax urceolata. 1 ✿
COLTSFOOT, WAND FLOWER. A perennial hardy in all zones, the wand flower makes a good ground cover for shady, moist areas with acidic, humus-rich soil. White flowers are borne on short, erect, spikes. Slow growing but worth the effort. Large, shiny, heart-shaped leaves are often used in flower arrangements.

Galium odoratum (Asperula). 2 ✿
SWEET WOODRUFF. Hardy perennial that thrives in cool climates, Galium makes a good ground cover in shady, moist areas.

Galtonia candicans. 2 ✿
SUMMER HYACINTH. Bulbs for shady, moist areas in zones 8 to 10. Fragrant white flowers on 3-foot-tall stems.

Galvezia speciosa. 2 ✿
ISLAND BUSH SNAPDRAGON. Native to the California coastal islands, and hardy to zone 8, this evergreen shrub has red flowers that resemble snapdragons. It grows best in full sun near the coast or in partial shade farther inland.

GAMMA GRASS. See *Tripsacum*.

Gamolepis chrysanthemoides. 5
Fast-growing evergreen subshrub with many bright yellow daisylike flowers. Similar in many respects to Euryops but more winter hardy. Very easy to grow and somewhat drought-resistant.

Garcia. 8
Two species of shrubs or small trees native to Mexico. Both species can cause allergy.

Garcinia mangostana. 4
MANGOSTEEN. An evergreen fruit tree from the tropics, very popular in Indonesia and the Philippines. Many claim that a fresh mangosteen is the best-tasting fruit in the world. A handsome tree, growing to 30 feet, with thick, leathery, glossy green leaves. Unfortunately, trees fail to fruit outside of the tropics.

GARDEN VERBENA. See *Verbena*.

Gardenia. 4
Evergreen shrubs with shiny, dark green leaves and large, highly fragrant white flowers. An extremely attractive plant when well grown. Gardenia is hardy to zone 8 and is often grown as a greenhouse or container plant in all zones. They thrive in rich, acid, moist soil with fast drainage and plenty of humus, in full sun close to the coast or partial shade farther inland. Heavy feeders, requiring an acid-based fertilizer, Gardenias may become chlorotic in soil that is too alkaline. Low-growing *G.* 'Radicans' is occasionally used as a ground cover for a small area. The heavy fragrance of Gardenia, so pleasant to many, may be too much for some who are odor-sensitive.

GARLIC, FLOWERING. See *Allium*.

Garrya. MALES 7, FEMALES 1 ✪
SILK TASSEL. Evergreen shrubs native to western coastal ranges. Hardy to zone 7 and very drought-tolerant. The plants are separate-sexed and the males have the showiest flowers, hence most selected varieties are male. Females are perfect allergy-free choices; males are not. Unfortunately, almost all the plants sold now appear to be clonal males.

GAS PLANT. See *Dictamnus albus*.

Gaultheria. MALES 5, FEMALES 1 ✪
CHECKERBERRY, SALAL, TEABERRY, WINTERGREEN. Evergreen shrubs for zones 7 to 10 that require partial shade and moist, acid soil. Small white flowers resemble the blossoms of blueberry and are sometimes followed by small edible but tasteless black or red fruits. *G. procumbens* is hardy to zone 4 and can be used as a ground cover under deciduous trees.

Gaura lindheimeri. 2 ✪
GAURA. Hardy perennial for full sun in all zones. Drought-tolerant natives of the Southwest, plants grow 3 feet tall and have pink buds and white flowers. Easy to grow and long-lived.

Gaussia. 7
Several species of palms from Puerto Rico and Cuba, sometimes grown in Florida.

GAYFEATHER. See *Liatris*.

Gazania. 4
Ground cover perennials in zones 9 to 10. Easy-to-grow plants come in a wide selection of hybrid colors. May naturalize in mild winter areas.

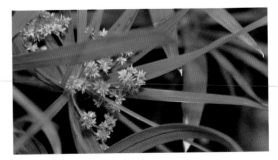

Geijera parviflora. 5
AUSTRALIAN WILLOW, WILGA. (Pictured above.) Common evergreen landscape tree in California, covered with tiny white flowers when in bloom. Not a true willow.

Gelsemium sempervirens. 4
CAROLINA JESSAMINE. Evergreen vine with tubular yellow flowers. All parts of this jessamine are extremely poisonous.

GENIPE. See *Melicoccus*.

Genista. 4
BROOM, SPANISH BROOM. Deciduous subshrubs with green stems and yellow flowers. Poisonous.

GENTIAN. See *Eustoma grandiflorum*; *Gentiana*.

Gentiana. 1 ✪
GENTIAN. Low-growing, spreading perennial for all zones. Thrives in full sun or partial shade, in moist, fast-draining, acidic soil. A good rock garden plant, with bright blue flowers held upright above foliage.

GERALDTON WAXFLOWER. See *Chamelaucium uncinatum*.

Geranium. 3
CRANESBILL, TRUE GERANIUMS. Low-growing, spreading perennials hardy into zone 3. Not to be confused with the showier related pot plant or greenhouse geranium (Pelargonium), true geraniums produce many small flowers in shades of rose, purple, white, red, or blue, and their leaves lack the strong scent of the Pelargonium. Fine plants for the perennial border or rock garden, Geraniums require constant moisture and do best in cool summer climates. A few species may be separate-sexed and female plants would be pollen-free.

GERANIUM, CALIFORNIA. See *Senecio*.

Gerbera jamesonii. 5
TRANSVAAL DAISY. Perennial hardy in zones 9 to 10, grown as annuals elsewhere. Very large, fancy daisy

flowers that make long-lasting cut flowers. Full sun with good soil; needs heat to thrive.

GERMAN IVY. See *Senecio.*

GERMAN VIOLET. See *Exacum.*

GERMANDER. See *Teucrium.*

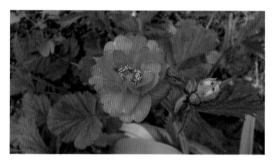

Geum. 2 ✪

(Pictured above.) Perennials hardy in all zones. Sun or part shade, needs good drainage. Flowers are yellow, copper, or orange; 'Mrs. Bradshaw' is a popular double red variety.

GIANT HYSSOP. See *Agastache.*

GIANT REED. See *Arundo donax.*

GIANT SEQUOIA. See *Sequoiadendron giganteum.*

Gilia. 3

BIRD'S EYES, BLUE THIMBLE FLOWER, YARROW GILIA. Tall western native annual for full sun.

Gillenia trifoliata. 2 ✪

BOWMAN'S ROOT. Native perennial for zones 3 to 8, best on the East Coast in moist, acid soils. Best in partial shade, gets 3 feet tall and 3 feet wide; many cute white flowers. Easy to grow.

GINGER. See *Alpinia; Asarum; Zingiber officinale.*

GINGER LILY. See *Hedychium.*

GINGERBREAD PALM. See *Hyphaene.*

Ginkgo biloba. MALES 7, FEMALES 2 ✪

CHINESE MAIDENHAIR TREE. Deciduous trees hardy to zone 4. Ginkgo are separate-sexed trees; mature female trees produce large, malodorous fruits that contain an edible seed. Oil from these seeds can cause skin rash, as can handling the ripe fruit. Because most find the fruit objectionable, male trees are commonly used in landscaping.

The female Ginkgo trees grow broader than the males and are often more handsome. A good tree for very large landscapes where it can be planted far from the house. There are at least three female cultivars sold: 'Golden Girl' has outstanding bright yellow fall color; 'Liberty Splendor' is a tall, wide tree of perfect form; and 'Santa Cruz' is a low-spreading tree.

Ginkgo extract is used to improve memory and also for certain heart conditions. Pollen from male trees is motile and can move on its own.

GINNALA MAPLE. See *Acer ginnala.*

GINSENG. See *Panax.*

Gladiolus. 3

GLADS. Corms that are hardy only to zone 7; elsewhere they must be lifted and stored for winter. They do best in full sun and well-drained soil. Tall, colorful stalks of lilylike flowers make these popular as cut flowers.

Glaucium. 3

HORNED POPPY, SEA POPPY. Perennials or annuals for full sun. Red or orange flowers on gray-leafed, shrubby plants.

Glechoma hederacea. 2 ✪

GROUND IVY. A member of the mint family, this low-growing perennial is hardy in all zones. Its small blue flowers and bright green round leaves make it a good ground cover for small areas in full sun to partial shade. Uncontained, it may become an invasive weed.

Gleditsia triacanthos. BISEXUAL 4, MALES 7, FEMALES 1 ✪

HONEY LOCUST, MORAINE LOCUST. Fast-growing, thorny, deciduous trees hardy for all zones; tolerant of desert conditions. Pendant clusters of small yellow or white flowers followed by long messy seedpods. Grafted varieties are thornless and produce fewer seedpods. Some of these "seedless" trees are males; however, Gleditsia trees may be perfect-flowered, monoecious, or dioecious. Huge numbers of male honey locust trees have been planted in many northern cities. Pollen from these trees can cross-react with other legume allergies such as soy or peanut allergy.

GLOBE AMARANTH. See *Gomphrena globosa.*

GLOBE FLOWER. See *Trollius.*

GLOBE THISTLE. See *Echinops exaltatus.*

GLORIOSA DAISY. See *Rudbeckia.*

Gloriosa rothschildiana. 3

CLIMBING LILY, GLORY LILY. Tuberous perennial hardy only in the mildest areas of zone 10. This African native climbs to 6 feet, with tendrils on the tips of the leaves, and covers itself with bold red and yellow flowers. Poisonous.

GLORY BUSH. See *Tibouchina urvilleana*.

GLORY LILY. See *Gloriosa rothschildiana*.

GLORY-OF-THE-SNOW. See *Chionodoxa*.

GLORYBOWER. See *Clerodendrum*.

GLOXINIA. See *Sinningia*.

Glyptostrobus lineatus. 6
CHINESE SWAMP CYPRESS, CHINESE WATER PINE. Deciduous conifer hardy to zone 9. Tolerant of wet soils.

GOATNUT. See *Simmondsia*.

GODETIA. See *Clarkia*.

GOLD DUST PLANT. See *Aucuba japonica*.

GOLD MEDALLION TREE. See *Cassia*.

GOLD VINE. See *Hibbertia*; *Stigmaphyllon*.

GOLDBACK FERN. See *Pityrogramma*.

GOLDEN BELLS. See *Forsythia*.

GOLDEN CANDLE. See *Pachystachys lutea*.

GOLDEN CREEPER. See *Stigmaphyllon*.

GOLDEN CUP. See *Hunnemannia*.

GOLDEN DROPS. See *Onosma tauricum*.

GOLDEN EARDROPS. See *Dicentra*.

GOLDEN FLEECE. See *Dyssodia tenuiloba*.

GOLDEN HEATHER. See *Hudsonia*.

GOLDEN LARCH. See *Pseudolarix kaempferi*.

GOLDEN RAGWORT. See *Senecio*.

GOLDEN TRUMPET TREE. See *Tabebuia*.

GOLDEN WATTLE. See *Acacia*.

GOLDENCHAIN TREE. See *Laburnum*.

GOLDENRAIN TREE. See *Koelreuteria paniculata*.

GOLDENROD. See *Solidago*.

GOLDFISH PLANT. See *Alloplectus nummularia*.

Gomphrena globosa. 4
GLOBE AMARANTH. Small annual for full sun. The globe-shaped pink, white, or violet flowers resemble clover blooms.

GOOSE PLANT. See *Asclepias*.

GOOSEBERRY. See *Ribes*.

GOOSEFOOT. See *Chenopodium*.

GOPHER PLANT. See *Euphorbia*.

GORDONIA. See *Franklinia alatamaha*.

Gossypium hirsutum. 3
COTTON. Annual or perennial subshrub. This is the cotton plant of commerce. Grown as a garden curiosity, cotton is easy to grow in full sun with plenty of fertilizer and water. Flowers resemble those of hollyhock and are followed by pods containing seeds and cotton. The cotton plant poses no real allergy potential; the fields in which it is grown, however, are among the most heavily fertilized and chemically sprayed of all land. For this reason, refrain from using cottonseed meal fertilizer on your vegetable garden. Leaves are poisonous.

GOUTWEED. See *Aegopodium*.

GRAIN SORGHUM. See *Sorghum*.

GRAMA GRASS. See *Bouteloua gracilis*.

GRAND FIR. See *Abies*.

GRAPE HYACINTH. See *Muscari*.

GRAPE IVY. See *Cissus*.

GRAPEFRUIT. See *Citrus*.

GRAPE. See *Vitis*.

Graptopetalum. 1 ✿
Succulent for zones 9 to 10.

GRASS NUT. See *Triteleia*.

GRASS PALM. See *Cordyline*.

GRASS TREE. See *Xanthorrhoea*.

GRAY SANTOLINA. See *Santolina*.

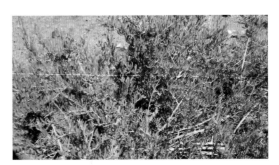

Grayia spinosa. MALES 7, FEMALES 1 ✿
HOPSAGE BUSH. (*Grayia spinosa*, female, pictured above.) An extremely drought-tolerant native shrub that is separate-sexed. Small gray leaves and attractive red, hoplike flowers on female plants. Male plants are allergenic. Look for the new female cultivar 'Hopsage

Sally'. Best in full sun in neutral to alkaline soils. Good desert plant, hardy in zones 6 to 10.

GREASEWOOD. See *Salvia*; *Senecio*.

GRECIAN LAUREL. See *Laurus nobilis*.

GREEN CARPET. See *Herniaria*.

GREEN SANTOLINA. See *Santolina*.

GREENBRIER. See *Smilax*.

GREENLEAF DAISY. See *Euryops*.

Grevillea. 5
SILK TREE. *G. noellii* is an evergreen shrub; *G. robusta* is a large, fast-growing evergreen tree from Australia. Both are hardy in zones 9 and 10. Bright yellow flowers attract tanagers and orioles that feed on the nectar. There are also a number of useful Grevillea species that are shrubs and subshrubs, and all are useful and drought-tolerant. Contact with leaves and flowers has been known to trigger itch and rash.

Grewia occidentalis. 5
LAVENDER STARFLOWER. A fast-growing, easy, evergreen shrub for zones 9 to 10. The small lavender flowers with yellow centers do not drop cleanly after blooming, leaving the bush looking dirty.

Griselinia. MALES 8, FEMALES 1 ✪
Evergreen shrubs native to New Zealand for zones 9 to 10, popular in California and Europe. The thick, shiny, attractive round leaves are sometimes variegated. Griselinia grow very well in coastal areas and are very drought-tolerant and insect- and disease-free. Can be used as hedge materials. Female plants are preferred, and there are several new cultivars now; see this listing in chapter 4.

GROUND CEDAR. See *Lycopodium*.

GROUND CHERRY. See *Physalis*.

GROUND IVY. See *Glechoma hederacea*.

GROUND PINE. See *Lycopodium*.

GROUSEBERRY. See *Viburnum*.

GRU-GRU PALM. See *Acrocomia*.

GUADALUPE FAN PALM. See *Brahea edulis*.

Guaiacum sanctum. 3
LIGNUM-VITAE. Evergreen shrub or tree used in zones 9 to 13. This tree has some of the hardest and heaviest wood of any tree in the world. Attractive leaves and flowers, the plant is good for seaside plantings. Flowers are usually purple or blue.

GUATEMALAN HOLLY. See *Olmediella betschlerana*.

GUAVA. See *Feijoa*; *Psidium*.

GUAYULE. See *Hevea*; *Parthenium argentatum*.

GUELDER ROSE. See *Viburnum*.

GUINEA GOLD VINE. See *Hibbertia*.

GUM MYRTLE. See *Angophora costata*.

GUM TREE. See *Eucalyptus*; *Liquidambar*.

GUMBO-LIMBO TREE. See *Bursera*.

GUMMY ACACIA. See *Robinia*.

Gunnera. MALES 6, FEMALES 1 ✪
Large perennial with giant leaves, up to 8 feet across; thrives in moist, rich, well-drained soil. Best in cool summer areas of zones 7 to 11.

GUTTA PERCHA TREE. See *Eucommia ulmoides*.

GUZMANIA. See *Bromelia*.

Gymnocladus dioica. MALES 8, FEMALES 1 ✪
KENTUCKY COFFEE TREE. Deciduous tree, hardy to zone 5. Interesting large compound leaves. These are separate-sexed trees; the grafted cultivars are male. Female trees produce large seedpods and do not cause allergy, although they can be messy. 'Expresso' is a male Gymnocladus sold as a "seedless" landscape tree. Seedpods are poisonous.

Gynura aurantiaca. 5
PURPLE VELVET PLANT. Houseplant with soft, pretty, hairy leaves and large clusters of malodorous yellow flowers in early summer. Used outside in zones 10 to 13; as a houseplant it might well be a good idea to keep the smelly yellow flowers clipped off, as they have many exposed stamens and will shed some pollen. Poisonous.

GYP CORN. See *Sorghum*.

Gypsophila. 6
BABY'S BREATH. Annuals or small perennials for all zones. Small white or pink flowers. Florists often develop allergy to baby's breath. Also implicated in asthma. Not recommended for floral bouquets.

Allergy Index Scale: 1 is Best, 10 is Worst.
✪ for 1 and 2   ✿ for 9 and 10
No matter what the ranking, always read the full plant description carefully and take note of any warnings.

HACKBERRY. See *Celtis*.

HAEMANTHUS. See *Hippeastrum*.

HAIRY LYCHEE. See *Nephelium lappaceum*.

Hakea. 5
PINCUSHION TREE, SEA URCHIN, SWEET HAKEA. Evergreen shrubs or small trees from Australia. Stiff leaves and fluffy, fragrant red or white flower clusters. Used for hedges and screens in zones 9 to 10.

Halesia. 3
OPPOSSUMWOOD, SILVERBELL TREE, SNOWDROP TREE. Several species of deciduous shrubs and trees native to the eastern United States and China. Attractive trees reach 50 to 60 feet, but grow slowly. Good show of flowers in late spring.

Halimiocistus sahucii. 3
Dense, small evergreen shrub hardy to zone 7. Covered with small yellow flowers; drought-tolerant.

Halimium. 2 ✪
Small, low-growing, spreading shrublets with bright yellow flowers resembling sunrose (Helianthemum). Thrives in full sun with good drainage.

Hamamelis. 6
WINTERBLOOM, WITCH HAZEL. Very early flowering deciduous trees or shrubs. Common witch hazel is hardy to zone 2. Bare branches are often brought inside in late winter where they will soon flower; when used in flower arrangements they may cause allergy.

Hardenbergia. 3
Easy-to-grow evergreen vines for zones 9 to 13. Bears purple flowers in long, loose clusters.

HARDTACK. See *Ostrya*.

HARDY RUBBER TREE. See *Eucommia ulmoides*.

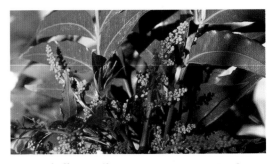

Harpephyllum caffrum. MALES 8, FEMALES 2 ✪
KAFFIR PLUM. (Pictured above.) Large separate-sexed evergreen tree for zones 9 to 13. Related to poison ivy, the female trees bear small edible red fruits. Male trees resemble Brazilian pepper trees and shed allergenic

pollen in late summer. Not sold sexed. Contact with leaves and sap may cause skin rash.

Harpullia. 8
Group of thirty-five species of trees and shrubs native to tropical Asia, Australia, and Madagascar, all with high potential for causing allergy.

HART'S-TONGUE FERN. See *Phyllitis scolopendrium*.

HAT PALM. See *Sabal*.

HAT TREE. See *Brachychiton discolor*.

HAW. See *Viburnum*.

HAWTHORN. See *Crataegus*.

HAWTHORN-LEAF MAPLE. See *Acer crataegifolium*.

HAZELNUT. See *Corylus*.

HE HUCKLEBERRY. See *Cyrilla racemosa*.

HEAL-ALL. See *Prunella*.

HEATH. See *Erica*; *Daboecia*.

HEATHER. See *Calluna*; *Erica*.

HEAVENLY BAMBOO. See *Nandina domestica*.

Hebe. 2 ✪
VERONICA. Evergreen shrubs, some hardy to zone 7. Hebe grow best near the coast and do not thrive in hot, dry areas. The many small flowers are blue, purple, lavender, or white. Easy to grow under the right conditions and with ample moisture.

HEDERA GENUS

Hedera. INDIVIDUALLY RANKED
IVY. All Hedera pose serious allergy potential unless kept small and grown in containers. The sap is known to cause occasional severe skin rash and the pollen can bring on sudden, intense allergic reactions. Ivy blooms only on old wood, so that if it is pruned hard each year there is much less chance of exposure to the pollen. Occasionally, ivy grows up the trunks of trees, eventually killing them and, in rare cases, forming an "ivy tree." A good substitute for Hedera is perennial Vinca. The leaves are poisonous if eaten and the black seed heads are especially toxic. Birds, however, particularly robins, will eat ivy fruit in early spring when there is little else to consume.

H. canariensis. 8
ALGERIAN IVY. Big-leafed subtropical vine, occasionally appearing in a variegated form. Much used in zones 9 to 13 as a ground cover. May be invasive and difficult to remove.

H. colchica. 8
PERSIAN IVY. Hardy in zones 8 to 10. Has larger leaves than *H. canariensis*.

H. helix. 7
ENGLISH IVY. The hardiest, most common, and most popular of the ivies, used as a ground cover, houseplant, or hanging basket plant. *H. helix* 'Baltica' is the hardiest of all small-leafed English ivies.

HEDGE APPLE. See *Maclura pomifera*.

HEDGE FERN. See *Polystichum*.

HEDGE MAPLE. See *Acer campestre*.

Hedycarya arborea. MALES 8, FEMALES 1 ✪
Evergreen tree from New Zealand occasionally grown in California, with 5-inch-long, leathery, toothed leaves and small red, olive-shaped fruits on female trees. Separate-sexed, but not sold sexed. Males pose allergy problem.

Hedychium. 5
GINGER LILY. Very tall perennials for zone 10. Big leaves and large flower spikes.

Hedyscepe canterburyana. 8
UMBRELLA PALM. Medium-size palm tree hardy only in zone 10.

Heimia salicifolia. 3
SUN OPENER. Woody perennial from Jamaica, hardy in zones 9 to 10. Yellow flowers, medicinal plants with psychoactive properties. Easy to grow.

Helenium autumnale. 9 ✎
FLOWERING SNEEZEWEED. A tall perennial hardy in all zones. The name says it all! The leaves and flowers of Helenium may cause skin rashes. All parts of the plant are poisonous if eaten.

Helianthemum nummularium. 3
SUNROSE. Slow-growing, sun-loving perennial hardy to zone 4. Attractive small flowers in many bright colors cover this small, spreading rock garden plant. Will not take overwatering.

Helianthus. 1 ✪ TO 6 DEPENDING ON CULTIVAR AND SPECIES
SUNFLOWER. Annuals and perennials. Big, bold, handsome flowers in many sizes and colors. Unfortunately, sunflowers are related to ragweeds, and cross-allergenic reactions are not uncommon. There are now quite a few garden sunflower cultivars that are sold as pollen-free plants, and these are attractive and nonallergenic.

Helichrysum. 4
EVERLASTING, STRAWFLOWER. Annuals used as dried flowers. Easy to grow from seed.

Heliconia. 2 ✪
FALSE BIRD-OF-PARADISE, LOBSTER-CLAW. Large group of tropical evergreens grown as greenhouse plants for their big leaves and showy flowers.

Heliopsis helianthoides scabra. 5
OX-EYE DAISY. Hardy perennial for cooler zones.

HELIOTROPE, GARDEN. See *Valeriana officinalis*.

HELIOTROPE, WILD. See *Phacelia distans*.

Heliotropium arborescens. 5
COMMON HELIOTROPE. Perennial that may form a shrubby evergreen in zone 10. Grown as annual in colder climates. Big clusters of strongly fragrant flowers are usually purple, occasionally white. Intense fragrance. Poisonous.

Helipterum roseum. 4
Annual daisy for full sun; easy to grow from seed. Used as a dried flower.

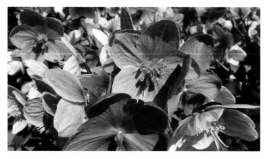

Helleborus. 4
CHRISTMAS ROSE, HELLEBORE, LENTEN ROSE. (Pictured above.) Perennials hardy in all zones. With their unusually colored small fragrant flowers, hellebores grow best in moist, shady areas. The scent of hellebores can cause allergy in some individuals. The sap can cause skin rash. All parts of this plant are extremely poisonous. For another very poisonous plant known as hellebore or false hellebore, see Veratrum.

Hemerocallis. 6
DAYLILY. Hardy, easy-to-grow perennial. Many possible flower colors. Thrives in sun or partial shade, with ample moisture. Daylily is one of the prime garden plants for triggering "lily rash," which one can get from actual skin contact with the leaves or flowers, especially during hot, sunny weather. Daylilies are not problematic per their pollen, but the potential for skin rash is high, and often the itch associated with this rash never completely goes away. All gardeners, allergic or not, would be wise to wear long-sleeved shirts and gloves when working with daylilies. Poisonous.

Hemigraphis. 1 ✪
WAFFLE PLANT. Houseplants grown for their attractive, heart-shaped leaves.

Hemiptelea davidii. MALES 10 ✎, FEMALES 1 ✪
A hardy deciduous tree from Korea, eastern Mongolia, Manchuria, and China, occasionally used in zones 5 to 8 as a small landscape tree or as a fast-growing, thorny hedge. An elm relative, the separate-sexed flowers on male plants are tiny but numerous and produce abundant, very allergenic pollen.

HEMLOCK, HEMLOCK SPRUCE. See *Tsuga*.

HEMP TREE. See *Vitex*.

HENS-AND-CHICKS. See *Echeveria*; *Sempervivum*.

Hepatica. 2 ✪
LIVERLEAF. Very hardy small perennial for all zones, but best in cool summer areas. Large, pretty, three-lobed leaves and violet or pink flowers on early spring-blooming plants for shady, moist spots. Whole plant is poisonous.

HERALD'S TRUMPET. See *Beaumontia grandiflora*.

HERCULES' CLUB. See *Zanthoxylum*.

Heritiera. 8
A group of about thirty trees from Australia or the tropics, all with high allergy potential.

Hermannia verticillata (Mahernia). 2 ✪
HONEY BELL. Evergreen perennial often sold in hanging baskets. Yellow, bell-shaped flowers. Poisonous.

Hernandia ovigera. MALES 8, FEMALES 1 ✪
Evergreen tree from subtropics (zones 11 to 13) occasionally grown in zone 10. Large rounded leaves, 8 inches long. Male tree has high allergy potential.

Herniaria. 2 ✪
GREEN CARPET, RUPTURE WORT. Very hardy evergreen spreading ground cover. Will stand some light traffic.

Hesperaloe parviflora. 1 ✪
Perennial native of Texas and Mexico. Tall spikes of pink flowers emerge from rosette of leaves. Drought-tolerant desert plant.

Hesperis matronalis. 4

DAME'S ROCKET, SWEET ROCKET. Perennial or hardy annual for all zones, bearing panicles of lavender or white flowers on 3-foot stems. Fast growing from seed.

Heterocentron elegans (Schizocentron). 2 ✪

SPANISH SHAWL. Trailing perennial for hanging baskets or as ground cover in shady areas of zones 9 to 10. Reddish leaves and red flowers.

Heteromeles arbutifolia. 3

CALIFORNIA HOLLY, CHRISTMAS BERRY, TOYON. Evergreen native tree of western coastal areas, hardy to zone 7. Small leaves; white flowers followed by clusters of small red berries. Drought-tolerant. Can be pruned into large shrub. Often used along freeways in California.

Heterospathe. 6

SAGISI PALM. Subtropical palm common in southern Florida.

Heuchera. 1 ✪

CORAL BELLS. Low-growing perennials, some species hardy in all zones. Easy to grow in sun or partial shade with plenty of water. Red flowers rise up from low basal foliage. Good rock garden plants.

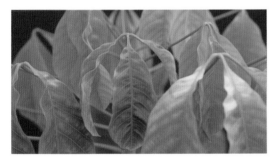

Hevea brasiliensis. MALES 10 🔪, FEMALES 3

RUBBER TREE. (Pictured above.) A large tropical tree grown commercially for the production of rubber. Both the pollen and the sap are highly allergenic for many people. Hevea is a member of the spurge or Euphorbia family, a large group infamous for causing many serious contact allergies, including swelling, rash, itching, burning, and in some cases, death.

Allergy to rubber (also called para rubber), or latex, is on the rise, because of the increased use of latex gloves by medical personnel, food service personnel, police, and emergency workers. The allergy often takes months or years of repeated exposure to emerge. Reaction can then be swift and often severe; there are reported cases of fatalities occurring when rubber dental implements, catheters, and other medical devices have been placed in contact with sensitive individuals. Severe rashes and other allergic responses to the wearing of latex gloves, or from inhaling the powdery dust found on the gloves, are also possible.

In addition to Hevea, *Parthenium argentatum*, or guayule, is occasionally used in the production of natural rubber. This desert shrub is related to ragweed, and it is quite possible that cross-allergic reactions will occur with increased use of guayule-based natural rubber. This is especially true because guayule rubber is being touted as a safe alternative to rubber from *Hevea brasiliensis*.

HIBA ARBORVITAE. See *Thujopsis dolabrata*.

HIBA CEDAR. See *Thujopsis dolabrata*.

Hibbertia (Candollea cuneiformis). 3

GUINEA GOLD VINE. Yellow-flowered evergreen shrubs and vines for zone 9 to 10.

Hibiscus. 3

ALTHEA, MALLOW, ROSE-OF-SHARON. A large group of more than 200 species of annuals, perennials, herbs, shrubs, and trees mostly grown as ornamentals. Common Hibiscus relatives are hollyhocks, okra, and cotton. Most members of this group have large, highly colored flower petals that are well designed by nature for pollen transfer by insects; thus, although most Hibiscus flowers have exposed pollen, few if any members of this group cause allergy. *H. syriacus*, rose-of-sharon or shrub althea, is a tall, hardy shrub. *H. moscheutos*, the rose mallow, is a large-flowered perennial that dies back in winter but regrows from a fleshy hardy rootstock. *H. rosa-sinensis*, the Chinese hibiscus, is a popular shrub in zones 10 to 13, with many beautiful hybrids in a wide array of colors. All Hibiscus are easy-to-grow plants in good sun with average soil and ample water.

HICKORY. See *Carya*.

HIMALAYAN POPPY. See *Meconopsis*.

HINDU-ROPE PLANT. See *Hoya*.

Hippeastrum. 3

AMARYLLIS, BLOOD LILY, HAEMANTHUS, VALLOTA. South American native bulb for zones 10 to 13; in colder zones the bulbs are dug and stored over winter. Very large, showy, trumpet-shaped flowers on sturdy stalks, arising from a base of strap-shaped leaves. Many fine hybrid varieties available in dozens of color combinations. Often grown in pots, amaryllis are popular flowering pot plants for sunny windows. They do best when fed lightly every few weeks during the bloom period. With all lily family relatives, such as amaryllis, there is always the potential of lily rash from too much contact with the leaves or bulbs.

Hippocrepis comosa. 2 ☻
Perennial leguminous ground cover for zones 9 and 10, resembling vetch. Thrives in full sun; drought-tolerant but benefits from regular watering. May be mowed after the pealike yellow flowers bloom. Tolerates light foot traffic—a good lawn substitute in smaller areas.

Hippophae. MALES 7, FEMALES 1 ☻
BUCKTHORN, SEA BUCKTHORN. Several species of small-leafed, thorny, European deciduous shrubs or small trees. Many buckthorns are separate-sexed, but are rarely sold sexed; male plants can contribute to allergy; females (fruiting) plants do not. Some species of Hippophae are winter hardy to zone 3. If a ratio of one male plant per three or more female plants is used, the potential for allergy is low. Many species bear small, vitamin-rich, orange fruits or berries in late summer; these are occasionally eaten but may be poisonous in large quantities. These same berries have possible value as anticancer agents.

HOG PLUM. See *Pleiogynium.*

Hoheria. 3
LACEBARK, MOUNTAIN RIBBONWOOD. Evergreen trees and deciduous shrubs and trees from New Zealand for zones 9 to 10. Thrives in full sun with ample moisture.

Holcus. 8
VELVET GRASS. A European species used in the western United States. An important allergy grass.

HOLLY FERN. See *Cyrtomium*; *Polystichum.*

HOLLY, MOUNTAIN. See *Nemopanthus.*

HOLLYHOCK. See *Alcea.*

HOLLYLEAF CHERRY. See *Prunus ilicifolia.*

HOLLYLEAF REDBERRY. See *Rhamnus.*

HOLLYLEAF SWEETSPIRE. See *Itea ilicifolia.*

Holodiscus. 6
CREAM BUSH, OCEAN SPRAY. Deciduous shrubs related to and resembling Spiraea. Hardy to zone 4, Holodiscus grows best in dry, sunny spots. The native cream bush produces long clusters of small creamy white flowers that birds like to eat.

Holoptelea. MALES 9 ✎, FEMALES 1 ☻
AFRICAN ELM, INDIAN ELM. Two species of deciduous trees, one from India and the other from Africa, both elm relatives.

HOLY THISTLE. See *Silybum.*

HOLY TREE. See *Melia.*

Homalanthus. MALES 10 ✎, FEMALES 3
About forty species of shrubs and trees with allergenic milky sap, native to tropical Asia and Africa. None is frost hardy, but some species are grown in the United States in zone 10 or in greenhouses as ornamentals. One species, *H. populifolius*, the Queensland poplar, is used to make a commercial black dye that is probably a potent allergen. Many species of Homalanthus are separate-sexed; the male plants can be depended on to release extremely toxic pollen. Euphorbia relatives.

H. populifolius. MALES 10 ✎, FEMALES 3
QUEENSLAND POPLAR. Evergreen trees from Pacific islands to Ceylon.

Homalocladium platycladum. 4
CENTIPEDE PLANT, RIBBON BUSH. Odd-looking novelty plant usually grown in pots or outdoors in zones 9 to 13. Leafless with small red berries.

HONESTY. See *Lunaria annua.*

HONEY BELL. See *Hermannia verticillata.*

HONEY LOCUST. See *Gleditsia triacanthos.*

HONEY MYRTLE. See *Melaleuca.*

HONEY PALM. See *Jubaea.*

HONEY TREE. See *Hovenia dulcis.*

HONEYBERRY. See *Melicoccus.*

HONEYBUSH. See *Melianthus.*

HONEYSUCKLE. See *Lonicera.*

HOP BUSH. See *Dodonaea viscosa.*

HOP HORNBEAM. See *Ostrya.*

HOP TREE. See *Ptelea.*

HOPS. See *Humulus.*

HOPSEED. See *Dodonaea viscosa.*

Hordeum. DOMESTIC VARIETY 4, WEED SPECIES 9 ✎
BARLEY. Pollen from barley is heavier than that of most grasses and poses less of an allergy problem. Pollen from the weedy varieties like *H. jubatum*, or foxtail barley, provokes allergy.

HOREHOUND. See *Marrubium vulgare*.

HORNBEAM. See *Carpinus*.

HORNBEAM MAPLE. See *Acer carpinifolium*.

HORNED MAPLE. See *Acer diabolicum*.

HORNED POPPY. See *Glaucium*.

HORSE CHESTNUT. See *Aesculus*.

HORSEMINT. See *Monarda*.

HORSERADISH. See *Armoracia rusticana*.

HORSETAIL RUSH. See *Equisetum hyemale*.

HORSETAIL TREE. See *Casuarina*.

HOSEDOUP. See *Mespilus*.

Hosta. 1 ✪
FUNKIA, PLANTAIN LILY. Very hardy perennials, members of the lily family, grown for their large, ornamental leaves. Hosta grow best in rich, moist soil in partial shade, and are especially beautiful when planted under trees. The large leaves are frequently damaged by snails and slugs. Many hybrid varieties are available. White, pink, or pale lavender, the sometimes fragrant flowers are held up above foliage on long, slender stalks.

HOT-DOG CACTUS. See *Senecio*.

HOTTENTOT FIG. See *Carpobrotus*.

HOUSELEEK. See *Sempervivum*.

Hovenia dulcis. MALES 6, FEMALES 1 ✪
HONEY TREE, JAPANESE RAISIN TREE. Asian native shade tree with small, edible raisinlike fruit. Separate-sexed but not usually sold sexed. A member of the buckthorn family.

Howea. 7
KENTIA PALM, PARADISE PALM, SENTRY PALM. Houseplant palms used outside in zones 10 to 13. As houseplants they are frequent hosts to spider mites, which can cause allergy. When used outdoors, if in bloom, the pollen can also cause allergy.

Hoya. 3
HINDU-ROPE PLANT, WAX FLOWER, WAX PLANT. Houseplants for sunny rooms, with thick leaves and clusters of pink flowers that look as though they're made of wax. The flowers are very fragrant and last for months. Not a pollen problem, but some may find the heavy, sweet fragrance intolerable.

HUCKLEBERRY. See *Vaccinium*.

HUCKLEBERRY, HE. See *Cyrilla racemosa*.

Hudsonia. 5
GOLDEN HEATHER, POVERTY GRASS. Three species of small, evergreen shrubby plants, native to the northeastern United States, used in some landscapes in cold winter areas. Hardy to zone 2. May cause occasional limited allergy.

Humata tyermannii. 4
BEAR'S FOOT FERN. Slow-growing, Chinese native fern for partial shade in frost-free zones.

HUMMINGBIRD FLOWER. See *Zauschneria*.

Humulus. MALES 7, FEMALES 1 ✪
HOPS. Annual and perennial, hardy, fast-growing vines. *H. lupulus* is used to flavor beer. Hop vines are separate-sexed; male vines infrequently are the cause of allergy. Commercial hops fields use only female plants because these make larger flowers, which are preferred for brewing beer. As a result, these large hop-growing areas present no pollen problems at all. There now are some female cultivars available; look for one with an OPALS #1 tag.

Hunnemannia. 4
GOLDEN CUP, MEXICAN TULIP POPPY. Short-lived perennial poppy for bright, sunny areas. Fast growing from seed; long-lasting flowers. Poisonous.

Hura. 9 ✺
MONKEY PISTOL, SANDBOX TREE. Two species of tropical trees from Central America occasionally used in zone 10. Sap from either can cause severe rash.

HYACINTH. See *Hyacinthus*; *Galtonia candicans*.

HYACINTH BEAN. See *Dolichos*.

HYACINTH, WILD. See *Dichelostemma*.

Hyacinthus. 3
HYACINTH. Hardy bulbs for all zones. Very fragrant flowers may cause odor challenges when planted en masse. Bulbs are poisonous.

Hybophrynium braunianum. 1 ✪
Tall houseplant grown for its unusual foliage. Grows best with regular fertilizer and water, in partial shade.

Hydnocarpus. 8
Many species of tropical trees. The seeds of *H. kurzii*, a large tree, yield chaulmoogra oil, which is used in the treatment of leprosy.

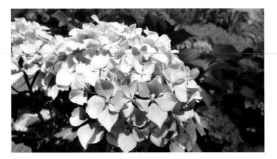

Hydrangea. INDIVIDUALLY RANKED
(Pictured above.) Many species of deciduous shrubs or vines, many hardy to zone 3. All Hydrangeas grow best in good soil with ample moisture, and none is drought-tolerant. In cooler climates, they thrive in full sun, but in hot summer areas, appreciate partial shade. The large floral panicles, in white, pink, red, or blue, are formed of many small flowers clustered together. Hydrangea leaves contain a natural sweetener, but because the leaves also contain toxic compounds, they should not be eaten.

Hydrangea flowers are pH sensitive—rather like a natural litmus paper. Blue flowers can be changed to pink with the addition of limestone to sweeten or raise the pH of the soil. Conversely, pink flowers can be changed to blue by lowering the pH or acidifying the soil with sulfur.

H. anomale. 6
CLIMBING HYDRANGEA. This one can climb 30 to 50 feet up a wall. Can be very attractive, but if used it should be placed so that it does not come too close to any bedroom windows that are ever opened.

H. macrophylla. 3
BIG-LEAF HYDRANGEA. May reach 12 feet outdoors in mild climates. Most often sold as a potted plant. Broad leaves and large, flat flower heads in pink, blue, or white.

H. paniculata. 5
PEE-GEE HYDRANGEA. Among the hardiest of the Hydrangeas, the pee-gee can withstand winters in zone 3. Large panicles of white flowers are borne in midsummer.

H. quercifolia. 6
OAK-LEAF HYDRANGEA. Large, deeply lobed leaves characterize the oak-leaf hydrangea. Forms a fairly large shrub in areas of adequate moisture. Implicated in some contact skin rash and itch from contact with the leaves.

Hydrastis canadensis. 2 ✪
GOLDENSEAL. A hardy native perennial for shady, moist soils in zones 3 to 7, goldenseal is an important medicinal plant.

Hymenanthera. MALES 6, FEMALES 1 ✪
Several species of evergreen trees and shrubs native to New Zealand and Australia. Some are grown outside in California. All are separate-sexed and the male plants can on occasion cause allergy.

Hymenocallis (Ismene). 3
BASKET FLOWER, PERUVIAN DAFFODIL, SPIDER LILY. Frost-tender native bulbs, producing lilylike flowers in midsummer. Poisonous.

Hymenosporum flavum. 3
SWEETSHADE. Small evergreen tree from Australia for zones 9 to 10. A nice tree with few bad habits.

Hypericum. 5
KLAMATHWEED, ST. JOHN'S WORT. Hardy perennial that is often used as a drought-tolerant ground cover that will grow in either sun or shade. In the Pacific Northwest this plant has naturalized and is known as klamathweed. It is the bane of livestock who eat it, because it causes photosensitivity; many cattle die from the resulting sunburn. St. John's wort also contains natural calmative compounds and is used in herbal medicine as a mood enhancer.

Hyphaene. 7
DOUM PALM, GINGERBREAD PALM. Several species of separate-sexed palms occasionally grown in Hawaii and Florida.

HYPOCYRTA NUMMULARIA. See *Alloplectus nummularia*.

Hypoestes phyllostachya. 1 ✪
PINK POLKA-DOT PLANT. With its dark green leaves splashed in pink, Hypoestes makes a good plant for shade in zones 10 to 11, and is a popular houseplant in colder zones. Easy to grow and propagate from seeds or cuttings, it is kept compact through constant pinching back.

HYSSOP. See *Agastache*; *Hyssopus officinalis*.

Hyssopus officinalis. 3
HYSSOP. Hardy ornamental herb for sun or shade in all zones with handsome large leaves and white, rose, or red flowers. A member of the mint family.

Allergy Index Scale: 1 is Best, 10 is Worst.
✿ for 1 and 2   ❧ for 9 and 10
No matter what the ranking, always read the full plant description carefully and take note of any warnings.

Iberis. 2 ✿

CANDYTUFT. Annuals and perennials. Annual candytuft is usually grown from direct seedings. Perennial Iberis is a small, frost-hardy, low-growing, evergreen plant with a good show of very bright white flowers in spring.

ICEPLANT. See *Carpobrotus*; *Cephalophyllum*; *Delosperma*; *Drosanthemum*.

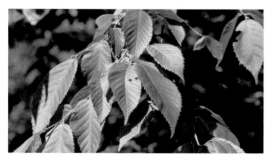

Idesia polycarpa. MALES 6, FEMALES 1 ✿

WONDER TREE. (Pictured above.) Large heart-shaped leaves on this small deciduous Asian native, hardy to zone 7. Separate-sexed, the female trees produce small, ornamental orange fruits. The males pose limited allergy problem.

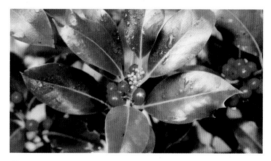

Ilex. MALES 7, FEMALES 1 ✿

HOLLY. (*Ilex*, female, pictured above.) Many species; most are hardy evergreen shrubs or small trees, although some are deciduous. All hollies are separate-sexed, and the male plants present potential for some airborne allergy. A great number of named, sexed cultivars are available for sale. To produce their characteristic red, white, yellow, or black berries, female hollies of certain species or cultivars must be pollinated; one male plant can pollinate many females. There are other forms, though (see chapter 4), that will set a good crop of fruit without pollination from males.

Landscapers frequently use all-male varieties as hedge plants, and in this situation they pose serious allergy potential. Allergy from holly pollen is not well documented, but is worthy of further research. Fruit is mildly poisonous but not fatal.

Illicium anisatum. 3
ANISE TREE, JAPANESE ANISE TREE. Broadleaf evergreen tree with fragrant leaves, small white flowers, and star-shaped seed cluster capsules, for zones 8 to 10. Poisonous seed.

IMMORTELLE. See *Xeranthemum annuum*.

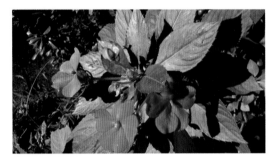

Impatiens. 1 ✪
BALSAM, BUSY LIZZY, TOUCH-ME-NOT. (Pictured above.) A tender annual for all zones, with shade and ample moisture. All Impatiens were once tall and white-flowered, but through selective breeding, there are hundreds of compact, dwarf, multiflowered, and multicolored varieties available at almost any nursery. Impatiens are easy to root from cuttings stuck in small pots of potting soil and kept well watered in the shade for a few weeks. As an annual for shady areas, Impatiens are the top bedding plant used in the United States; they're easy to grow and dependable.

From an allergy point of view, Impatiens are one of our best annual flowers. The petals are large and highly colored, and the pollen-producing parts are few and deeply hidden well inside the flower. They are not known to cause any rashes nor do they have any close allergenic relatives.

The yellow- and orange-flowered wild Impatiens grows along the margins of woodlands in much of North America. The juice from its soft stems is a time-honored remedy for rashes caused by stinging nettle and poison ivy, which usually thrive under similar cultural conditions.

Both the Latin name of Impatiens and the common name of touch-me-not refer to the fact that the ripe, oval-shaped seedpods eject their seeds forcefully when even lightly touched or slightly squeezed.

Incarvillea delavayi. 2 ✪
Large perennial hardy to zone 6. The fleshy roots may be dug and stored over winter north of zone 6. Needs good drainage and sun or part shade to produce bold, trumpet-shaped purple flowers with yellow throats.

INCENSE CEDAR. See *Austrocedrus*; *Calocedrus decurrens*.

INCHWORM. See *Senecio*.

INDIA HAWTHORN. See *Rhaphiolepis indica*.

INDIAN BEAN TREE. See *Catalpa*.

INDIAN CHERRY. See *Rhamnus*.

INDIAN CURRANT. See *Symphoricarpos*.

INDIAN MOCK STRAWBERRY. See *Duchesnea indica*.

INDIAN PINK. See *Silene*.

INDIAN PLUM. See *Oemleria cerasiformus*.

INDIAN POKE. See *Veratrum*.

INDIGO, WILD. See *Baptisia australis*.

INSIDE-OUT FLOWER. See *Vancouveria*.

Inula ensifolia. 3
HORSEHEAL. Hardy, easy-to-grow perennial for full sun in zones 4 to 9; bright yellow daisylike flowers are attractive to butterflies.

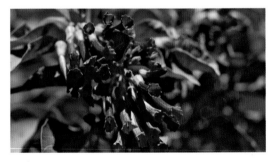

Iochroma cyaneum. 3
(Pictured above.) Tall evergreen shrub for full sun in zones 9 to 10. Produces clusters of long tubular purple flowers that are very attractive to hummingbirds.

Ipheion uniflorum. 2 ✪
SPRING STAR FLOWER. Bulb for zones 7 to 10. Easy to grow; frequently naturalizes.

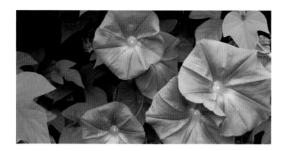

Ipomoea (Calonyction; Quamoclit). 4

BLUE DAWN FLOWER, CARDINAL CLIMBER, MOON FLOWER, MORNING GLORY. (Pictured above.) Perennial or annual vines for full sun or partial shade. Very fast growing when well adapted. In zones 9 to 13, morning glory can become rampant and overgrow fences, shrubs, and sheds. Annual varieties reseed readily. Flowers come in many colors, but perhaps the most impressive is the very large flowered annual 'Heavenly Blue'. All morning glory leaves are capable of causing skin rash in sensitive individuals.

The individual flowers of the morning glory have little exposed pollen and do not present much problem as an inhalant allergen. However, when growing strongly, the sheer mass of blooms may present an overwhelming fragrance for perfume-sensitive individuals; will often reseed and can indeed become weedy.

The seeds of Ipomoea contain a powerful hallucinogen similar to the drug LSD.

Ipomopsis. 3

SCARLET GILIA. Short-lived perennials or annuals for any zone. Slender plants are several feet tall and do best in groups. Direct seed in full sun. Long, tubular, red or red-and-yellow flowers. One species is native to the southern United States and can grow to 6 feet.

Iresine herbstii. MALES 6, FEMALES 1 ✪

BEEF PLANT, BLOOD-LEAF. Shade plant in zone 10 or houseplant in other zones. Frost-tender foliage plant with large green leaves with deep red veins. Fast growing from cuttings. Separate-sexed.

Iris. 1 ✪ TO 4 DEPENDING ON CULTIVAR OR SPECIES

A large group of rhizomatous or bulbous perennials. The rhizomatous varieties are very hardy and easy to grow, given full sun and well-drained soil. Bulbous varieties prefer moist soil and may even be grown as bog plants. In the mild winter areas, large bearded or German Iris are grown in clay pots that can be set aside when the short bloom period is over. Orris root, a fixative for perfumes, powders, and potpourris, is made from Iris roots. Allergy to orris root is very common, and skin rash from handling Iris roots is also not uncommon. Odor-sensitive individuals may be allergic to the fragrance of the Iris. There are a few native species of Iris that are dioecious; none of these is especially allergenic, but still it would be fun to be able to buy all-female Iris (I have some of these myself).

IRISH MOSS. See *Sagina subulata*.

IRONBARK. See *Eucalyptus*.

IRONWEED. See *Verbesina*; *Vernonia*.

IRONWEED, YELLOW. See *Verbesina*.

IRONWOOD. See *Cyrilla racemosa*; *Lyonothamnus floribundus*; *Olneya tesota*; *Parrotia*.

ISLAND BUSH SNAPDRAGON. See *Galvezia speciosa*.

ISMENE. See *Hymenocallis*.

ISOTOMA FLUVIATILIS. See *Laurentia*.

ITALIAN MAPLE. See *Acer opalus*.

ITCHWEED. See *Veratrum*.

Itea ilicifolia. 5

HOLLYLEAF SWEETSPIRE. Evergreen shrub with long drooping clusters of small white fragrant flowers, for zones 6 to 9. Needs plenty of soil moisture.

ITHURIEL'S SPEAR. See *Triteleia*.

Iva. 10 ◗

A group of common tall allergenic weeds usually growing in wet areas in most zones. A dwarf form of Iva is now being used in some "native" landscapes, a trend that should be discouraged.

IVY. See *Hedera*.

IVY-LEAFED MAPLE. See *Acer cissifolium*.

IVY, WATER. See *Senecio*.

Ixia. 3

AFRICAN CORN LILY. Corms are hardy in zones 8 to 10.

Ixiolirion. 3

An Asian native bulb hardy in zones 8 to 10. Blue flowers in spring.

Jacaranda mimosifolia. 4

JACARANDA. A large deciduous tree from Brazil that puts on a glorious display of small, tubular, sky-blue flowers. Cold-hardy only to about 20°F, Jacaranda is grown in mild winter areas around the world. On some city blocks the entire block has been lined with Jacaranda trees, which makes for a glorious burst of blue color when they bloom, but is a serious potential allergy problem for anyone with an existing sensitivity to legumes or legume pollen.

JACOBAEA. See *Senecio*.

JACOBINIA. See *Justicia*.

JACOB'S LADDER. See *Polemonium; Smilax*.

Jacquemontia. 4

Large group of mostly tropical vines with blue flowers, occasionally grown in zone 10.

Jacquinia. 6

BARBASCO. Tropical shrubs and trees with small red, white, or yellow flowers followed by small orange fruits used by South American natives to poison fish. Several species of Jacquinia are grown in Florida.

JADE PLANT. See *Crassula*.

JAMBU. See *Syzygium*.

JAPAN PEPPER. See *Zanthoxylum*.

JAPANESE ANISE TREE. See *Illicium anisatum*.

JAPANESE ARALIA. See *Fatsia japonica*.

JAPANESE CARPET. See *Zoysia*.

JAPANESE CEDAR. See *Cryptomeria japonica*.

JAPANESE EUONYMUS. See *Euonymus*.

JAPANESE FELT FERN. See *Pyrrosia lingua*.

JAPANESE MAPLE. See *Acer japonicum*.

JAPANESE NUTMEG TREE. See *Torreya*.

JAPANESE POINSETTIA. See *Pedilanthus tithymaloides*.

JAPANESE RAISIN TREE. See *Hovenia dulcis*.

JAPANESE SNOWBELL. See *Styrax*.

JAPANESE SPURGE. See *Pachysandra*.

JAPANESE VARNISH TREE. See *Firmiana simplex*.

JAPANESE ZELKOVA. See *Zelkova*.

JASMINE BOX. See *Phillyrea decora*.

Jasminum. 7

JASMINE. Several hundred species of evergreen or deciduous flowering vines and shrubs. Members of the olive family. Flowers, usually strongly fragrant, are white, yellow, or pink. The flowers present allergy potential both from their intense fragrance and for their pollen, which is similar to that of olives, a well-known and potent allergen.

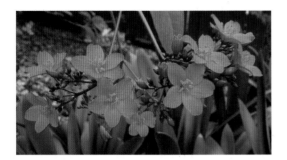

Jatropha. **MALES 8 TO 10 🌰, FEMALES 3**
AUSTRALIAN BOTTLE PLANT, BARBADOS NUT, CORAL PLANT, PEREGRINA, PHYSIC NUT. (Pictured above.) Large group of subtropical plants occasionally planted in zones 10 to 13 and in greenhouses. All plants in this group present numerous allergy potential. Several species have attractive yellow fruit, which is poisonous if eaten. Jatropha is a type of Euphorbia, and as such the sap is highly allergenic; pollen from male plants is also very allergenic.

JAVA APPLE, JAVA PLUM. See *Syzygium.*

JAVAN GRAPE. See *Tetrastigma.*

JELLY PALM. See *Butia capitata.*

JERUSALEM ARTICHOKE. See *Helianthus.*

JERUSALEM CHERRY. See *Solanum.*

JERUSALEM SAGE. See *Phlomis fruticosa*; *Pulmonaria.*

JERUSALEM THORN. See *Parkinsonia aculeata.*

JESSOP. See *Ledebouria socialis.*

JEWEL VINE. See *Derris.*

JEWISH MYRTLE. See *Ruscus.*

JIMSON WEED. See *Datura.*

Joannesia. **9 🌰**
Several species of large trees from Brazil, occasionally used in zones 9 to 10.

JOB'S TEARS. See *Coix lacryma-jobi.*

JOE-PYE WEED. See *Eupatorium.*

Johannesteijsmannia. **1 ✿**
Four species of small palm trees from Borneo and Sumatra, occasionally grown in Florida.

JOHNNY-JUMP-UP. See *Viola.*

JOHNSON GRASS. See *Sorghum.*

JOINT FIR. See *Ephedra.*

JOJOBA. See *Simmondsia.*

JONQUIL. See *Narcissus.*

JOSHUA TREE. See *Yucca.*

JOSTABERRY. See *Ribes.*

JOVE'S FRUIT. See *Lindera.*

Juania. **MALES 8, FEMALES 1 ✿**
CHONTA PALM. Tall dioecious palm trees from Chile.

Jubaea. **7**
CHILEAN WINE PALM, COQUITO PALM, HONEY PALM. A large palm tree from Chile, hardy to 20°F.

Jubaeopsis caffra. **7**
Palm tree used in California and Florida.

Juglans. **8 TO 9 🌰**
BLACK WALNUT, BUTTERNUT, ENGLISH WALNUT, MADEIRA NUT, WALNUT. Large deciduous nut-bearing trees, some species hardy in all zones. All walnuts produce airborne pollen and allergy, but some are worse than others. By far the most problematic in number and intensity of attack is the California black walnut, a large native tree. The butternut and English walnut are slightly less potent allergens. Allergy is also reportedly triggered by the odor of rotting husks that surround the nuts. On some occasions this odor allergy is more severe than that to the pollen.

JUJUBE. See *Ziziphus.*

JUNEBERRY. See *Amelanchier laevis.*

JUNIPERUS GENUS

Juniperus. **MONOECIOUS 9 🌰, MALES 10 🌰, FEMALES 1 ✿**
CEDAR, HABBEL, JUNIPER, MOUNTAIN CEDAR, OZARK WHITE CEDAR, RED CEDAR, WHITE CEDAR. Hardy, drought-tolerant, easy-to-grow, common coniferous evergreen shrubs and trees, which are related to cypress, not true Cedar (Cedrus). Juniper berries are used to flavor gin, and are also used in herbal medicine as a natural diuretic and decongestant; large doses may be poisonous.

Juniper is one of the primary causes of allergies in many parts of the world. In numerous areas of the United States, juniper is *the* primary cause of allergic asthma and hay fever. Cross-allergenic reactions are common between juniper and all species of cypress.

The different species bloom in different ways: The very worst are the males of the separate-sexed species (dioecious); monoecious species always present allergy problems as well; the female plants of separate-sexed species, however, are fine for allergy-free landscapes.

Most junipers bloom from early winter into late spring, sometimes releasing so much pollen that the shrubs appear to smoke. A few species of mostly western junipers bloom from September to November. Other species bloom sporadically throughout the year, creating an almost constant level of airborne pollen in many landscaped areas. In zones 7 to 10 in particular, junipers, especially male plants, may bloom several times each year.

In Arkansas, Missouri, Oklahoma, Texas, and parts of Mexico the most common juniper is *J. ashei*, the Ozark white cedar, which is a juniper, despite its name. All of these are separate-sexed.

In New Mexico, Arizona, parts of Texas, and into Mexico the most common species is the alligator juniper, *J. deppeana*, also separate-sexed.

In the eastern United States the most common species is the red cedar, *J. virginiana*, again a separate-sexed species.

In much of the Rocky Mountain area the predominant juniper is the Colorado red cedar, *J. scopulorum*, another separate-sexed species.

In parts of California, there is a common monoecious juniper, the California juniper, *J. occidentalis*. This species is also sometimes separate-sexed. All other junipers native to California are all separate-sexed.

In separate-sexed juniper species, only the pollen-free female plants produce the round juniper berries. Plants without berries are male.

Each male juniper bush or tree produces enough pollen to fertilize thousands of female plants. In some areas of the United States, during the early spring or late fall and early winter months of the juniper bloom, there is so much pollen in the air that every person living there is inhaling hundreds of juniper pollen grains with every breath.

The relative humidity of an area has much to do with the actual amount of allergy to juniper pollen. In humid areas there is less allergy; in warm, dry areas, typical of much of the western United States, juniper pollen floats easily in the air, causing a great deal of allergy. Juniper pollen can also irritate the skin and is capable of causing contact dermatitis as well as severe inhalant allergy.

In certain geographical locations where cities are surrounded by hills full of wild junipers, the only effective measure may be to selectively remove many of the wild male junipers growing close to the urban areas; males are easy to identify because they are the ones with no berries.

Alas, I have been told numerous times now that in the wild lands surrounding many cities in Arizona, New Mexico, and large parts of Texas, that the firewood cutters have all developed allergies (and often asthma) to juniper pollen. They have discovered that often when they cut down a tree without any berries on it (a male) they start to feel sick. As a result, they all too often only cut down juniper trees that have berries! The end result of this terrible practice, where millions of female juniper trees (that produce no pollen and also trap pollen) have been selectively removed, is that in these wild lands everything is sexually out of balance, and allergy and asthma are increasing dramatically. The state governments of these areas should remedy this situation.

Throughout America there are many millions of imported, nonnative juniper trees, shrubs, and ground covers, most of which are separate-sexed; the female plants of these species can be used in allergy-free landscapes. One notable exception is the Himalayan juniper (*J. recurva*), which is monoecious and, like all plants bearing unisexual flowers on the same tree, sheds allergenic pollen.

Over the years landscapers have preferred to plant junipers without berries to reduce the amount of litter produced by each plant, and wholesale nurseries have propagated many millions of these pollen-producing male selections, all of which cause allergy. The net result has been a steady increase in urban *Juniperus* pollen and related allergic reactions. The answer is to identify and use female-only junipers in all future landscaping applications. Listed below are sexed junipers, of which many are female clones.

J. chinensis.

CHINESE JUNIPER. Female Chinese juniper cultivars include 'Blue Point', 'Excelsior', 'Femina', 'Foemina', 'Iowa', 'Keteleeri Beissn', 'Mountbatten', 'Obelisk', 'Oblong', 'Olympia', and 'Pyramidis Variegata'.

Male named varieties include 'Armstrong', 'Aurea', 'Blue Pfitzer', 'Columnaris Glauca', 'Leena', 'Pendula', 'Pfitzeriana Glauca', 'Pyramidalis', and 'Story'.

Some cultivars are monoecious, bearing flowers of both sexes on one plant. Avoid using 'Hornibrook', 'Robusta Green', and 'Sphoerica'.

J. c. 'Torulosa', the Hollywood juniper, is a very common tall, twisted juniper. The plants are usually female (identified by their berries), although some cultivars of this variety are male and should be avoided. If you don't see berries on it, don't buy it!

J. communis.
COMMON JUNIPER, ENGLISH JUNIPER, POLISH JUNI-
PER, SWEDISH JUNIPER. All plants of this species are
separate-sexed. Use only female plants, which are identifiable by their berries. 'Hornibrookii' is a female shrub
and is a good choice for allergy-free landscapes.

J. davurica.
'Expansa' is a named male cultivar.

J. deppeana.
ALLIGATOR JUNIPER. Separate-sexed; look for berries
indicating female plants.

J. drupacea.
All known cultivars of this species are males.

J. flaccida.
This variety bears flowers of both sexes, each on separate branches. Do not use.

J. horizontalis.
CREEPING JUNIPER, PROSTRATE JUNIPER. 'Admi-
rabilis' is a male plant and should be avoided. Good
female cultivars for allergy-free landscapes include 'Bar
Harbor', 'Filicina', 'Glenmore', and 'Viridis'.

J. × media.
'Globosa' and 'Hetzii' are female plants and good allergy-
free choices; 'Pfitzeriana' and 'Plumosa' are male.

J. occidentalis.
CALIFORNIA JUNIPER. A monoecious species that
should be avoided.

J. oxycedrus.
A separate-sexed species. Look for berries that indicate
safe female plants.

J. phoenicea.
A monoecious species that should be avoided.

J. recurva.
HIMALAYAN JUNIPER. A monoecious species that
should be avoided.

J. rigida.
A separate-sexed species. Look for berries that indicate
allergy-free female plants.

J. sabina 'Cupressa'.
The named cultivar 'Femina' is an allergy-free female.
'Arcadia', 'Blue Danube', 'Broadmore', 'Buffalo', 'Savin',
'Scandia', and 'Tamariscifolia' (tam juniper) are all male
plants and should be avoided.

J. scopulorum.
COLORADO RED CEDAR. A separate-sexed species.
Allergy-free female cultivars include 'Admiral', 'Blue

Heaven', 'Blue Moon', 'Cologreen', 'Gracilis', 'Platinum',
'Spearmint', 'Sutherland', and 'Welchii'. Male cultivars
include 'Emerald' or 'Emerald Green', 'Gray Gleam', 'Sky-
rocket', 'Steel Blue', and 'Wichita Blue'. *J. s.* 'Moonglow'
can be either a male or a female. Don't buy 'Moonglow'
unless it has the berries that indicate a female plant.

J. silicicola.
SOUTHERN JUNIPER. A separate-sexed species. Look
for berries that indicate allergy-free female plants.

J. squamata.
'Meyeri' is an allergy-free female cultivar.

J. virginiana.
EASTERN RED CEDAR. A separate-sexed species, allergy-
free female cultivars include 'Canaertii', 'Chamberlaynii',
'Pendula Chamberlaynii', and 'Pendula Virdis'. Male
cultivars to be avoided include 'Burkii', 'Cupressifolia',
'Filifera', 'Hillspire', 'Prostrata Silver', 'Silver', and 'Tri-
partita'. Some *J. virginiana* may be of either sex; look for
berries indicating female plants on 'Glauca', 'Manhat-
tan Blue', 'Pendula', and 'Reptans' or 'Pendula Reptans'.

J. wallichiana.
BLACK JUNIPER. A separate-sexed species. Look for
berries indicating allergy-free female plants.

JUPITER'S BEARD. See *Centranthus ruber.*

Jurinea. 5
Large group of daisylike annuals and perennials often
grown from seed.

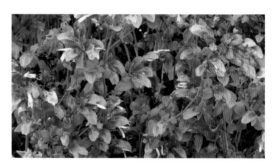

Justicia (Beloperone; Jacobinia). 1 ✪
CHUPAROSA. (*Justicia brandegeana* pictured above.) A
very large group of herbs and shrubs from the subtropics into temperate North America. The most commonly
used is *J. brandegeana*, the shrimp plant. This unusual-
looking flowering shrub grows best in sunny locations
in zones 10 to 13, and produces drooping yellow or
reddish flowers that look like large shrimps.

K

Allergy Index Scale: 1 is Best, 10 is Worst.
✿ for 1 and 2   ❧ for 9 and 10
No matter what the ranking, always read the full plant description carefully and take note of any warnings.

Kadsura japonica. **MALES 7, FEMALES 1** ✿
Evergreen vine for zones 9 to 13.

KAFFIR LILY. See *Clivia.*

KAFFIR PLUM. See *Harpephyllum caffrum.*

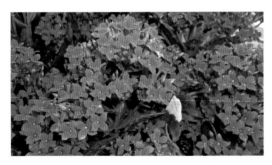

Kalanchoe. **2** ✿
MATERNITY PLANT. (Pictured above.) Succulents used as houseplants.

KALE. See *Brassica.*

Kalmia. **8**
CALICO BUSH, MOUNTAIN LAUREL. Hardy evergreen shrubs or small trees with large clusters of showy flowers in many colors. Hardy to zone 5, Kalmia grows best in moist, well-drained, acid soil in the partial shade of large deciduous trees. Kalmia produces a large amount of pollen and allergy to it is common. All parts are highly poisonous, including the pollen. Never plant Kalmia near any doors or bedroom windows.

Kalmiopsis leachiana. **3**
Oregon native evergreen shrub, hardy to zone 7, producing quantities of small pink flowers in spring. Thrives only where soil is moist, shady, and acidic.

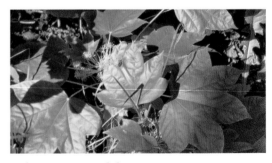

Kalopanax septemlobus. **4**
CASTOR OIL TREE. (Pictured above.) Large deciduous tree, hardy to zone 5, produces small white flowers in spring. Native of China. Needs moist soil to thrive.

KANGAROO PAW. See *Anigozanthos.*

KAPOK. See *Chorisia.*

KARO. See *Pittosporum*.

KATSURA TREE. See *Cercidiphyllum japonicum*.

KAVA-KAVA. See *Piper*.

KAWA-KAWA. See *Macropiper*.

Keckiella. 2 ✪

Many species, all native to the U.S. and most of the West; most are hardy to zone 7 and do well in warm, sunny areas. Drought-tolerant and attractive shrubs, subshrubs and vines, depending on species; all of them attract hummingbirds.

KEI APPLE. See *Dovyalis hebecarpa*.

KENTIA PALM. See *Howea*.

KENTUCKY COFFEE TREE. See *Gymnocladus dioica*.

KENYA IVY. See *Senecio*.

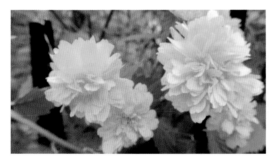

Kerria japonica. 2 ✪

(Pictured above.) Deciduous shrub for partial shade to zone 3. An easy-to-grow member of the rose family, its flowers resemble little double yellow roses.

Keteleeria. 3

Several species of tall evergreen trees, hardy to zone 8. Native to Asia and related to pines, Keteleeria are often grown in California. In the wild, they may reach 160 feet.

KEY PALM. See *Thrinax*.

KHAT. See *Catha edulis*.

KIKUYUGRASS, KIKUYU GRASS. See *Pennisetum clandestinum*.

KING PALM. See *Archontophoenix*.

KINNIKINNICK. See *Arctostaphylos*.

Kirengeshoma palmate. 4

WAXBELLS. A large, 4-foot-tall and as wide perennial for shady areas in zones 4 to 9 in slightly acid soils, with good moisture and a deep mulch. Blooms late in the season with bell-shaped yellow flowers. Related to Hydrangea.

KIWI. See *Actinidia*.

KLAMATHWEED. See *Hypericum*.

KLEINIA. See *Senecio*.

Knautia macedonica. 5

Short-lived perennials for zones 4 to 9 with very attractive flowers. Best not to use these as cut flowers, as they may shed more pollen if brought indoors.

Kniphofia uvaria (Tritoma). 4

POKER PLANT, RED-HOT POKER, TORCH LILY. Perennial hardy to zone 4 and easy to grow. Tall spikes of red-orange-yellow flowers. Direct sniffing of these red flowers can trigger allergy.

KNOTWEED. See *Polygonum*.

Kochia. 6

BURNING BUSH, SUMMER CYPRESS. Annuals grown in all zones.

Koeleria. 8

WESTERN JUNE GRASS. A forage grass in the western United States.

Koelreuteria paniculata. 4

GOLDENRAIN TREE, VARNISH TREE. Large deciduous tree native to Asia, grown for its pendant, fragrant yellow flowers, followed by long-lasting clusters of seedpods shaped like Chinese lanterns. Common in California and hardy to zone 7.

KOHUHU. See *Pittosporum*.

Kolkwitzia amabilis. 3

BEAUTY BUSH. Deciduous shrub hardy to zone 4. Pink honeysuckle-like flowers with yellow throats bloom in early summer; the flowers are followed by bristly pink fruits.

KOREAN VELVET GRASS. See *Zoysia*.

KOWHAI. See *Sophora*.

KUDZU. See *Pueraria lobata*.

KUMQUAT. See *Citrus*; *Fortunella*.

K

Allergy Index Scale: 1 is Best, 10 is Worst.
✪ for 1 and 2   ✎ for 9 and 10
No matter what the ranking, always read the full plant description carefully and take note of any warnings.

LABIATAE. See *Mentha.*

Laburnum. 7

GOLDENCHAIN TREE. Deciduous tree, hardy to zone 4. Produces long chains of pealike yellow flowers. The three-lobed leaflets resemble clover leaves. Often confused with another yellow flowering deciduous tree, *Koelreuteria paniculata,* the goldenrain tree. The trees produce a quantity of seeds and pods, and this seed is very poisonous if eaten. All parts of the Laburnum are highly toxic. Children have been poisoned from simply sucking on fresh Laburnum flowers. Pollen can trigger legume allergy.

LACEBARK. See *Hoheria.*

LACEBARK, QUEENSLAND. See *Brachychiton discolor.*

Lachenalia. 2 ✪

CAPE COWSLIP. Bulb for zone 10.

LADIES'-TOBACCO. See *Antennaria.*

LADY FERN. See *Athyrium.*

LADY PALM. See *Rhapis.*

LADY SLIPPER. See *Cypripedium.*

LAELIA. See *Orchids.*

Lagerstroemia indica. 5

CRAPE MYRTLE. Hardy to zone 6, crape myrtle does best where summer days are bright and hot. Crape myrtle is not related to the true myrtles, and allergy to its flowers is not well documented, despite the fact that it produces a huge number of small flowers, each bearing an unusually high number (up to 200) of stamens (the male pollen parts). In cooler areas it blooms, but is susceptible to mildew, which may in itself contribute to allergy. Do not plant in shady areas.

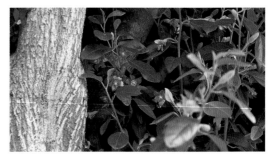

Lagunaria patersonii. 9 ✎

COW ITCH TREE, PATERSON PLUM, PRIMROSE TREE. (Pictured above.) An upright evergreen tree, hardy to zone 9. It bears attractive purple primroselike flowers, which are followed by seedpods filled with incredibly itchy, tiny hairlike fibers. Just opening one of these pods spreads the irritating hairs to hands, face, neck, and eyes, producing sudden, severe contact irritation.

Not a tree to spread a picnic blanket under. I once found a very large Lagunaria tree growing as a shade tree in the lunch area of an elementary school; a terrible choice of a tree for this spot.

LAMB'S EAR. See *Stachys byzantina*.

LAMIACEAE. See *Mentha*.

Lamiastrum galeobdolon. 3
FALSE LAMIUM, YELLOW LAMIUM. A yellow-flowered perennial, hardy to zone 5. It has become a serious invasive plant in the northwestern U.S.

Lamium. 5

Lamium maculatum. MALES 6, FEMALES 1 ✪
DEAD NETTLE. Perennial hardy to zone 3, occasionally used as a hanging basket plant or ground cover. May become weedy. Thrives in moist soil and partial shade. Many cultivars but rarely sold sexed.

Lampranthus. 3
ICEPLANT, REDONDO CREEPER.

LANCEPOD. See *Lonchocarpus*.

LANCEWOOD. See *Pseudopanax*.

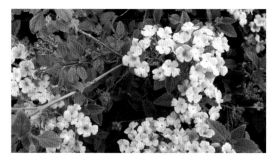

Lantana. 2 ✪ TO 6 DEPENDING ON CULTIVAR
(Pictured above.) Evergreen or deciduous shrubs or ground covers, hardy only in warm winter areas. The prickly leaves may cause skin rash for a few individuals. The odd scent of the flowers or crushed leaves also may make a few people nauseous. The green berries are highly poisonous. A few of the newer cultivars of Lantana are male-sterile and produce no pollen. The trailing purple form is a low-pollen plant.

Lapageria rosea. 2 ✪
CHILEAN BELLFLOWER. Evergreen vine hardy to zone 8. National flower of Chile, with large, rosy red flowers. Needs shade and ample water to thrive.

LARCH. See *Larix*.

Larix. 2 ✪
LARCH, TAMARACK. Deciduous conifer that loses its needles in winter. Hardy to coldest zones 1 and 2, larch does not tolerate warm climates. Slow growing and very long-lived, it will thrive in damp, poorly drained areas. The golden autumn color and attractive soft green of the emerging springtime foliage make the larch an attractive tree for most of the year.

LARKSPUR. See *Consolida ambigua*; *Delphinium*.

Larrea tridentata. 6
CREOSOTE BUSH. Evergreen shrub native to hot, desert areas. It produces small yellow flowers. The odd smell of these shrubs will bother some and the pollen affects others. Skin rash is possible from contact with the sap. In hot desert areas, far better choices for desert landscape shrubs would be native female selections of Grayia, Atriplex, or Forestiera (see all).

Latania. MALES 8, FEMALES 1 ✪
LATAN PALM. Three species of very attractive fan palms common to Florida. Separate-sexed; males cause allergy. Oval, brownish green fruit on female trees.

Lathyrus. 3
SWEET PEA. Lathyrus is fast growing from seed planted very early in the season and does best in cool summer areas. In warmer zones, the best stands of sweet pea are had by planting the seed in September, in loose soil in a sunny spot next to a fence or other support structure. *L. odoratus* is the common annual sweet pea. *L. littoralis* is a perennial vine that grows profusely all along the coast from Northern California to Washington. As a cut flower, the intense fragrance of some sweet peas may bother a few odor-sensitive individuals. Sweet peas are *not* to be confused with vegetable garden peas—all parts of Lathyrus are poisonous.

LAUREL. See *Antidesma*; *Laurus*; *Prunus*; *Umbellularia*.

LAUREL SUMAC. See *Rhus*.

Laurelia. MALES 8, FEMALES 1 ✪
Two species of tall evergreen trees from Chile grown in California. The 3-inch-long, rounded leaves are very glossy. Male plants are much more common than females.

Laurentia (Isotoma) fluviatilis. 1 ✪
BLUE STAR CREEPER, ISOTOMA. Very low-growing perennial for zones 7 to 11. Related to Lobelia, its tiny leaves and blue, star-shaped flowers make a beautiful ground cover for fall. Requires regular feeding and ample water to thrive.

Laurophyllus. MALES 10 🟢, FEMALES 1 ⊕
Small evergreen tree or shrub from South Africa.
Dioecious, but not sold sexed.

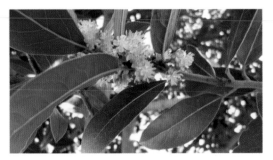

Laurus nobilis. MALES 9 🟢, FEMALES 1 ⊕
BAY, GRECIAN LAUREL, ROMAN LAUREL, ROYAL BAY,
SWEET BAY, SWEET LAUREL. (*Laurus nobilis*, male,
pictured above.) A large, fairly slow-growing evergreen
tree (or shrub) with aromatic leaves that are used in
cooking. Hardy to zone 6, the sweet bay is a popular
large container plant. The males of these separate-sexed
trees produce abundant allergenic pollen. Allergy to the
pollen is fairly common, and cross-reaction allergies
caused by eating foods flavored with the leaves are also
not uncommon. Laurus is not usually sold sexed except
for the cultivar 'Saratoga', which is a male and should
not be used. Several new female cultivars are now in
initial production and eventually will be sold with
#1 ranked OPALS tags on them (see chapter 4). Female
trees can be planted close together to make a thick
evergreen pollen-free hedge. Quite drought-tolerant,
it will grow in sun or shade, and is sometimes used in
cold winter areas as a houseplant.

LAURUSTINUS. See *Viburnum*.

Lavandula. 5
LAVENDER. Several species of evergreen, gray-leafed
shrubby plants with fragrant leaves and flowers used in
sachets and for perfumes. Although the pollen is rarely
allergenic, lavenders are a common cause of allergy in
those who are sensitive to perfumes and other strong
odors and is therefore not highly recommended. Oil
of lavender, made from the fresh flowers and leaves, is
known to cause skin rash. Plants and products from
these plants are quite estrogenic.

Lavatera. 3
TREE MALLOW. Annuals and subshrubs grown as
perennials in zones 9 to 13, and as fast-growing annuals or pot plants elsewhere. The rosy pink or lavender
flowers resemble hollyhock and are attractive to
hummingbirds. All mallows are easy to grow and
not fussy about soil or water.

LAVENDER. See *Lavandula*.

LAVENDER COTTON. See *Santolina*.

LAVENDER MIST. See *Thalictrum*.

LAVENDER STARFLOWER. See *Grewia occidentalis*.

Lawns.
Lawns are a leading factor in allergy in the United
States because of the pollen that they produce when
flowering, the airborne mildew and mold spores that
often thrive in turf, and the host of pollen-producing
weeds that are often part of the average lawn.

When selecting grass for a lawn, choose slow-
growing, disease-resistant varieties that do not flower
when kept mowed short. Tall fescues are good choices
for many areas because they do not bloom while short.
Ordinary (common) Bermuda grass lawns, on the other
hand, flower at almost any length and are constant,
year-round sources of potent allergenic pollen. Hybrid
Bermuda grass, however, grows more slowly, flowers
much less, and is a far better choice.

To keep a lawn in good shape it is necessary to
fertilize it regularly with high-nitrogen fertilizer, water
it frequently if needed, and keep it mowed weekly during the growing season. With some lawns (bent grass
or Bermuda, for instance), it may be necessary to mow
every two or three days. Keeping the blades on the
lawn mower sharp is always a good idea, too. (A note
about lawn fertilizer: Some lawns in warm areas may
benefit from as much as 8 pounds of actual nitrogen
per year per 1,000 square feet. To simplify this, with
a common high-nitrogen fertilizer like ammonium
sulfate [21-0-0], these lawns could use up to 40 pounds
annually on a section of lawn that measures about
35 by 30 feet.)

Most lawn grasses release their pollen in the early
morning, and it is best to mow later in the day to reduce
the amount of pollen scattered by the mower blades. Do
not mow grass when it is still damp from dew or rain
because this can cause fungus diseases to spread. Many
people who are allergic to grass pollen will also be allergic to the gases (VOCs) given off during mowing. If you
are highly allergic to grass, get someone else to cut it for
you, or consider planting a low-allergy ground cover.

Spraying or spreading chemical insecticides on
your lawn is not recommended, because in many cases
these lawn chemicals cause allergies themselves.

Likewise, the products that fertilize grass and kill dandelions at the same time ("weed & feed") are not safe either. They have been implicated as causing leukemia in cats and dogs that play on treated lawns. If they can cause cancer in cats and dogs, they can't be all that good for kids or adults either.

If bald spots occur in a good lawn they should be worked up and replaced with new sod; or seed, fertilizer, and mulch should be sprinkled on the problem spot. When trying to grow a lawn from seed it is good policy to cover the seed with at least ¼ inch of old manure or similar mulch. If bare spots are left in a lawn, they are usually quickly filled with broadleaf weeds or with annual bluegrass (*Poa annua*), which blooms at almost any height and causes allergy.

The development of all-female and low-pollen-producing lawn grass cultivars offers much promise for allergy-free lawns of the future. For further information on lawn grasses, see Agropyron (quackgrass); *Arrhenatherum elatius* (tall oatgrass); Bromus (brome grass); *Buchloe dactyloides* (buffalo grass); Distichlis (saltgrass), *Pennisetum clandestinum* (kikuyugrass), and Poa (bluegrasses). Look for lawn grasses sold with an OPALS #1 ranked female tag. It is perfectly possible to now have all-female lawns, and even all-female pastures.

LAWSON CYPRESS. See *Chamaecyparis*.

Layia platyglossa. 3
TIDYTIPS. California native flowering annual. Fast-growing in sunny areas.

LEATHERLEAF. See *Viburnum*.

LEATHERLEAF FERN. See *Rumohra adiantiformis*.

Lechea. 5
A wildflower native to the northeastern United States and related to the rockrose, the seed is occasionally used in wildflower mixes. Suspected of causing limited allergy, Lechea grows best in dry, sandy soils.

Ledebouria socialis. 2 ✪
JESSOP. Bulbous, succulent-leafed houseplants that need bright light to grow well.

Ledum. 4
Hardy shrubs for cold, damp areas. Related to heather.

Leitneria floridana. MALES 6, FEMALES 1 ✪
CORKWOOD. Small separate-sexed, deciduous trees or shrubs, native to wet forest areas of the southeastern United States.

LEMAIREOCEREUS THURBERI. See *Cactus*.

LEMON. See *Citrus*.

LEMON VERBENA. See *Aloysia triphylla*.

LEMONADE BERRY. See *Rhus integrifolia*.

LENTEN ROSE. See *Helleborus*.

Leonotis. 5
LION'S EAR, LION'S TAIL. Orange flower spikes on tall, erect, frost-tender perennials. Odd-smelling (but not unpleasant) leaves. A member of the mint family. Possible contact allergy problems.

Leontopodium alpinum. 5
EDELWEISS. Low-growing woolly leafed hardy perennial, usually with white flowers.

LEOPARD FLOWER. See *Belamcanda chinensis*.

LEOPARD PLANT. See *Ligularia*.

LEOPARD'S BANE. See *Doronicum*; *Senecio*.

Lepechinia. 2 ✪
PITCHER SAGE. Large shrubby perennials best in zones 7 to 11, with some shade in hottest areas. Fairly drought-tolerant and easy to grow, *L. fragrans* is native to California and is pollinated by bumblebees. Salvia-like flowers on these Salvia relatives.

Lepidorrhachis. 7
Subtropical palm trees common in Florida.

Lepidozamia. MALES 8, FEMALES 1 ✪
Palmlike plants from Australia, grown in zone 10. Dioecious, but not sold sexed.

Leptinella squalida. 5
BRASS BUTTONS. A small, low-growing perennial hardy to zone 5. White flowers appear to have some potential for allergy.

Leptodermis oblonga. 2 ✪
Perennials from China hardy to zone 4, many lilac-pink flowers on tidy plants that attract butterflies. Easy to grow in full or partial sunny spots. A high-nectar, low-pollen plant.

Leptospermum. 4
MANUKA, TEA TREE. Small native Australian tree bearing many tiny, attractive flowers. Best in zones 9 to 11.

Lespedeza bicolor. 5
SHRUBBY LESPEDEZA. Nonnative flowering perennial in the pea family. Very high potential for becoming invasive. Not recommended.

L

Leucaena pulverulenta. 4

A south Texas native flowering tree, hardy only in warmest parts of zone 10, and also in zones 11 to 13.

Leucodendron. MALES 6, FEMALES 1 ✪

SILVER TREE. Large group of evergreen shrubs and trees from South Africa, often used as landscape plants in coastal California. These are separate-sexed, but not usually sold sexed. Look for some female selections with OPALS #1 tags. Hardy only to zone 9.

Leucojum. 2 ✪

SNOWFLAKE. Hardy spring-blooming bulbs.

Leucophyllum frutescens. 2 ✪

TEXAS RANGER. Native Texas tall desert shrub with gray leaves and rosy purple bell-shaped flowers. Drought-tolerant.

Leucospermum. 3

PINCUSHION. Shrubby Protea relative with long clusters of showy tubular flowers; difficult to grow outside of zones 10 to 13.

Leucothoe. 4

FETTERBUSH, SIERRA LAUREL. Evergreen shrub native to southeastern United States, hardy to zone 5. Needs moist, acid soil with good drainage and partial shade to thrive. Produces tall spikes of white flowers. All parts of plant are extremely poisonous.

Levisticum officinale. 3

LOVAGE. Hardy perennial herb grows to 6 feet. Aromatic seeds.

Lewisia. 1 ✪

BITTERROOT. Hardy perennials with succulent-like leaves and clusters of white, pink, or red flowers; good choice for rock gardens. Plants need perfect drainage.

Liatris. 4

BLAZING STAR, GAYFEATHER. Tall, showy perennials with spikes of white- or rose-colored flowers. Many fine species of hardy natives, hardy to zone 3, and all of them make excellent pollinator plants.

LIBOCEDRUS. See *Calocedrus decurrens*.

LICHI NUT. See *Litchi chinensis*.

Licuala. 1 ✪

A large group of small palm trees, some hardy into zone 9. They are good in containers and occasionally used as houseplants.

LICURI PALM. See *Syagrus*.

LIGNUM-VITAE. See *Guaiacum sanctum*.

Ligularia (Farfugium). 5

LEOPARD PLANT. Foliage plant hardy in zones 6 to 10; elsewhere a houseplant grown for its long, leathery, thick leaves.

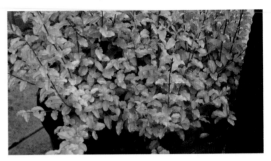

Ligustrum. 9 (SEE EXCEPTION) ✪

PRIVET. (Pictured above.) Deciduous or evergreen shrubs or small trees, often used as hedges in all parts of the United States. Privet is among our most common landscape shrubs, but as members of the olive family, it presents several serious allergy problems. The fragrance of the many small white flowers may cause allergy in odor-sensitive people, and the pollen from the flowers also causes an often severe reaction, especially in people already allergic to olive pollen. Keep privet hedges low and well pruned to discourage blooming. Plants and seeds are poisonous and plants are often highly invasive.

Exception: There is a new evergreen privet, the golden leaf 'Ligustrum Sunshine', now sold through the Sunset Magazine Western Garden Collection, and it is nonflowering, so it has very little allergy potential, if any.

LILAC. See *Syringa*.

Lilium. 4

LILY. Numerous varieties of bulbous perennials, hardy in most zones. Like most bulbs, they require fertile, well-drained soil to thrive. Allergy to lily pollen is not common, despite the fact that it is held on exposed stamens and easily contacted. The pollen is heavy and not designed by nature to travel far in the air, and the petals of all lilies are large, highly colored, and attractive to insect pollinators. There are now a few pollen-free selections of lilies being sold. People handling large numbers of lily bulbs, especially those working in fields or packing houses, frequently develop contact rashes from the bulbs. As cut flowers the fragrance of some lilies can be slightly offensive. Many lilies are poisonous if eaten.

LILLY-PILLY TREE. See *Acmena smithii; Syzygium.*

LILY. See *Lilium.*

LILY-OF-THE-NILE. See *Agapanthus.*

LILY-OF-THE-VALLEY. See *Convallaria majalis.*

LILY-OF-THE-VALLEY BUSH. See *Pieris.*

LILY-OF-THE-VALLEY TREE. See *Clethra arborea; Crinodendron; Liriope; Oxydendrum.*

LILYTURF. See *Liriope.*

LIME. See *Citrus.*

LIME TREE. See *Tilia.*

LIMELEAF MAPLE. See *Acer distylum.*

Limonium. 3
SEA LAVENDER, STATICE. Annuals and perennials, some hardy to zone 3. Easy to grow, these make good long-lasting dried flowers.

Linanthus. 3
Group of annuals and a few perennials, some California natives.

Linaria. 1 ✿
TOADFLAX. Annuals and perennials, with flowers resembling those of snapdragon.

LINDEN. See *Tilia.*

Lindera. MALES 6, FEMALES 1 ✿
BENJAMIN BUSH, JOVE'S FRUIT, SPICEBUSH. Many species of small trees and shrubs, most from Asia but some native to the U.S. and Canada, hardy in zones 4 to 10, depending on species. Separate-sexed, the males can cause limited allergies. Females are identified by the small, black, single-seeded berries that change from green, to red, to black. Plants grow well in shade to semi-shade, in moist, acid soils.

LINGONBERRY. See *Vaccinium.*

Linnaea borealis. 1 ✿
TWINFLOWER. Small evergreen subshrub hardy to zone 2. Bears small, twinned, tubular rose or white flowers. Thrives in moist, peaty, acidic soil. This is the only plant that the great Swedish botanist Carl Linnaeus, developer of the binomial system of biological nomenclature, named for himself.

Linum. 4
FLAX. Blue-flowered (some ornamental ones are red) annuals and perennials. These are mostly the field crops grown in cool areas for their oil-producing seed and for the fiber used to produce linen. Allergy to flax flowers is usually limited to those living close to large fields of blooming flax, and even then is uncommon.

LION'S EAR, LION'S TAIL. See *Leonotis.*

LIPPIA. See *Phyla nodiflora.*

LIPSTICK PLANT. See *Aeschynanthus.*

Liquidambar. 6
SWEET GUM. Large, deciduous trees, native to the eastern United States and Asia. Very popular street trees in many cities, sweet gum is hardy in zones 5 to 10. They are prized for their brilliant scarlet autumn color, in which they resemble maples; but unlike maples, sweet gums produce a quantity of small, prickly round seed capsules in late summer.

The trees are monoecious, having both sexes on the same tree but not in the same flowers, and thus rely on the wind for pollination. Allergic reaction to Liquidambar pollen is usually not severe.

Sap from the Asian sweet gum is used to make aromatic storax, which is used in incense and perfumes. Allergy to storax itself is not uncommon. These trees can drop considerable moderately allergenic pollen almost directly underneath them; do not plant them where this pollen will be tracked into the house.

Liriodendron. 3
TULIP POPLAR, TULIP TREE, YELLOW POPLAR. A handsome, large, fast-growing native deciduous tree, hardy in zones 3 to 10. The tulip tree has large, beautiful lyre-shaped leaves, grows to 100 feet, has deep roots, and is tolerant of a very wide array of soil and weather conditions, including city environments. It has good fall color and attractive, large, yellow-orange, tulip-shaped flowers in the spring. Tulip trees do not transplant easily and are not as commonly used as they might well be. Good, low-allergy city trees, tulip poplars should be used much more than they are now.

Liriope. 3
LILY-OF-THE-VALLEY-TREE, LILYTURF, MONDO GRASS. Grassy evergreen flowering perennials, some hardy to zone 3. Members of the lily family, and similar to the genus *Ophiopogon*, they produce spikes of small, showy lilac or white flowers and grow best in partial shade.

LISIANTHUS. See *Eustoma grandiflorum.*

Litchi chinensis. 4
LICHI NUT, LYCHEE NUT. Evergreen tree only suitable for the warmest, mildest winter areas of zone 10. It

grows best in moist, acid soil. The fruit is popular in Asian cuisine and has a sweet, unusual taste.

Lithocarpus densiflorus. 6

TANBARK OAK. Evergreen tree native to the West Coast and not hardy north of zone 7. An oak relative, the male flowers of Lithocarpus are malodorous, although rarely a serious allergen.

Lithodora diffusa (Lithospermum). 2 ✪

Low, shrubby small perennial for partial shade in zones 7 to 12. Its leaves and stems are covered with fine hairs and the plant bears small, tubular, very bright, intense blue flowers.

Lithops. 1 ✪

FLOWERING STONES, LIVING STONES, STONEFACE. Unusual succulents best grown in pots and kept dry in cool weather. Plants look like small rocks and the flowers are surprisingly large for the size of the plants.

LITHOSPERMUM. See *Lithodora diffusa.*

Lithrea. 10 🌱

Three species of subtropical trees and shrubs from South America, used in zones 9 to 13, especially in California. Relatives of poison ivy, Lithrea bears creamy yellow lustrous flowers that produce highly allergenic pollen. One species in particular, *L. caustica*, is especially toxic. The flowers and seeds of this plant are poisonous, the pollen becomes airborne and is highly allergenic, and the sap can cause severe and painful skin rashes and swelling. Plants are dioecious but neither sex is desirable due to the potential for allergy and asthma.

Litsea. MALES 7, FEMALES 1 ✪

A large group of several hundred Laurel-related species of deciduous or evergreen, subtropical and tropical trees and shrubs, mostly from Australia and Asia. Popular landscape plants in zones 9 to 10. Dioecious but not yet sold sexed.

LITTLELEAF LINDEN. See *Tilia.*

LIVE FOREVER. See *Dudleya.*

LIVERLEAF. See *Hepatica.*

LIVING STONES. See *Lithops.*

LIVINGSTONE DAISY. See *Dorotheanthus bellidiformis.*

Livistona. 1 ✪

CHINESE FOUNTAIN PALM. Small- to medium-size Chinese and Australian fan palms, for zones 9 to 10. They are attractive trees with no allergy problems.

Loasaceae. 8

A large group of herbs used as ornamentals. All members of this species can cause skin irritation.

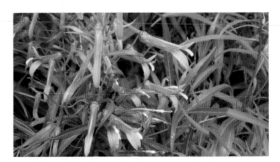

Lobelia. BISEXUAL 2 ✪, MALES 4, FEMALES 1 ✪

CARDINAL FLOWER. (*Lobelia laxiflora*, pictured above.) Popular perennials or annual bedding plants for full sun or partial shade in all zones. One species is a tall, red-flowered perennial for shady areas in zones 3 to 7. The annuals flower in shades of purple or blue. Lobelia is poisonous if eaten, but is occasionally used as an aid to quit smoking. Some of the tall perennial Lobelia species are dioecious, but they're not yet sold sexed.

LOBIVIA; LOBIVOPSIS. See *Cactus.*

LOBSTER-CLAW. See *Heliconia.*

Lobularia maritima. 5

SWEET ALYSSUM. A fast-growing annual or short-lived perennial with thousands of tiny white, pink, or purple flowers. Plants will not overwinter outside of zones 9 to 10 but will often reseed themselves. Alyssum is heavily fragrant in hot weather, and the smell can cause allergy for some. The leaves and flowers of sweet alyssum also are known to sometimes cause skin rash. Alyssum may spread and become weedy in certain locations. A few alyssum in the garden is not much of a problem, but don't overdo this one.

LOCOWEED. See *Datura; Oxytropis.*

LOCUST. See *Robinia.*

Lodoicea. MALES 8, FEMALES 1 ✪

DOUBLE COCONUT PALM. A tall palm, rare in cultivation; separate-sexed with males capable of causing allergy.

LOGANBERRY. See *Rubus.*

Logania. 4

Large group of mostly Australian herbs and shrubs used in zones 8 to 10.

Lolium. 9 ✺

DARNEL, RYEGRASS. There are several types of rye-grasses: *L. perenne*, or perennial ryegrass, *L. multiflorum*, or Italian ryegrass, and a hybrid of the above two species. Ryegrass pollen is a common, widespread, and often severe allergen in all parts of the United States. Most of this pollen, however, is not coming from lawns: ryegrass must usually be over a foot tall before it flowers and most lawns never reach that height. Almost all ryegrass allergy comes from plants escaped as weeds or grown in pastures as forage crops. Nonetheless, because allergy to ryegrass pollen is so common, cross-allergic reactions to the volatile oils released when ryegrass lawns are mowed are also reported.

A great deal of the world's supply of ryegrass seed is produced in central Oregon; this seed crop is, of course, allowed to flower, and early summer allergy to ryegrass in this area is intense.

In many areas of the southern United States it is common practice to overseed dormant Bermuda grass lawns with annual ryegrass, and these lawns, if not mowed often, can contribute to wintertime grass allergy in these areas. (Note: Ryegrass is not the same as rye, *Secale cerale*, a grain crop.)

Lomandra. MALES 7, FEMALES 1 ✪

Large attractive clumping ornamental grasses. At the time of this writing all the named cultivars appear to be male, but seedling plants are also sold, and they could be either sex. *L. hystrix* 'Tropic Belle' is a male. *L. confertifolia* 'Seascape', *L. longifolia* 'Breeze', and *L. longifolia* 'Nyalla' are also male plants.

LOMARIA. See *Blechnum*.

Lonas annua. 5

Annual for all zones. Umbel-shaped flowers on erect stems resemble yarrow.

Lonchocarpus. 4

LANCEPOD. Evergreen tropical trees from which the botanical insecticide rotenone is derived. One species, *L. violaceus*, has long leaves covered in translucent dots and drooping chains of long tubular flowers that are white on the outside and purple on the inside. It is a common plant in Florida. Lonchocarpus is a member of the legume family.

Lonicera. 5 TO 6

HONEYSUCKLE, TWINBERRY, WOODBINE. Many species of evergreen and deciduous shrubs and vines, some hardy to zone 3. Because it is such a common landscape plant, and large numbers of people have long been exposed to the sweet, pervasive scent, allergy to the fragrance is not uncommon. Pollen from honeysuckle has also occasionally been implicated in allergy but is fairly rare. In some southern states *L. japonica*, the Japanese honeysuckle, has become invasive, naturalized, and is rapidly taking over large areas of native woodland plants. This evergreen honeysuckle has a slightly higher potential (6) for allergy than other species.

LOOSESTRIFE. See *Lythrum*.

Lophomyrtus. 5

Smaller evergreen shrubs from New Zealand for zones 9 to 10; they look quite similar to small-leafed Coprosma plants, but are not dioecious.

Lophophora. 1 ✪

MESCAL BUTTON, PEYOTE. Small spineless cacti, native to Texas and northern Mexico. The crowns of these succulent plants yield the hallucinogenic alkaloid known as peyote, used by Native Americans of these areas.

Lophostemon confertus. 5

BRISBANE BOX. Evergreen tree for zones 9 to 13, white flowers, related to Eucalyptus but not as allergenic as most Eucalyptus.

LOQUAT. See *Eriobotrya*.

Loropetalum chinense. 4

Evergreen shrubs bearing small clusters of greenish white, pink, or red flowers; hardy in zones 7 to 10. Many different cultivars, some with reddish or bronze-colored foliage.

Lotus. 3

PARROT BEAK, TREFOIL. Many species of evergreen shrubs and herbs. *L. berthelotii*, parrot beak, is a spreading red-flowered, frost-tender perennial. *L. corniculatus*, bird's-foot trefoil, is a low-growing, very cold-hardy perennial with yellow flowers resembling pea blossoms; it is used as a ground cover or as a pasture legume.

LOVAGE. See *Levisticum officinale*.

LOVE APPLE. See *Solanum*.

LOVE-IN-A-MIST. See *Nigella damascena*.

LOVE-LIES-BLEEDING. See *Amaranthus*.

LOVEJOY. See *Episcia*.

LUCKY TREE. See *Thevetia*.

LULO. See *Solanum*.

Luma apiculata (Myrtus luma). 4

AMOMYRTUS. Large evergreen shrub or small tree for zones 9 to 10. Related to the myrtles, which it resembles.

Lunaria annua. 4

HONESTY, MONEY PLANT. Easy-to-grow biennial for sun or shade in all zones. Honesty bears purple flowers on erect stalks that are followed by paper-thin, translucent pods that are often used for dried flower arrangements. On rare occasions people are allergic to these dried flowers, although almost no one is allergic to the flowers themselves in the garden. Dried leaves of silver-dollar Eucalyptus are also sometimes sold as "money plant" and these too can on occasion trigger allergy from their odor.

LUNGWORT. See *Pulmonaria*.

Lupinus. 3

LUPINE. Annuals, perennials, or subshrubs of the legume family. All lupines need good drainage and full sun. When used as cut flowers, the pollen may pose an allergy problem. All parts of the plant are poisonous if eaten. As with any flowering legume relative, it is not a good idea to use these as cut flowers inside the house if there are any people living there who have soy or peanut allergies.

LYCASTE. See *Orchids*.

LYCHEE NUT. See *Litchi chinensis*.

Lychnis (Viscaria). 3

CAMPION, CATCHFLY, MALTESE CROSS, MULLEIN PINK. Easy-to-grow annuals and perennials for sunny areas. Related to Dianthus, a few species are dioecious but are never sold sexed.

Lycium. 5

MATRIMONY VINE. Large group of deciduous or evergreen vines and shrubs of the potato family. Some species are separate-sexed but not sold sexed.

Lycopersicon lycopersicum. 3

TOMATO. Tomato plants are not an important allergy problem for many. A few people are bothered by the smell of tomato leaves and, in rare cases, develop rashes upon contact with the leaves.

Lycopodium. 10 🚫

CLUB MOSS, GROUND CEDAR, GROUND PINE, PRINCESS PINE, RUNNING MOSS, RUNNING PINE. Native species used as ground cover for moist, shady areas. Occasionally used in hanging baskets. These are not flowering plants but spore-bearing mosses that produce a vast number of spores. Lycopodium spores are gathered for many industrial uses; as a result, exposure to Lycopodium is quite common. The spores are still used in some cosmetics and, because of their high flammability, in fireworks. Swags of bright green Lycopodium are often brought indoors at Christmas time to use as decorations. Allergic response to Lycopodium spores is fairly common and often unusually severe, typical of which are hay fever and serious rash from contact. Those suffering an allergy to molds and spores should be careful around fireworks, and check all cosmetics to see whether Lycopodium is listed as an ingredient. Poisonous if eaten.

LYCORIS. See *Lilium*.

Lygodium japonicum. 4

Climbing ferns for shady areas of zones 8 to 10. They need ample moisture to thrive.

Lyonia. 7

Shrubs grown in cool, moist soils of zones 6 to 10. All parts of Lyonia are poisonous if eaten, making the plants dangerous to livestock. Contact with the leaves and sap may cause skin rash.

Lyonothamnus floribundus. 4

CATALINA IRONWOOD. Evergreen native shrub or tree, to 60 feet. Needs good drainage and grows best near the coast. The clusters of small white flowers do not drop off cleanly after blooming. Drought-tolerant.

Lysiloma thornberi. 5

FEATHER BUSH. An Arizona native fernlike shrub or small tree for desert areas of zones 8 to 12; deciduous in the desert but may be semievergreen elsewhere. It bears small white flowers.

Lysimachia ciliata. 2 ✪

FRINGED YELLOW LOOSESTRIFE. A 3-foot-tall perennial, well adapted to wet soils, hardy in zones 2 to 7. Not an allergy problem plant, but all species of Lysimachia have some potential to be invasive. This species is unusual because it uses an oil rather than nectar to draw pollinators. Pollinated by honeybees, bumblebees, and other native bees. Not related to purple loosestrife (see below).

Lythrum. 4

PURPLE LOOSESTRIFE. Hardy, very invasive tall perennials for bogs and wetlands.

Maackia. 3
Easy-to-grow Asian native deciduous shrubs or trees,
hardy to zone 3. They bear clusters of pealike white
flowers.

Macadamia. 3
MACADAMIA NUT TREE, QUEENSLAND NUT. Easy-to-
grow tree wherever there is little frost, as in zone 10.
Fast-growing from seed. Leaves are sharp-toothed and
resemble holly. It bears small white flowers in winter,
followed by the edible nuts.

MACARTHUR PALM. See *Ptychosperma*.

Macfadyena unguis-cati (*Doxantha*). 3
CAT'S CLAW, YELLOW TRUMPET VINE. Drought-tolerant
perennial vine for zones 8 to 10 that grows best with
good summer heat. Bears bright yellow, trumpet-
shaped flowers and large, round, deep green leaves.
Claw-shaped tendrils make it able to cling to masonry.
Can grow to 30 feet.

Macleaya microcarpa. 4
CORAL PLUME POPPY. A very large perennial with tall
spikes of coral-colored flowers. Hardy to zone 3, this big
perennial poppy does best in moist, well-drained sandy
soils in part shade.

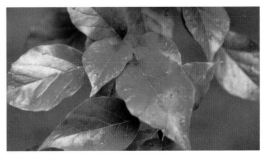

Maclura pomifera. MALES 9 ✎, FEMALES 2 ✪
BOWDOCK, BOWWOOD, HEDGE APPLE, OSAGE
ORANGE. (Pictured above.) A thorny, deciduous separate-
sexed tree, occasionally used for large hedges, common
throughout the eastern United States. The wood is used
to make strong, supple archery bows. Female Osage
orange bears large, softball-size, round, inedible fruits
called Osage apples or hedge apples, which are used to
repel cockroaches. These female trees, which produce no
pollen, make good choices for the allergy-free landscape.

The milky sap of Maclura is a contact allergen and
the pollen is also allergenic. A member of the mulberry
family, Osage orange is very easy to grow and transplant. Male trees can be identified by the flowers, which
are small, dull yellow balls on short stalks. Female trees
bear larger, round, green ball-shaped flowers. There are
a few selected, asexually grown clones, such as 'Fan
d'Arc' and 'Altamont', but these are all pollen-producing
males. Leaves are poisonous.

Macropiper. **MALES 7, FEMALES 1 ☮**
KAWA-KAWA, PEPPER TREE. Attractive shrubs or small trees from New Zealand. Rare in the United States.

Macrozamia. **MALES 8, FEMALES 1 ☮**
A group of separate-sexed palms from Australia, grown in zone 10.

MADAGASCAR JASMINE. See *Stephanotis.*

MADAGASCAR PERIWINKLE. See *Catharanthus roseus.*

MADAGASCAR PLUM. See *Flacourtia.*

MADEIRA NUT. See *Juglans.*

MADEIRA VINE. See *Anredera.*

Madhuca indica. **7**
BUTTER TREE, MAHUA TREE. Large evergreen tree native to India and the source of considerable pollen allergy there. Zones 10 to 13.

MADRONE, MADRONO. See *Arbutus.*

MAGIC FLOWER. See *Cantua buxifolia.*

Magnolia. **LARGE DECIDUOUS 6, EVERGREEN AND SMALL DECIDUOUS 4 TO 5**
Evergreen or deciduous trees and shrubs, for zones 3 to 11, depending on species.

M. acuminata, the cucumber tree or sweet bay, is a very large, tall, common deciduous shade tree hardy in zones 4 to 10. This species is ranked 6, and causes allergies where it is used to line entire city blocks.

M. denudata, the large Chinese white magnolia or lily tree, bears very large white flowers and is hardy in zones 3 to 10.

M. grandiflora, the common bull bay or southern magnolia tree, is a common evergreen tree that gets quite tall and wide and bears large, cup-shaped fragrant white flowers. It is hardy in zones 5 to 10.

M. soulangiana, the saucer magnolia or tulip tree, is a deciduous, often shrubby small tree that puts on a big display of flowers early in spring before the leaves appear. It is good for areas where late frosts are a problem.

Allergy to Magnolia is only occasional and allergic response to the pollen is usually moderate, not severe. Those who live on a block lined with big Magnolias, or who have a large Magnolia in their own yard, have a much greater chance of becoming hypersensitive than others.

Because deciduous Magnolias produce most of their flowers abundantly early in the year, their total bloom is much heavier than that of the evergreen varieties, which bloom off and on throughout much of the year.

The fragrance from some of the deciduous Magnolias, especially the cucumber tree, may cause negative odor challenges for some individuals.

MAGNOLIA VINE. See *Schisandra.*

MAHERNIA. See *Hermannia verticillata.*

Mahoberberis miethkeana. **2 ☮**
Hardy evergreen shrubs related to barberry. Its dense growth habit, thick, round leaves, and sharp spines make it useful as a barrier shrub.

MAHOGANY. See *Swietenia.*

MAHOGANY, MOUNTAIN. See *Cercocarpus.*

Mahonia aquifolium. **2 ☮**
CALIFORNIA HOLLY GRAPE, OREGON GRAPE. Evergreen shrubs for zones 5 to 10, with thick, glossy leaves and edible (but tasteless) fruits.

MAIDENHAIR FERN. See *Adiantum.*

MAIDENHAIR TREE. See *Ginkgo biloba.*

MAIDEN'S WREATH. See *Francoa ramosa.*

MALABAR PLUM. See *Syzygium.*

MALAY APPLE. See *Syzygium.*

Malcolmia maritima. **1 ☮**
VIRGINIAN STOCK. A fast-growing, unscented annual for full sun. (See also *Matthiola.*)

MALE LINDEN. See *Tilia.*

MALLEE. See *Eucalyptus.*

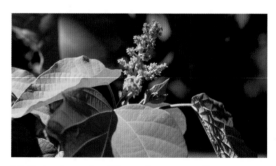

Mallotus japonica (Croton). **MALES 9 ☙, FEMALES 1 ☮**
(Pictured above.) A small, evergreen, separate-sexed tree from China and Japan, hardy only in zone 10. Large green leaves start out as red, resembling poinsettia bracts. Male flowers are yellowish green; female

flowers are reddish. Pollen from males is quite potent. Some potential for skin rash from contact.

MALLOW. See *Hibiscus*; *Lavatera*, *Malvaviscus drummondii*.

Malpighia glabra. 4
ACEROLA, BARBADOS CHERRY, WEST INDIAN CHERRY. An evergreen shrub occasionally raised commercially, especially in southern Florida. Hardy in zones 9 to 13, the bushes grow to 15 feet and produce high yields of a small fruit that has the highest content of vitamin C of any fruit—3,300 milligrams per 100 grams of fruit, almost 100 times more vitamin C than in an orange. The fruits, or cherries, may be red, purple, yellow, or orange, depending on the strain of seed used. Highly productive cultivars can be bought occasionally; there is great variability among the seedling-grown trees. Some trees bear leaves with tiny stinging hairs that can cause rash.

MALTESE CROSS. See *Lychnis*.

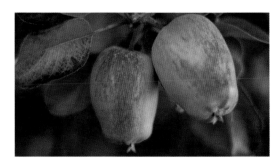

Malus. 3 TO 4 DEPENDING ON CULTIVAR
APPLE, CRABAPPLE. (Pictured above.) Apples and crab-apples are hardy in most zones and make handsome additions to the landscape.

Apple trees are not known to cause much allergy, but those living in or next to orchards may well develop hypersensitivity to the pollen. People who are allergic to roses have a greater chance of developing allergy to apple blossom pollen because they are both in the rose, or *Rosa*, family.

Apple pollen is heavy and does not travel far from the tree, so if planted away from the house, apples and crabapples present few allergy problems. Leaves and seeds are poisonous. A few strictly flowering crabapple cultivars are pollen-free.

Malvaviscus drummondii. 3
TEXAS SUPERSTAR. A red-flowered (sometimes pink) large perennial native to Texas, hardy to zone 7.

Bright-colored flowers on an easy-to-grow plant for sunny spots. Very drought-tolerant.

Mammea americana. 5
MAMEY. A tropical American fruit that looks, smells, and tastes much like an apricot. Large evergreen trees, they can occasionally be found in southern Florida. The leaves and sap of the mamey tree can cause rashes and serious swelling.

MAMMILLARIA. See *Cactus*.

MANCHURIAN MAPLE. See *Acer mandshuricum*.

MANDARIN ORANGE. See *Citrus*.

Mandevilla (Dipladenia). DECIDUOUS 4, EVERGREEN 2 ☻
Evergreen and deciduous vines. The evergreen vines are beautiful but are difficult to grow in most areas, even in milder parts of zone 10. The allergy potential from the evergreen Mandevilla is very low. The deciduous *M. laxa*, or Chilean jasmine, is much hardier (zones 7 to 10), has very fragrant white flowers, and is easier to grow than the evergreen species. It has a somewhat higher allergy potential because of the possibility of negative odor reactions.

Mangifera indica. COMPLETE-FLOWERED 5, MALES 10 ❧, FEMALES 3
MANGO. A tropical fruit tree for the mildest frost-free coastal areas of zone 10. It produces large, attractive, sweet fruit. Mango is an especially interesting allergy plant; the trees bear three kinds of flowers—male only, female only, and complete flowers with both male and female parts in the same flower. As a result of this system, some highly allergenic pollen becomes airborne.

As a relative of poison ivy and poison sumac, contact with the sap also may cause a rash. Typical of the allergic reactions to members of this group (Anacardiaceae), the onset of symptoms is delayed for several hours after exposure. Those who have already been overexposed to poison ivy or poison oak may well develop a cross-allergic reaction to eating mango.

MANGOSTEEN. See *Garcinia mangostana*.

MANGROVE PALM. See *Nypa*.

MANILA GRASS. See *Zoysia*.

MANILA PALM. See *Veitchia*.

MANUKA. See *Leptospermum*.

MANZANITA. See *Arctostaphylos*.

MANZANOTE. See *Olmediella betschlerana*.

MAPLE. See *Acer*.

Maranta leuconeura. 1 ✪
PRAYER PLANT. A houseplant, good in terrariums, that needs filtered light, warmth, and regular water.

MARGUERITE DAISY. See *Anthemis*; *Chrysanthemum*.

MARIGOLD. See *Tagetes*.

MARIPOSA LILY. See *Calochortus tolmiei*.

MARJORAM. See *Origanum majorana*.

MARKING-NUT TREE. See *Semecarpus*.

MARLOCK. See *Eucalyptus*.

MARMALADE BUSH. See *Streptosolen jamesonii*.

Marrubium vulgare. 2 ✪
HOREHOUND. Hardy perennial herb of the mint family.

MARSH GRASS. See *Spartina*.

MARSH MARIGOLD. See *Caltha palustris*.

MASCARENE GRASS. See *Zoysia*.

MASTERWORT. See *Astrantia*.

MATERNITY PLANT. See *Kalanchoe*.

MATILIJA POPPY. See *Romneya coulteri*.

Matricaria recutita. 5
CHAMOMILE. Plants smell like pineapple when crushed. The tea has been known to occasionally trigger anaphylactic shock, especially in those who already have existing ragweed allergies (both plants are composites, Sunflower family). See also *Chamaemelum nobile*.

MATRIMONY VINE. See *Lycium*.

Matthiola. 5
STOCKS. Perennial usually grown as annual. Erect flower stalks with many fragrant individual flowers of purple, white, rose, blue, or yellow. The pollen is of little concern. Common cut flowers, stocks have a powerful fragrance, and those with hypersensitivity to perfumes may be allergic to them.

MATTRESS VINE. See *Muehlenbeckia complexa*.

Mauritia flexuosa. MALES 8, FEMALES 1 ✪
MORICHE PALM. Tall fan palm tree from Trinidad. An exception to most fan palms, most of which are perfect-flowered and completely insect-pollinated, making them fine allergy-free landscaping choices. The moriche palm, however, is separate-sexed, and the pollen-producing males can cause allergy. Male moriche palms are identified by their taller and thinner trunks; females are stockier and produce small fruits.

MAYBUSH, MAYDAY TREE. See *Prunus padus*.

MAYFLOWER. See *Claytonia*.

MAYPOP. See *Passiflora*.

Maytenus boaria. 6
MAYTEN TREE. Small evergreen tree grown widely in zones 9 to 11. Resembling willows in appearance, they are related to Euonymus. These trees, when in full bloom, have numerous inconspicuous tiny, white-greenish flowers.

MAZARI PALM. See *Nannorrhops*.

Mazus reptans. 1 ✪
Hardy perennial ground cover with small clusters of flowers, blue with markings of yellow and white. A good rock garden plant that will not stand up to foot traffic.

MEADOW RUE. See *Thalictrum*.

MEADOW SAFFRON. See *Colchicum autumnale*.

MEADOWSWEET. See *Filipendula*.

Meconopsis. 3
HIMALAYAN POPPY. Many species, all with large, brightly colored flowers. Some species are long-lived, quite hardy perennials, while others will grow for a year or two and then will die soon after flowering (monocarpic). Best grown in zones 3 to 7.

MEDITERRANEAN FAN PALM. See *Chamaerops humilis*.

MEDLAR. See *Mespilus*.

MEEHANIA CORDATA. See *Mentha*.

Melaleuca. 7
BOTTLEBRUSH, CAJEPUT TREE, HONEY MYRTLE. Popular landscape trees and shrubs from Australia, used often in zones 9 to 13. Brushy flower stalks may be red, yellow, white, purple, or cream and, like true bottlebrush (Callistemon), the flowers have many exposed male stamens. Melaleuca occasionally has a strong smell and this may cause allergy in odor-sensitive people. *M. alternifolia* oil, claimed to cure almost anything, is widely marketed and may cause allergy. Cross-reactive responses between Melaleuca and Callistemon are common. Can be invasive in southern states. Because of their shape, this pollen will not travel far in the wind, but is a problem close to the plants themselves (proximity pollinosis).

Melampodium. 5

Perennial, frost-hardy daisy, native to southwestern United States and Mexico.

Melia. 4

ARBOR SANCTA, BEAD TREE, CHINA BERRY, FALSE SYCAMORE, HOLY TREE, PATERNOSTER TREE, PERSIAN LILAC, PRIDE OF CHINA, PRIDE OF INDIA, SYRIAN BEAD TREE, TEXAS UMBRELLA TREE. A wide deciduous tree, hardy in zones 7 to 10. The Melia produces quantities of poisonous seeds that are used for making rosaries. People have been poisoned by chewing on these rosaries, and even a small number of seeds can be fatal to children.

Melianthus. 5

HONEYBUSH. Frost-tender ornamental and medicinal herb for zone 10. Leaves give off foul odor when crushed.

Melicoccus. MALES 8, FEMALES 1 ✪

GENIPE, HONEYBERRY, SPANISH LIME. Tall (to 60 feet) dioecious tree for zones 10 to 13, commonly used in Florida. Female Melicoccus produce an edible green fruit, yellow inside. Not sold sexed, the males produce allergenic pollen, but the females are fine choices for the frost-free allergy-free landscape.

Melilotus. 5

SWEET CLOVER. Tall, bushy varieties of clover that bear small stalks of white or yellow flowers. These cause more allergy than low-growing, creeping varieties of clover.

Meliosma. 4

Rare, hardy tree from China. Scented flowers are greenish yellow.

MELITTIS MELISSOPHYLLUM. See *Mentha.*

Menispermum. MALES 6, FEMALES 2 ✪

MOONSEED, YELLOW PARILLA. Native woody vines, grown for their foliage. Moonseed is separate-sexed, and the males could cause allergy. Female vines can be recognized by their black fruits. Menispermum can be propagated by cuttings, and only the females, which are choices for the allergy-free landscape, should be encouraged. All parts are highly poisonous.

Mentha. 3

MINT, PENNYROYAL, PEPPERMINT. Hardy, grown for their intensely scented, sometimes flavorful foliage. All mints require ample moisture to thrive. Sometimes invasive herbs for all zones.

Recently, allergies to mint have started to show up around the world; this is probably related to the fact that so many consumer products, from mouthwash and toothpaste to shampoo and cough syrup, and a host of other products, all now include some form of mint. In the garden the mints and their relatives are normally marvelous plants, attractive to many pollinators, easy to grow, hardy, and low producers of pollen (relying instead on considerable nectar sources). However, perhaps due to this overexposure to mint for so many people, contact with mint family leaves and flowers is now slightly suspect, as is eating mint products and using mint in other forms. Once a mint allergy starts, then one can quickly become allergic to all the mint relatives.

Sometimes the allergic symptoms from mint exposure are very asthmalike, and can on occasion be considered dangerous. Most at risk would be people working with cut flowers from various members of Lamiaceae or Labiatae. I recently heard from a large cut flower company where workers cutting Caryopteris (a mint relative) flowers were breaking out with asthmalike symptoms along with headaches.

In addition to the above cautions, it is worth mentioning that mint (and also lavender), as a food or tea or as used in toiletries, has a highly phytoestrogenic potential. In this day and age when we are bombarded with xenoestrogens from plastics and from pesticides and other chemicals, we might all be wise to take a second look at our mint consumption. There is also evidence that too much estrogen can aggravate allergies, asthma, and autoimmune diseases. It is also suspect in breast cancer and prostate cancer, and in obesity.

Mentzelia. 2 ✪

BLAZING STAR, EVENING STAR. Hardy annuals and perennials for desert areas in full sun, with well-drained soil. Mentzelia grows to about 3 feet in some species and has large, bright yellow flowers with orange centers.

MERATIA. See *Chimonanthus.*

MERCURY. See *Chenopodium.*

Mertensia. 1 ✪

CHIMING BELLS, GIANT FORGET-ME-NOT, MOUNTAIN BLUEBELL, VIRGINIA BLUEBELL. Tall, blue-flowered, very hardy, shade-loving plants that need acid soil and ample moisture.

M

Meryta sinclairii. MALES 7, FEMALES 1 ✿
PUKA. Houseplant grown for its attractive large leaves, Meryta is occasionally grown outside in mild parts of zone 10 and in zones 11 to 13, where the plant may become a small tree. Native to New Zealand, the females of this separate-sexed species are a good choice for allergy-free households. Female plants make small, fleshy black fruits.

MESCAL BEAN. See *Sophora secundiflora.*

MESCAL BUTTON. See *Lophophora.*

Mespilus. 3
HOSEDOUP, MEDLAR. A thorny tree that bears white or pink blossoms followed by small, pear-shaped fruits that are picked green and allowed to ripen off the tree, where they develop a flavor similar to spiced applesauce. Budded trees are often grafted onto quince, pear, or hawthorn rootstocks.

MESQUITE. See *Prosopis.*

MESSMATE. See *Eucalyptus.*

Metasequoia glyptostroboides. 4
DAWN REDWOOD. A large, fast-growing deciduous conifer. A beautiful but messy tree that drops litter year-round. Related to cypress and with a flowering system seemingly well designed to produce allergy, this tree is, nonetheless, rarely implicated in allergy. The dawn redwood was long considered by botanists to be extinct until a few living trees were found in a small, isolated valley in China in the early 1950s. Seeds were brought to the United States, and trees are now fairly common. A big dawn redwood tree is growing at my house, and it is said to be the largest one in the United States.

Metrosideros. 6
POHUTUKAWA, NEW ZEALAND CHRISTMAS TREE. Evergreen trees or big shrubs native to New Zealand and common in zone 10 of California. They do best near the coast, where they produce red flowers. Source of some localized allergy.

MEXICAN BLUE PALM. See *Brahea armata.*

MEXICAN BUCKEYE. See *Ungnadia.*

MEXICAN BUSH SAGE. See *Salvia.*

MEXICAN FAN PALM. See *Washingtonia robusta.*

MEXICAN FIRE PLANT. See *Euphorbia.*

MEXICAN FLAME VINE. See *Senecio.*

MEXICAN GRASS TREE. See *Nolina longifolia.*

MEXICAN ORANGE. See *Choisya ternata.*

MEXICAN PALO VERDE. See *Parkinsonia aculeata.*

MEXICAN STAR. See *Milla biflora.*

MEXICAN SUNFLOWER. See *Tithonia rotundifolia.*

MEXICAN TEA. See *Chenopodium.*

MEXICAN TULIP POPPY. See *Hunnemannia.*

MICHAELMAS DAISY. See *Aster.*

Michelia. 3
BANANA SHRUB. Evergreen shrubs or trees for zone 10; their large, white flowers, which resemble those of Magnolia, smell like ripe bananas. They need fertile soil, ample water, and partial shade to grow well.

Microcachrys. MALES 7, FEMALES 1 ✿
CREEPING PINE. An evergreen shrub, native to Tasmania, and grown in zones 8 to 11. It is related to Podocarpus (not to pine). Female plants make strawberry-like red fruits.

Microcoelum (Lytocaryum). 6
WEDDEL PALM. Short palms from Brazil, grown in zones 9 to 10.

Microcycas. MALES 7, FEMALES 1 ✿
PALMA CORCHO. Medium-size palms from Cuba and used in zone 10.

Microlepia. 3
Shade-loving, dry-soil fern for zone 10.

MICROMERIA. See *Satureja.*

MIGNONETTE. See *Reseda odorata.*

MILK BARREL. See *Euphorbia.*

MILKBUSH. See *Euphorbia.*

MILKWEED. See *Asclepias.*

MILKWORT. See *Polygala.*

Milla biflora. 2 ✿
MEXICAN STAR. Bulbs for full sun in zones 9 to 10. The flat, star-shaped flowers are white with green stripes.

MILLET. See *Panicum.*

MILO. See *Sorghum.*

MILTONIA. See *Orchids.*

MIMOSA. See *Acacia; Albizia julibrissin.*

MIMOSA, PRAIRIE. See *Desmanthus.*

Mimosa pudica. **2** ✿

SENSITIVE PLANT. Small, fast-growing houseplant or annual. A slight touch on the little leaves and the leaves quickly fold up, to reopen later. It needs a bright window when grown inside.

Mimulus (Diplacus). **1** ✿

STICKY MONKEY FLOWER. Hardy native Californian subshrub that bears yellow or orange flowers that resemble monkey faces. An easy-to-grow, loosely structured plant that requires good drainage.

Mimusops elengi. **7**

INDIAN CHERRY TREE. A large, evergreen semitropical tree, the source of considerable pollen allergy in several countries, including India.

Mina lobata (Quamoclit). **4**

SPANISH FLAG. A perennial vine for zone 10; of the morning glory family, it has heart-shaped leaves and long red flowers that fade to yellow, then white. Fast growing from seed soaked overnight in warm water. Possible contact rash from the leaves.

MINER'S LETTUCE. See *Montia.*

MING ARALIA. See *Polyscias.*

MINIATURE FAN PALM. See *Rhapis.*

MINT. See *Mentha.*

Mirabilis jalapa. **3**

FOUR O'CLOCK. Drought-tolerant perennials from Peru, useful in zones 7 to 10, but grown as annuals elsewhere. Tuberous roots can be dug and stored in cold winter areas. The 2-inch, trumpet-shaped, red, yellow, or white flowers remain closed until afternoon. Four o'clocks are pollinated by night-flying moths, drawn in by the fragrance of the flowers. This same rich fragrance may affect odor-sensitive individuals. Roots are said to be hallucinogenic.

MIRACULOUS FRUIT. See *Synsepalum dulcificum.*

MIRROR PLANT. See *Coprosma repens.*

MIST FLOWER. See *Eupatorium.*

MISTLETOE. See *Phoradendron serotinum; Viscum cruciatum.*

MOCCASIN FLOWER. See *Cypripedium.*

MOCK ORANGE. See *Murraya paniculata; Philadelphus; Pittosporum.*

Mold.

Although not true plants, molds are common in gardens and landscapes, where they are both infectious agents for some plants and beneficial catalysts in the process of natural decomposition and decay. Allergy to mold (or especially to the spores of mold) is very common and contact should be avoided. Fruit, especially if left in plastic bags, will mold quickly, and handling moldy fruit releases quantities of airborne spores.

Fresh air and sunlight are the natural enemies of most molds. In the garden, limit mold growth with judicious watering, pruning, and thinning of overhead trees to allow direct sunlight to penetrate the canopy, and by planting to encourage good air circulation. Compost heaps often harbor molds and sensitive individuals should let someone else turn the heap. Plants infested with molds or mildews should be discarded, not composted.

Natural fertilizers, especially cow manure, often harbor many mold spores. Often when new lawns are planted and allergies erupt, the lawn grass is blamed when actually it is mold spores in the manure that trigger the reaction.

Plants that fail to thrive in the garden will often become targets for insects. Mold spores will land on the "honeydew" left from insects, quickly germinate, and grow rapidly. Soon the entire plant (and this can happen to trees, too) will look dirty. Actually, it is dirty, covered with mold spores and hence very allergenic. Such plants should be removed and trashed. All species of mold spores are allergenic.

MOLE PLANT. See *Euphorbia.*

Moluccella laevis. **2** ✿

BELLS OF IRELAND. Annuals grown for their unusual green flowers, borne on tall spikes.

Monadenium. **8**

Group of about fifty species of succulent subshrubs or herbs from eastern Africa, seldom seen in the United States. Allergenic pollen and caustic, allergenic sap.

Monarda. **3**

BEE BALM, HORSEMINT, OSWEGO TEA. Easy to grow in full sun or partial shade, these tall perennials are hardy in all zones. Large clusters of puffy, rosy red flowers are fragrant and attractive to butterflies and hummingbirds. The pungently scented leaves are used in tea. Pollen is not a problem, but the fragrance may affect a few.

MONDO GRASS. See *Liriope.*

MONEY PLANT. See *Lunaria annua.*

MONGOLIAN LINDEN. See *Tilia.*

MONK'S-PEPPER TREE. See *Vitex.*

MONKEY FLOWER. See *Mimulus.*

MONKEY PISTOL. See *Hura.*

MONKEY-HAND TREE. See *Chiranthodendron pentadactylon.*

MONKEY-PUZZLE TREE. See *Araucaria.*

MONKSHOOD. See *Aconitum.*

Monstera (Philodendron pertusum). 4
SPLIT-LEAF PHILODENDRON, SWISS CHEESE PLANT.
Frost-tender evergreen tropical and subtropical vines
for shady, protected areas of zones 9 and 10, and as
houseplants elsewhere. Easy to grow, these large-leafed
plants rarely flower indoors, but when they do, their
pollen may trigger reactions. Outside, these plants present little allergy potential. The sap of these tropicals
may also cause contact rash. All parts are poisonous.

Montanoa. 6
DAISY TREE. Large group of flowering shrubs or small
trees, native to Mexico and the New World tropics.
Hardy only in warmest parts of zone 10.

MONTBRETIA. See *Crocosmia*; *Tritonia triacanthos.*

MONTEZUMA CYPRESS. See *Taxodium.*

Montia. 1 ✿
MINER'S LETTUCE. Small herbs, many native, for moist,
shady areas or full sun along the coast. Very common
forest herb in the redwood areas. The edible leaves have
a spicy, peppery taste.

MOON CACTUS. See *Selenicereus.*

MOON FLOWER. See *Ipomoea.*

MOONSEED. See *Cocculus laurifolius*; *Menispermum.*

MOOSEBERRY. See *Viburnum.*

MORAEA. See *Dietes.*

MORAINE LOCUST. See *Gleditsia triacanthos.*

MORICHE PALM. See *Mauritia flexuosa.*

Moringa oleifera. 5
DRUMSTICK TREE. Tropical species (zones 11 to 13)
will not take any frost. Fast-growing tree from India
with many medicinal uses.

MORNING COCKLE. See *Silene.*

MORNING GLORY. See *Ipomoea.*

MORTON BAY CHESTNUT. See *Castanospermum australe.*

MORTON BAY FIG. See *Ficus.*

MORUS GENUS

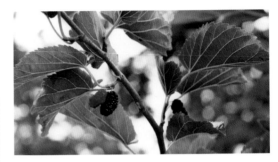

Morus. INDIVIDUALLY RANKED
MULBERRY. (Pictured above.) This large group of
deciduous trees, shrubs, vines, and herbs is very
important in the study of allergy. Different species
of Morus have distinct flowering systems, producing
varying degrees of allergy potential. Allergic reaction
to Morus pollen is often severe, and in some western
cities it is the primary cause of springtime asthma and
hay fever. Most species of Morus are separate-sexed,
and male trees are exceptionally allergenic and also
trigger considerable allergic asthma. All mulberry trees
are easily grown from dormant cuttings. They are also
quite easy to cleft-graft, and it is simple enough to graft
a male mulberry tree to scion wood from a female tree,
which will result in a sex change and, of course, a fruiting, nonpollinating tree. The highest pollen count
ever recorded in the U.S., more than 60,000 grains per
cubic yard of airspace, was from male (fruitless) mulberry trees, planted in an elementary school yard in Las
Vegas, Nevada.

M. alba. MALES 10 ✸, FEMALES 1 ✿
SILKWORM MULBERRY, WHITE MULBERRY. Trees may
be either male or female or, in a few rare cases, both.
There are some varieties sold for their fruit and these
need further study before they can be ranked. More
than a dozen kinds of *M. alba* are sold as fruitless
mulberries; these all-male varieties are to be avoided.
Fruitless mulberry trees, which are usually *M. alba*
cultivars, are among our very worst allergy trees in the
United States. *M. alba* 'Chaparral' is a newer weeping

male clone. *M. alba* 'Pendula' is a very fine female weeping form that makes very little fruit.

M. alba × *rubra* 'Illinois Everbearing'. 2 ✪
A hybrid cross between white and red mulberry, developed for fruit production. This tree is hardy to -25°F.

M. australis. **NOT YET RANKED**
AINO MULBERRY, JAPANESE MULBERRY, KOREAN MULBERRY. Heavy pollen producers; avoid use of male trees. Female, fruiting trees should be fine.

M. bombycis. 7
CHINESE MULBERRY.

M. nigra. 2 ✪
BLACK MULBERRY. A large tree hardy in zones 4 to 10. These are fruiting trees and although quite messy, not nearly as allergenic as some other species.

M. platanifolia. 10 🍃
Most of these are all-male clones and are therefore to be avoided.

M. rubra. **MONOECIOUS 6, MALES 8, FEMALES 1** ✪
AMERICAN MULBERRY, PURPLE MULBERRY, RED MULBERRY. A common large tree of the eastern United States, red mulberry is almost always a fruiting tree.

MOSES-IN-THE-CRADLE. See *Rhoeo spathacea*.

MOSS CAMPION. See *Silene*.

MOSS ROSE. See *Portulaca grandiflora*.

MOTH MULLEIN. See *Verbascum*.

MOTH ORCHID. See *Orchids*.

MOTHER-IN-LAW'S TONGUE. See *Sansevieria trifasciata*.

MOUNT ATLAS PISTACHE. See *Pistache*.

MOUNTAIN ASH. See *Sorbus*.

MOUNTAIN BLUEBELL. See *Mertensia*.

MOUNTAIN CAMELLIA. See *Stewartia*.

MOUNTAIN HOLLY. See *Nemopanthus*.

MOUNTAIN LAUREL. See *Kalmia*.

MOUNTAIN MAHOGANY. See *Cercocarpus*.

MOUNTAIN RIBBONWOOD. See *Hoheria*.

MOUNTAIN SPRAY. See *Holodiscus*.

MOURNING BRIDE. See *Scabiosa*.

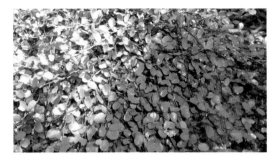

Muehlenbeckia complexa. **MALES 7, FEMALES 1** ✪
MATTRESS VINE, WIRE VINE. (Pictured above.) Fast-growing evergreen ground cover or hanging basket vines with wirelike stems and tiny green leaves, hardy in zones 6 to 10. Look for female wire vines sold with an OPALS #1 tag.

Mukdenia rossi. 2 ✪
A low-growing perennial deciduous ground cover for zones 4 to 9, does best in part shade. Green leaves turn bright red in fall. Small white flowers in spring and summer.

MUKU TREE. See *Aphananthe*.

MULBERRY. See *Broussonetia papyrifera*; *Morus*.

MULGA. See *Acacia*.

MULLEIN. See *Verbascum*.

MULLEIN PINK. See *Lychnis*.

Murraya paniculata. 6
MOCK ORANGE, ORANGE JESSAMINE. Evergreen shrubs or small trees for zone 10 in frost-free areas and partial shade. Fast-growing to 12 feet, the clustered white flowers have a jasmine fragrance and are very attractive to bees. Older shrubs bear small red fruits. The plants are used for big, loose hedges. The heavy fragrance may adversely affect odor-sensitive individuals. Pollen is allergenic.

Musa paradisiaca. 3
BANANA, PLANTAIN. Tall, frost-tender evergreen trees that produce bananas. To grow best they need ample water, fertile soil, warmth, and protection from wind. In cooler areas, bananas are grown in large pots and then moved inside when frost threatens. The flowers are eaten in many areas, usually boiled. The fruit should be left on the trees until almost ripe, and then picked and brought inside to ripen off the tree; bananas left to ripen on the tree often cause indigestion. Certain banana cultivars are pollen-free.

M

Muscari. 2 ✪

GRAPE HYACINTH. Bulbs hardy in all zones. The spring-blooming blue flowers are held on stalks rising above the grasslike foliage.

Mushrooms.

Mushrooms reproduce by spores, and spores, like pollen, may cause allergies. Large globe-shaped mushrooms called puffballs are common in many lawns and gardens. Stepping on these will release millions of airborne spores.

MUSTARD. See *Brassica*.

Myoporum. 2 ✪

Evergreen shrubs or trees mostly from New Zealand and Australia, for zones 9 to 10. Three species are commonly grown in Florida and California: *M. debile*, a low-growing ground cover; *M. laetum*, a fast-growing, drought- and salt-tolerant large shrub or small- to medium-size tree that attains its maximum size near the coast; and *M. parvifolium*, a tall ground cover for banks. All Myoporums are easy and fast growing, requiring initial watering until established, and then becoming quite drought-resistant. A leaf held up to the sun reveals the pores (myoporum) clearly. Wild birds eat the small reddish fruits.

Myosotis. 2 ✪

FORGET-ME-NOT.

Myrica. MONOECIOUS 6, MALES 9 ✇, FEMALES 1 ✪

BAYBERRY, CALIFORNIA WAX MYRTLE, CANDLEBERRY, COMPTONIA, PACIFIC WAX MYRTLE, SWAMP CANDLEBERRY, SWEET GALE, WAX MYRTLE. Evergreen or deciduous shrubs or trees, many native to the United States. All Myrica berries yield a wax that is used to scent candles and perfumes. Some people are sensitive to the smell of Myrica, and even more are allergic to the abundant pollen from the male plants. Many species of Myrica are separate-sexed, but female plants are hard to find. In the near future there will be some select all-female cultivars released of both northern and southern wax myrtle. These will be sold with an OPALS #1 ranked tag and will make great hedge plants. A heavy fruiting cultivar of California wax myrtle is also in the works. Wild birds eat the berries. Myrica is drought-tolerant once established, and also is generally pest-free.

    M. rubra, Chinese waxberry or strawberry tree, has edible fruit; dioecious, male plants are allergenic.

Myristica fragrans. MALES 7, FEMALES 1 ✪

NUTMEG. A large group of large tropical evergreen trees native to Indonesia, Grenada, and Australia, grown for their large brown seeds, which yield the spice nutmeg, and which are surrounded by a thin net or aril that is ground to yield the spice mace. Nutmegs are separate-sexed trees.

Myroxylon balsamum. 7

BALSAMO, PERU BALSAM TREE, QUINA. A large tropical tree from which the substance Peru balsam is made. This is used in many salves and creams and other products such as shampoo and soaps, and it is often quite allergenic. The tree itself is moderately allergenic. Not frost-tolerant, and also invasive in the tropics.

Myrrhis odorata. 4

SWEET CICELY. Hardy perennial, upright to 3 feet, sweet cicely roots are eaten fresh or cooked. The plants need fertile, moist soil and partial shade to thrive.

Myrsine. 1 TO 7, VARIES BY SPECIES AND SEX ✪

AFRICAN BOXWOOD, CAPE MYRTLE. A drought-tolerant shrub for zones 9 to 13, often used for foundation plantings and low hedges. The tiny (male) flowers cause allergy if the (male) plant is allowed to bloom. Most blooms are borne on older wood, so frequent shearing reduces the allergy potential. A good substitute shrub for Myrsine is female Podocarpus. Myrsine is a tough plant to rank because it may be perfect-flowered, monoecious, or dioecious. The most allergenic are dioecious males. All-female plants are allergy-free, and monoecious plants, if they make fruit, are in between. Finding fruit on existing plants should certainly be a plus. Most plants sold in California are male.

MYRTLE. See *Cyrilla racemosa*; *Luma apiculata*; *Myrica*; *Myrsine*; *Myrtus communis*; *Umbellularia californica*; *Vinca*.

MYRTLE, HONEY. See *Melaleuca*.

MYRTLE, JEWISH. See *Ruscus*.

Myrtus communis. 5

TRUE MYRTLE. An easy-to-grow, drought-tolerant evergreen shrub or small tree (to about 16 feet), for zones 8 to 11. Very small, dark green leaves and small, white flowers makes this an attractive plant for full sun, but it may get leggy in the shade. Because it is easily shaped by shearing, it is often used for foundation plants, screens, tub plants, topiary, and hedges.

Allergy Index Scale: 1 is Best, 10 is Worst.
✿ for 1 and 2   ◊ for 9 and 10
No matter what the ranking, always read the full plant description carefully and take note of any warnings.

NAKED LADY. See *Amaryllis belladonna*.

NAMAQUALAND DAISY. See *Venidium*.

Nandina domestica. 1 ✿
HEAVENLY BAMBOO, EVERGREEN SUBSHRUB. The plants are completely hardy in zones 7 to 10, and the roots are hardy to zone 6. There are many dwarf varieties available, and all Nandina make fine landscaping plants. Although it resembles bamboo, it is not related; Nandina plants have clusters of white flowers, followed by bright red, round, fleshy-coated little seeds, which persist on the plants for months. Easy to grow and very drought-tolerant in sun or partial shade; the color of the leaves is best in good light.

NANKING CHERRY. See *Prunus tomentosa*.

Nannorrhops. 1 ✿
MAZARI PALM. Four species of small- to medium-size slow-growing palms from India, Afghanistan, and Iran, hardy in zones 8 to 10.

NANNYBERRY. See *Viburnum*.

Narcissus. 4
DAFFODIL. Trumpet-shaped yellow, white, or pale green flowers on these spring-blooming bulbs. Daffodils will persist and naturalize where conditions are perfect—fertile, fast-draining soil with ample moisture.

Allergic reactions are reported from handling daffodil bulbs, but this is most common in bulb-packing sheds or with workers digging the bulbs. People working at cutting Narcissus for the commercial cut-flower trade also experience allergy to daffodil pollen, sap, and foliage.

For the average gardener, or for those who buy an occasional bunch to bring indoors, the allergy potential is very small. However, allergy is well documented and some caution is advised. The bulbs and all parts of Narcissus contain toxic calcium oxylate crystals.

NASTURTIUM. See *Tropaeolum*.

NATAL IVY. See *Senecio*.

NATAL PLUM. See *Carissa*.

NAUPKA. See *Scaevola*.

NECTARINE. See *Prunus persica*.

NEEDLE PALM. See *Rhapidophyllum hystrix*; *Yucca*.

NEEM, NEEM TREE. See *Azadirachta indica*.

Nelumbo. 1 ✿
WATER LILY. Hardy flowering pond plants.

Nemesia strumosa. 2 ✿
Easy-to-grow annuals from seed; for full sun. Some species of Nemesia are small, shrublike, heatherlike subshrub perennials for zones 7 to 10.

Nemopanthus. MALES 7, FEMALES 1 ✿

CATBERRY, MOUNTAIN HOLLY. Native deciduous shrub of the eastern United States, hardy to zone 5. It resembles holly (Ilex). Catberry needs moist soil and partial shade to grow well.

Nemophila. 1 ✿

BABY BLUE EYES. Fast-growing annuals from seed for full sun or part shade. Nemophila needs ample moisture.

Neolitsea. MALES 6, FEMALES 1 ✿

A group of about eighty evergreen trees native to Japan and Korea, all of which are separate-sexed; the males present limited potential for allergy. Trees grow 12 to 20 feet and females have small, usually black berries. *N. dealbata* is a tropical dioecious evergreen tree common in parts of Australia. Unlike most separate-sexed plants, *N. dealbata* is mostly insect-pollinated and makes a good choice for the allergy-free landscape.

Neopanax (Nothopanax). MALES 6, FEMALES 1 ✿

FIVE-FINGERS. Tall (to 25 feet) New Zealand native evergreen shrubs and trees, used in zone 10. Neopanax are characterized by their long, five-lobed, serrated leaves. The trees are separate-sexed and the males show potential for allergy. Females are identifiable by their small dark purple fruits.

NEOREGELIA. See *Bromelia*.

NEPAL CAMPHOR TREE. See *Cinnamomum camphora*.

Nepenthes. NOT YET RANKED.

A family of separate-sexed carnivorous herbs or vines from the Philippines. Rarely seen in this country.

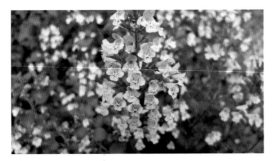

Nepeta. 2 ✿

CATMINT, CATNIP. (Pictured above.) Perennial hardy members of the mint family. They thrive in moist soil, in full sun to partial shade. Very fine pollinator plants.

Nephelium lappaceum. MALES 6, FEMALES 1 ✿

HAIRY LYCHEE, RAMBUTAN. Large, tall, separate-sexed evergreen tropical fruit trees. Related to mangosteen, the female trees bear delicious fruit.

Nephrolepis. 3

SWORD FERN. A group of easy-to-grow, long-lived ferns. One species, *N. exaltata* 'Bostoniensis', the Boston fern, and the more compact *N. exaltata* 'Bostoniensis Dallas', the Dallas fern, are popular houseplants. All ferns have spores, and spores can cause allergy, so with this in mind do not hang houseplant or patio ferns directly over chairs or tables. In the garden, however, sword ferns pose little allergy risk. They thrive in shady areas with good soil moisture.

Nephrosperma. 6

VAN HOUTTAN PALM. A tropical palm, to 30 feet, used in equatorial landscapes.

NEPHTHYTIS. See *Syngonium podophyllum*.

Nerine. 2 ✿

A bulbous perennial bearing pink or red flowers, usually grown in pots but used outdoors in zones 7 to 10.

Nerium oleander. 6

OLEANDER. Very common evergreen landscape shrubs and small trees in zones 8 to 10. All parts of the oleander are exceptionally poisonous, as is the smoke from them when burned. In recent years a virus has been killing off many oleander hedges in Southern California, especially in some desert areas. There is no known cure for this virus and it is expected to spread. Oleanders are tough and drought-resistant; they flower well if pruned back occasionally. Pollen from oleander is not a well-documented allergy factor, despite the fact that the plants bloom profusely and the pollen-bearing stamens are well exposed. The sap is known to cause rash, and the odd fragrance is allergenic for some individuals. Oleanders planted in the shade will often become attacked by mealybugs, and mold spores will grow and proliferate on such branches, becoming quite allergenic.

Nertera granadensis. 2 ✿

BEAD PLANT. Tender houseplants or ground cover for small areas in zone 10; best in partial shade with good moisture.

NERVE PLANT. See *Fittonia*.

Nestegis. MALES 8, FEMALES 1 ✿

Evergreen trees or shrubs from New Zealand. Hardy only in zones 8 to 10. Related to olives, these plants are dioecious but not yet sold sexed.

NET BUSH. See *Calothamnus*.

NETTLE. See *Urtica*.

NEW MEXICAN PRIVET. See *Forestiera*.

NEW ZEALAND BRASS BUTTONS. See *Cotula squalida*.

NEW ZEALAND BUR. See *Acaena*.

NEW ZEALAND CHRISTMAS TREE. See *Metrosideros*.

NEW ZEALAND FLAX. See *Phormium tenax*.

NEW ZEALAND LACEBARK. See *Hoheria*.

NEW ZEALAND LAUREL. See *Corynocarpus laevigata*.

NEW ZEALAND SPINACH. See *Tetragonia*.

NEW ZEALAND TEA TREE. See *Leptospermum*.

NICHOL'S WILLOW-LEAFED PEPPERMINT TREE. See *Eucalyptus*.

Nicotiana. 3
FLOWERING TOBACCO. Frost-tender perennials for full sun, used as annuals in all zones.

NIDULARIUM INNOCENTII. See *Bromelia*.

Nierembergia. 1 ✪
CUP FLOWER. White- or purple-flowered perennials, for full sun with ample water, in zones 7 to 10. The plants must be sheared yearly to maintain their shape. Most species are low growing and mounded, but one is tall.

Nigella damascena. 3
LOVE-IN-A-MIST. Tall annuals with unusual blue flowers and large, light, 1-inch papery seedpods that are used in dried flower arrangements.

NIGHT JASMINE. See *Nyctanthes*.

NIGHT JESSAMINE. See *Cestrum nocturnum*.

NIGHT PHLOX. See *Zaluzianskya capensis*.

NIGHT-BLOOMING CACTUS. See *Cereus*; *Selenicereus*.

NIGHTSHADE. See *Solanum*.

NIKAU PALM. See *Rhopalostylis*.

NIKKO FIR. See *Abies*.

NINEBARK. See *Physocarpus*.

NIPA PALM. See *Nypa*.

NOBLE FIR. See *Abies*.

Nolana. 2 ✪
Annual vines that resemble morning glories, with bright, large flowers. They are difficult to grow well, requiring full sun and very well-drained soil.

Nolina longifolia. MALES 6, FEMALES 1 ✪
BEARGRASS, MEXICAN GRASS TREE. A desert relative of Yucca and Agave, many species and some are native; some can be almost treelike. Asparagus relatives. Drought-tolerant.

NORFOLK ISLAND PINE. See *Araucaria*.

Normanbya. 7
BLACK PALM. A tall (to 60 feet) Australian native, used in zones 10 to 13.

NORSE FIRE PLANT. See *Columnea*.

NORWAY MAPLE. See *Acer platanoides*.

Nothofagus. 5
A group of deciduous and evergreen trees related to beech, hardy only in zones 8 to 11. Native to New Zealand and Australia.

NOTHOPANAX. See *Neopanax*.

NUT GRASS. See *Cyperus*.

NUTGALL. See *Rhus*.

NUTMEG. See *Myristica fragrans*; *Torreya*.

Nyctanthes. 5
NIGHT JASMINE, TREE-OF-SADNESS. Small Asian trees or shrubs for zones 9 to 10, bearing fragrant white flowers that yield a perfume and an orange dye.

Nymphaea. 1 ✪
WATER LILY. Blooming aquatic plants hardy in all zones.

Nypa. 7
MANGROVE PALM, NIPA, NYPA PALM. Native to India and the Solomon Islands and occasionally planted in zones 10 to 13.

Nyssa. MALES 8, FEMALES 1 ✪
BEE GUM, PEPPERIDGE TREE, TUPELO, SOUR GUM, SWAMP GUM, WILD OLIVE. Native, winter-hardy deciduous tree with attractive leaves and often exceptionally beautiful fall color. Thrives in continually moist soils. Tupelos are separate-sexed trees; the males contribute to allergy, the females produce clusters of small, round blue berries on 2-inch stems. The cultivar 'Miss Scarlet' is a pollen-free female prized for its brilliant red fall color and ornamental blue fruit. Most other known named cultivars (at this time) are unfortunately male trees.

OAK. See *Quercus*.

OAK, TANBARK. See *Lithocarpus densiflorus*.

OAK-LEAF HYDRANGEA. See *Hydrangea quercifolia*.

OATS. See *Avena*.

OAXACA PALMETTO. See *Sabal*.

OBEDIENCE PLANT. See *Physostegia virginiana*.

OCEAN SPRAY. See *Holodiscus*.

Ochna serrulata. 2 ✪

BIRD'S-EYE BUSH, MICKEY MOUSE PLANT. Evergreen
shrub for zones 9 to 10. The large yellow flowers
appear in early summer and are followed by red sepals,
then black fruit that resembles a mouse's face and
ears. Thrives in partial shade and moist, acidic soil;
a good potted plant.

Ocimum. 2 ✪

BASIL. Annual culinary and decorative herb, fast growing from seed.

OCONEE BELLS. See *Shortia*.

OCOTILLO. See *Fouquieria splendens*.

OCTOPUS TREE. See *Brassica*.

ODONTOGLOSSUM. See *Orchids*.

Oemleria cerasiformis. MALES 6, FEMALES 1 ✪

INDIAN PLUM, OSO BERRY. A dioecious (separate-
sexed) member of the rose family, this large deciduous
shrub is native from British Columbia to California
and is used as an ornamental in zones 4 to 10. Only
the female plants have small blue-black fruits.
Drought-tolerant.

Oenothera. 3

EVENING PRIMROSE. Hardy perennials and biennials
for full sun, in all zones. *O. berlandieri*, or *O. speciosa*,
is the Mexican evening primrose, with large pink
flowers; it is fast spreading and reseeds easily, sometimes becoming invasive. *O. biennis* is a tall wildflower.
O. missourensis, the Missouri evening primrose, is a
very hardy, low-growing, yellow-flowered perennial.
Tall *O. tetragona*, or sun drops, opens its yellow blooms
in the daytime.

OIL PALM. See *Corozo*.

OKRA. See *Abelmoschus esculentus*.

OLD MAN. See *Artemisia*.

OLD MAN CACTUS. See *Cephalocereus senilis*;
Espostoa lanata.

OLD WOMAN. See *Artemisia*.

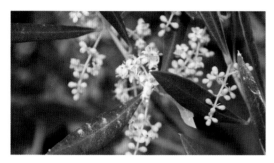

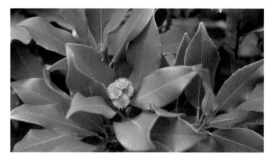

Olea europaea. 10 🖊

OLIVE. (*Olea europaea*, var. 'Swan Hill', pictured above.) Evergreen trees hardy in zones 8 to 10. Olives need good summer heat to make their best fruit. Olive trees are easy to transplant and, as urban sprawl has taken over orchards, many full-size trees have been moved into city landscapes. This is unfortunate because olive blossoms are a primary cause of severe allergy. The bloom on olives is heavy and the trees often are in bloom from April through June. The pollen is exceptionally light and buoyant and often becomes airborne. In many southern and western cities olives produce the worst early summer pollen. If olive trees are pruned hard each winter they will not bloom, but this is difficult if the trees are allowed to grow too tall.

One variety, 'Swan Hill', has been widely sold as an allergy-free, nonblooming tree, but I have been watching these trees for a decade now, and they do bloom and produce pollen. 'Swan Hill' is essentially an all-male tree. 'Majestic Beauty' is another of these so-called low-allergy or allergy-free trees, but it is really another male clone with allergenic pollen.

Also worth noting is the fact that olive trees will grow perfectly well in the tropics and subtropics but will almost never flower in these climates. In the tropics an olive tree might be a good choice, but in most other climates, it is anything but. Olive pollen is also a very strong trigger for asthma.

OLEANDER. See *Nerium oleander.*

OLEANDER, YELLOW. See *Thevetia.*

Olearia. 6

ASTER TREE, DAISYBUSH. Many species of shrubs and small trees mostly from New Zealand and Australia. Several species of Olearia are used as landscape material in California and Florida, but these ragweed relatives produce a heavy bloom and have allergy potential.

OLIVE. See *Olea europaea.*

Olmediella betschlerana. MALES 7; FEMALES 1 ☺

COSTA RICAN HOLLY, GUATEMALAN HOLLY, MANZAN-OTE. (Pictured above.) Small- to medium-size evergreen trees for zones 9 to 13. Separate-sexed, with male trees presenting some allergy potential. If pollinated, female trees produce hard, inedible green fruits the size and shape of a Japanese persimmon. Young trees are frost-tender but acquire more hardiness as they age. Trees grow to about 30 feet tall and nearly as wide, are pest-free, and have attractive large, glossy leaves that resemble those of holly. Not sold sexed.

Olneya tesota. 4

DESERT IRONWOOD. Leguminous evergreen tree for desert areas of zones 8 to 10.

Oncidium. 1 ☺ TO 3 DEPENDING ON SPECIES

DANCING-LADY ORCHIDS. A very large group of orchids from tropical South America. Greenhouse plants. (See also *Orchids.*)

ONION. See *Allium.*

Onoclea. 4

Tall, hardy ferns for moist, shady areas.

Onosma tauricum. 2 ☺

GOLDEN DROPS. Perennials for sun or shade, hardy in zones 3 to 10. Golden drops make excellent rock garden plants.

OPHIOPOGON. See *Liriope.*

OPPOSSUMWOOD. See *Halesia.*

OPUNTIA. See *Cactus.*

ORANGE. See *Citrus.*

ORANGE BROWALLIA. See *Streptosolen jamesonii.*

ORANGE CLOCK VINE. See *Thunbergia.*

ORANGE JESSAMINE. See *Murraya paniculata.*

O

Orbignya. 7
BABASSU, COHUNE PALM. Twenty species of subtropical palm trees from Central and South America, grown in zones 9 to 10. Some species reach 60 feet.

ORCHARD GRASS. See *Dactylis*.

ORCHID CACTUS. See *Epiphyllum*.

ORCHID PANSY. See *Achimenes*.

ORCHID TREE. See *Bauhinia*.

ORCHID VINE. See *Stigmaphyllon*.

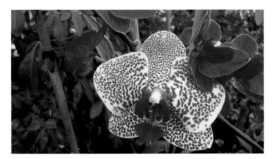

Orchid. 1 ✪
(Pictured above.) The largest group of plants in the world, orchids come in many sizes, shapes, and colors. Some are hardy into the coldest zones, while others thrive only in frost-free jungles. Many orchids, called epiphytic, live in trees and need no soil. Other terrestrial orchids grow in the ground. All orchids need good moisture, and most potted orchids are planted in containers of pure tree bark, or a mix of bark and sand; these require regular fertilizing every two weeks during the growing season. Most orchids do best in partial shade, and a lath house is a popular place in which to grow them. Because orchids often have some of the world's fanciest flowers and are well designed to attract insect pollinators, they rarely cause allergy. On a few occasions, orchids have been blamed for causing contact skin allergy, but this appears to be rare. Moth orchids (Phalaenopsis) often do well inside if they get decent light. Outside in a yard, in zones 9 to 13, Cymbidium orchids often will thrive. Plant these in a 5-gallon pot filled with chunks of fir bark, then plant the whole pot in the ground in a half-sun, half-shade spot.

OREGON BOXWOOD. See *Paxistima*.

OREGON GRAPE. See *Mahonia aquifolium*.

OREGON MYRTLE. See *Umbellularia californica*.

ORGANPIPE CACTUS. See *Cactus*.

ORIENTAL ARBORVITAE. See *Platycladus orientalis*.

Origanum majorana (Amaracus). 3
SWEET MARJORAM. Perennial culinary herb with strongly scented leaves, for moist, shady areas. Oil of marjoram is known to cause skin rash.

ORNAMENTAL GRASS. See *Festuca*; *Pennisetum*.

ORNAMENTAL PEAR. See *Pyrus*.

Ornithogalum. 3
CHINCHERINCHEE, PREGNANT ONION, STAR OF BETHLEHEM. Bulbs for sun or partial shade in zones 7 to 10. The bulbs are poisonous.

Oryza. 7
RICE. A cultivated grain crop. Very few people are allergic to eating rice, and a common diet used to eliminate the possible causes of an unknown allergy is pears, lamb, and rice. The only exception is found among those living close to rice paddies; although self-pollinated and the pollen does not travel far, it is the cause of late fall severe asthma in localities where it is grown.

OSAGE ORANGE. See *Maclura pomifera*.

Oscularia. 1 ✪
Small, drought-resistant shrubby succulent plants for full sun in zone 10. They bear pink or purple flowers.

OSIER. See *Cornus*.

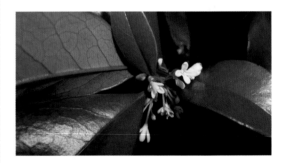

Osmanthus. MALES 6, FEMALES 1 ✪
SWEET OLIVE. (Pictured above.) About fifteen species of slow-growing, evergreen tall shrubs and small trees, some hardy to zone 6. Osmanthus grows best in partial shade with ample moisture. The tiny flowers have a powerful fragrance, suggestive of apricot, and this scent may trigger allergic reaction in odor-sensitive individuals. Some species are separate-sexed, but the male plants do not release much airborne pollen.

Osmanthus is related to olive and ash, but unlike them, male Osmanthus flowers have very few and very small male stamens.

Osmunda. 3
CINNAMON FERN, ROYAL FERN. Shade- and moisture-loving ferns, hardy to zone 3. The emerging fronds of Osmunda can be eaten, usually boiled.

OSO BERRY. See *Oemleria cerasiformis*.

Osteomeles. 4
Several species of deciduous and evergreen shrubs from China, New Zealand, and Hawaii, hardy to zone 7. The flowers of Osteomeles resemble those of hawthorn or Cotoneaster.

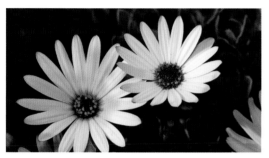

Osteospermum. 4
AFRICAN DAISY, CAPE MARIGOLD. (Pictured above.) Several species of spreading, sun-loving, easy-to-grow ground covers, hardy in zones 9 to 10.

Ostrya. 6
BEETLEWOOD, DEERWOOD, HARDTACK, HOP HORN-BEAM, STONEWOOD. Hardy deciduous trees of the birch family, prized for their fine yellow autumn color. Although all may cause early spring allergy, they have a relatively short bloom period that lessens their overall impact. An occasional hop hornbeam in the landscape is not much of a problem. The leaves of hop hornbeam resemble those of elm and they bear papery clusters of seeds that resemble ripe hops.

OSWEGO TEA. See *Monarda*.

OURICURI PALM. See *Syagrus*.

OX-EYE DAISY. See *Chrysanthemum*; *Heliopsis helianthoides scabra*.

Oxalis. 1 ☉
SHAMROCK, SORREL, SOUR WEED, WOOD SORREL. Many species of small, low-growing perennials and annuals characterized by their three- and four-lobed leaves, which resemble clover. Some of this genus are difficult-to-eradicate weeds, but a few are shade-loving ground covers. The plants contain oxalic acid, which gives the stems a pleasantly tart flavor. The leaves are considered poisonous.

Oxydendrum. 2 ☉
LILY-OF-THE-VALLEY TREE, SORREL TREE, SOURWOOD, TITI. A slow-growing, tall (to 80 feet) native deciduous tree of the eastern United States, hardy in zones 5 to 10. Oxydendrum grows best in moist, acid soils. The large leaves turn a bright scarlet red or orange in autumn, and in the springtime the tree bears tiny tubular white flowers that attract bees.

Oxytropis. 6
CRAZYWEED, LOCOWEED. Perennial members of the legume family, sometimes grown as ornamentals. Plants, seeds, and flowers are poisonous if eaten.

OZARK WHITE CEDAR. See *Juniperus*.

O

Allergy Index Scale: 1 is Best, 10 is Worst.
⊘ for 1 and 2   ◗ for 9 and 10
No matter what the ranking, always read the full plant description carefully and take note of any warnings.

Pachysandra. 6
JAPANESE SPURGE. Hardy in all zones, this common, spreading ground cover is widely used in zones 3 to 7, in moist areas of full sun to deep shade. Evergreen in the south and deciduous in the north, Pachysandra can cause allergies in any climate. A better choice for the allergy-free garden is *Vinca minor* in the north and *V. major* in the south. Skin rash is also very possible.

Pachystachys lutea. 2 ⊘
GOLDEN CANDLE. A houseplant, or grown outside in the mildest parts of zone 10. Related to Justicia, or shrimp plant, which it resembles. It grows best in partial shade, with good soil and ample water.

PACIFIC WAX MYRTLE. See *Myrica.*

Paeonia. FULL DOUBLES 1 ⊘, SINGLES 3
PEONY. Hardy, long-lived perennials that grow best in moist, sunny spots in zones 3 to 8. The plants bear large leaves and very large, showy red, pink, or white flowers. Peonies refuse to grow in hot, dry areas and are almost impossible to grow well in zones 9 to 13. Tree peonies are deciduous shrubs, some to 6 feet, that are hardy to zone 2; they produce exceptionally large flowers, often fully double. Most peonies are hybrids and there is a wide selection from which to choose.

PAINTED DAISY. See *Chrysanthemum; Pyrethrum.*

PAINTED FINGERNAIL PLANT. See *Bromelia.*

PAINTED TONGUE. See *Salpiglossis sinuata.*

PALM LILY. See *Yucca.*

PALMA CHRISTI. See *Ricinus communis.*

PALMA CORCHO. See *Microcycas.*

PALMA PITA. See *Yucca.*

PALMETTO. See *Sabal.*

PALMETTO THATCH. See *Thrinax.*

PALMYRA PALM. See *Borassus.*

PALO VERDE. See *Cercidium.*

PAMPAS GRASS. See *Cortaderia selloana.*

PANAMIGA, PANAMIGO. See *Pilea.*

Panax. 2 ⊘
GINSENG. Very winter-hardy perennial grown for its prized, medicinal roots. Ginseng is notoriously difficult to grow and requires moist, rather poor, acid soil, partial shade, and a deep mulch to thrive.

Pandanus. MALES 9 ◗, FEMALES 1 ⊘
PANDUS PALM, SCREW PINE. Very large group of Old World tropical shrubs and trees, all separate-sexed. The males cause widespread allergy in Myanmar, Sri Lanka,

and the Philippines. Some species are used in tropical and subtropical landscapes in the United States.

Pandorea. 2 ✿
BOWER VINE, WONGA-WONGA VINE. Large, vigorous evergreen vines for sun or shade in zones 9 to 10. They have large leaves and 2-inch, trumpet-shaped white, pink, or rose-colored flowers. Prune after blooming to encourage new growth.

PANDUS PALM. See *Pandanus.*

Panicum. 5
MILLET, PANIC GRASS. A common grain crop.

PANSY. See *Viola.*

PANSY ORCHID. See *Orchids.*

Papaver. 3
POPPY. Annuals and perennials for full sun. The red Flanders poppy or Shirley poppy is an annual variety that grows fast from seed. *P. orientale*, the Oriental poppy, is a perennial hardy to zone 2 and has very large, papery flowers in white, lilac, pink, red, or scarlet. *P. nudicale*, the Iceland poppy, is grown as an annual and flowers well during the winter months in zones 7 to 10. The bitter sap of all poppies is potentially poisonous.

PAPAYA. See *Carica papaya.*

PAPER MULBERRY. See *Broussonetia papyrifera*; *Morus.*

PAPERBARK MAPLE. See *Acer griseum.*

PAPHIOPEDILUM. See *Orchids.*

PAPYRUS. See *Cyperus.*

Parabenzoin. MALES 9 ✎, FEMALES 1 ✿
Two species of deciduous shrubs or small trees, native to Japan and China and used there in landscapes. Separate-sexed with males having high potential for allergy.

PARADISE PALM. See *Howea.*

PARADISE TREE. See *Simarouba.*

PARA NUT. See *Bertholletia excelsa.*

PARA RUBBER. See *Hevea brasiliensis.*

PARA-PARA. See *Pisonia.*

Parajubaea. 6
Two species of tall palms (to 20 feet) from the subtropics, used in zones 9 to 13.

Pardancanda norrisii. 3
CANDY LILY. Hardy perennial lilies for zones 5 to 9. Easy to grow and often self-seeding.

Parkinsonia aculeata. 5
JERUSALEM THORN, MEXICAN PALO VERDE. Drought-tolerant, thorny deciduous desert tree, to 30 feet, that bears yellow flowers. Sometimes the cause of limited local allergy. Drought-tolerant. Zones 8 to 10.

PARLOR IVY. See *Senecio.*

PAROUOT PALM. See *Acoelorrhaphe wrightii.*

PARROT BEAK. See *Clianthus puniceus*; *Lotus*; *Parrotia.*

Parrotia. 4
PARROT BEAK, PERSIAN IRONWOOD, PERSIAN WITCH HAZEL. Deciduous tree or large shrub for zones 8 to 9, prized for its autumn color.

PARSLEY PANAX. See *Polyscias.*

PARTHENIUM GENUS

Parthenium. INDIVIDUALLY RANKED
A group of domestic and wild perennial plants related to asters and daisies, all of them with some potential for both pollen and contact allergy. There are several other species of Parthenium besides the ones listed below, and all of them are, at best, suspect.

P. argentatum. 6
GUAYULE. Native to desert areas of the Southwest, guayule is raised as a domestic rubber-producing plant and is one of only two plants used commercially in natural rubber production (see also *Hevea brasiliensis*). A 3-foot-tall shrub with small white or yellowish flowers, guayule is drought-tolerant and needs fast-draining soil and high summer heat to grow well. Guayule is a ragweed relative, and it has allergenic pollen, but the rubber made from Guayule is not a latex, and it does not cause the same sort of dangerous allergic reactions as rubber made from *Hevea brasiliensis*.

P. hysterophorum. 10 ✎
POUND CAKE WEED. A common weed in the southern United States that causes severe skin rash and inhalant allergy.

P. integrifolium. 7
WILD QUININE. A hardy native plant, also highly suspect per allergies.

Parthenocissus. 4
BOSTON IVY, VIRGINIA CREEPER, WOODBINE. Several species of deciduous, long-lived clinging vines, some native to the United States and others to Asia. Allergies to Boston ivy or Virginia creeper are uncommon.

Members of the grape family, their grapelike fruits are mildly toxic if consumed. Some plants of Parthenocissus are dioecious, but none is sold sexed, yet.

Paspalum. 9 ✎
BAHIA GRASS, DALLIS GRASS. Perennial, fast-growing, spreading grasses used for pastures and hay crops. There are many species worldwide: *P. dilatatum*, or dallis grass, is a common forage grass in warmer parts of the United States, and it often escapes cultivation to become a large, crabgrass-like weed in lawns. In the lawn, dallis grass flowers when still short and produces large amounts of allergenic pollen. Bahia grass, another of this group, is used as a warm-climate lawn grass and also flowers when short.

Passiflora. 3
MAYPOP, PASSION FLOWER, PASSION FRUIT. Mostly evergreen, some deciduous vines for zones 8 to 10. *P. edulis* produces a rich, sweet, flavorful fruit that is said to be an aphrodisiac. The vines are easy to grow, easily propagated from cuttings, and have very unusual large flowers, the parts of which are said to represent the Passion of Jesus Christ. The best fruit is produced when there are several plants for cross-pollination. Leaves and unripe fruit are poisonous.

PATERNOSTER TREE. See *Melia*.

PATERSON PLUM. See *Lagunaria patersonii*.

Paulownia tomentosa. 4
EMPRESS TREE. Large, fast-growing deciduous tree with very large, heart-shaped leaves and many tubular, lilac-blue flowers in spring. Hardy in zones 7 to 10, the empress tree is a member of the trumpet vine family and bears clusters of fragrant, trumpet-shaped flowers, which are edible and eaten fresh in salads. The tree needs good soil, full sun, and ample water to thrive. The wood is prized by carvers for its close grain and density. Paulownia is named for Anna Paulowna, princess of Holland and daughter of the Russian czar Paul I. May become an invasive species in the southeastern United States.

PAUROTIS WRIGHTII. See *Acoelorrhaphe wrightii*.

PAW PAW. See *Asimina triloba*.

Paxistima. 2 ✪
OREGON BOXWOOD. A low-growing, Pacific Northwest native evergreen shrub used for low hedges and ground covers. It needs good drainage but is otherwise not hard to grow.

PEACH. See *Prunus persica*.

PEANUT. See *Arachis hypogaea*.

PEAR, ORNAMENTAL, FLOWERING, EVERGREEN. See *Pyrus*.

PEARLBUSH. See *Exochorda*.

PEARLY EVERLASTING. See *Anaphalis*.

PEAS, GARDEN. See *Pisum sativum*.

PEAS, SWEET. See *Lathyrus*.

PEASHRUB, SIBERIAN. See *Caragana arborescens*.

PEASHRUB, SWAN RIVER. See *Brachysema lanceolatum*.

PECAN. See *Carya illinoensis*.

Pedilanthus tithymaloides. 10 ✎
DEVIL'S BACKBONE, JAPANESE POINSETTIA, REDBIRD CACTUS, RIBBON CACTUS, SLIPPER PLANT. Houseplants or used outside in frost-free parts of zone 10. Not a type of cactus, but related instead to Euphorbia; the pollen is allergenic and the sap can cause severe skin rash.

PEDIOCACTUS. See *Cactus*.

PEE-GEE HYDRANGEA. See *Hydrangea paniculata*.

Pelargonium. 3
GERANIUM. These are the tender showy-flowered houseplants and warm-climate perennials that most people know as geraniums. They thrive in full sun and are remarkably drought-resistant. The large, soft, slightly fuzzy leaves have a characteristic pungent odor and are occasionally zoned with dark green or purple or variegation. Pelargoniums release little pollen, but their fragrance and the smell of their leaves may affect a few odor-sensitive individuals.

Ivy-leaf geraniums have waxy leaves without the characteristic odor. They tolerate some shade and, because of their lack of scent, are a better choice for the allergy-free garden.

Pellaea. 3
BIRD'S-FOOT FERN, CLIFF-BRAKE, COFFEE FERN. Shade- and moisture-loving ferns with attractive finely cut leaves, for zones 8 to 10.

Peltophorum. 6
A small group of frost-tender flowering trees. The source of considerable localized pollen-allergy in India. *P. pterocarpum*, yellow poinciana, is a very fast-growing evergreen tree with many bright yellow flowers. Easy to grow with few insect pests. Zones 10 to 13.

PENCIL BUSH, PENCIL TREE. See *Euphorbia*.

Pennisetum. INDIVIDUALLY RANKED

A large group of grasses, some very allergenic, some with great potential for becoming invasive, and also some excellent selections for the allergy-free landscape.

P. clandestinum. NOT YET RANKED

KIKUYUGRASS. A rapidly growing, sod-forming turf grass suitable for all southern areas. A South African male-sterile, female clone of this grass is a very low-pollen producer and may be a very useful low-allergy lawn grass. Flowering kikuyu is a known allergen, especially in South Africa, where it is native. In California it has become invasive in many areas.

P. purpureum hybrids. 1 ✪

The newer cultivars of ornamental Pennisetum, 'Princess Molly', 'Prince', 'Princess Caroline', 'First Knight', and 'Vertigo' are all interspecific hybrid pollen-free selections. These were all created by the plant breeder Dr. Wayne Hannah, from the University of Georgia. He is also working on a number of new, very interesting pollen-free selections of other grasses and some trees. Watch for his new introductions.

P. setaceum. 8

FOUNTAIN GRASS. This is a large ornamental clump grass, hardy in all zones; it may naturalize in milder areas. It produces tall purplish seed heads that are held well above the plant. These and other ornamental grasses are gaining in landscape popularity because of the ease with which they are grown. Fountain grass causes frequent allergy, and its further use is discouraged.

PENNYROYAL. See *Mentha.*

Penstemon. 2 ✪

BEARD TONGUE. A large group of flowering perennials, one an Asian import but most native; various species are hardy throughout the United States. Penstemon is easy to grow, long-lived, and easy to propagate from cuttings. Plants grow in clumps from 1 to 6 feet tall depending on species. In California, *P. heterophyllus* has become quite popular in recent years due to its good drought tolerance and wide range of flower colors.

PEONY. See *Paeonia.*

Peperomia. 3

EMERALD LEAF, WATERMELON PEPEROMIA. Several species of attractive houseplants, usually low and spreading. All like semi-shade and ample moisture.

PEPPER. See *Piper.*

PEPPER TREE. See *Drimys*; *Macropiper*; *Piper*; *Schinus*; *Vitex.*

PEPPER VINE. See *Piper.*

PEPPERIDGE TREE. See *Nyssa.*

PEPPERMINT. See *Eucalyptus*; *Mentha.*

PEPPERMINT TREE. See *Agonis flexuosa.*

PEPPERMINT WILLOW. See *Eucalyptus.*

PEPPERWOOD. See *Umbellularia californica*; *Zanthoxylum.*

PEREGRINA. See *Jatropha.*

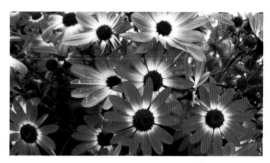

Pericallis. 4

(Pictured above.) A few species, most in the trade, are horticultural hybrids, closely related to Senecio and Cineraria. Perennials often treated as annuals. Full sun in all zones.

Perilla frutescens. 3

SHISO. Tall, big-leafed annual that resembles Coleus, with its large edible leaves that taste like mint. The long clusters of flower buds are also cooked in Japanese tempura batter. Perilla thrives in sun or partial shade with generous water.

PERIWINKLE. See *Catharanthus roseus*; *Vinca.*

Pernettya mucronata. 2 ✪

An evergreen shrub for zones 7 to 10. Pernettya produces tiny, pink, bell-shaped flowers followed by attractive bright purple, white, or black berries. It thrives in moist, acid soil, and needs partial shade in the hottest areas. A light yearly pruning keeps it compact.

Perovskia atriplicifolia. 1 ✪

RUSSIAN SAGE. A tall perennial or subshrub, hardy in almost any plant zone, drought-resistant, with small gray leaves, these plants are magnets for honeybees and also attract small butterflies and other pollinators. Perfect-flowered with a very small amount of pollen but

P

a generous supply of nectar, these are excellent allergy-free plants and also excellent choices for the pollinator garden. Those who are highly allergic to bee stings might not want this, though. The light blue flowers are very attractive not just to bees, but also to gardeners.

Persea. 3

AVOCADO. A large group of tender evergreen trees for zones 9 to 10. *P. americana*, the common edible avocado, is not frost-resistant and is most commonly grown as a houseplant outside of the warmest zones; 'Bacon' is among the hardiest cultivars. In fertile soil in areas with little frost, a mature avocado tree can grow to 70 feet. Because of its shallow roots, avocado requires summer irrigation and year-round mulch. The pollen is rarely implicated in allergy.

    P. borbonia, the red bay, shore bay, or swamp bay, is a large tree, native to the southeastern United States, that can reach 80 feet, although it is usually much smaller. It thrives in moist to wet soils in zones 8 to 10. *P. indica* is a smaller evergreen tree used mostly in California. Persea leaves are poisonous.

PERSIAN IRONWOOD. See *Parrotia*.

PERSIAN IVY. See *Hedera colchica*.

PERSIAN LILAC. See *Melia*.

PERSIAN RANUNCULUS. See *Ranunculus*.

PERSIAN VIOLET. See *Exacum*.

PERSIAN WITCH HAZEL. See *Parrotia*.

PERSIMMON. See *Diospyros*.

PERUVIAN DAFFODIL. See *Hymenocallis*.

PERUVIAN LILY. See *Alstroemeria*.

PETTICOAT PALM. See *Copernicia*.

Petunia. 2 ✪

Annuals and a few perennials that are very popular as container and bedding plants for full sun. Newer varieties, like the 'Carpet Series' (including 'Purple Wave'), grow low, spread, and have lots of flowers. Petunias need good soil, adequate moisture, and warm temperatures to grow well. Most require judicious deadheading to encourage continuous bloom. Petunia was one of the first flowers I used in inhalant testing many years ago, and I never found anyone allergic to it.

PEYOTE. See *Lophophora*.

Phacelia distans. 7

WILD HELIOTROPE. A small annual native to dry areas of the western United States, with fernlike leaves and coils of small, blue, bell-shaped flowers. It causes contact skin rash.

PHALAENOPSIS (moth orchid). See *Orchid*.

Phalaris. 8

CANARY GRASS, CANARY REED GRASS. A coarse, tall-growing forage grass for pastures.

Phaseolus. 4

BEANS. The flowers and fruit of beans are not of concern when it comes to allergies. However, contact with leaves can cause rash and old bean plants often have rust. Use care when pulling up old plants.

Phellodendron. MALES 7, FEMALES 1 ✪

AMUR CORK TREE, CORK TREE. Ten species of large deciduous trees, all with thick, corky bark, for zones 4 to 10. Cork trees are separate-sexed and the tall (to 80 feet) males shed large quantities of airborne pollen with allergy potential. Female trees produce small resin-scented black fruits. The compound leaves of Phellodendron resemble those of ash. 'His Majesty' and 'Macho' are male cultivars and should be avoided. No relation to Philodendron. There are no known female cultivars of cork tree, alas.

Philadelphus. DOUBLES 3, SINGLES 4

MOCK ORANGE. Many species of deciduous shrubs, most with fragrant white flowers, hardy in zones 3 to 10. Mock orange grows best in full sun or partial shade in hot areas. Not fussy about soil or watering, it should be pruned hard each year after blooming, thinning and removing the oldest wood to encourage new growth and continued bloom. *P. lewisii* is native to the northwestern United States and is the state flower of Idaho. *P. virginalis* is a hybrid with double flowers; the cultivar 'Minnesota Snowflake' is fully double and releases less pollen than single varieties. Certain kinds of Philadelphus are very fragrant, and these may affect some sensitive individuals.

Phillyrea decora. MALES 9 🔪, FEMALES 1 ✪

JASMINE BOX, PRIVET, SHARPBERRY TREE. An evergreen shrub or small tree from the Mediterranean area, hardy in zones 6 to 10. These are separate-sexed plants, and because they are members of the olive family, the tiny white flowers of the males have high potential for allergy. Female shrubs produce small red fruits that turn purple in late fall. Some of the plants appear to be androdioecious, meaning they always produce pollen even if they make fruit. With this in mind, it is difficult to recommend any Phillyrea. In some areas these have become invasive.

Philodendron. 3

Houseplants, used outside in frost-free parts of zones 9 to 10. Several hundred species of frost-tender evergreen perennials. Most of these plants seldom flower; the flowers of Philodendron, however, are designed to release airborne pollen, and in the tropics this group of plants contributes to allergy. As used in the United States, most Philodendrons are low-allergy-ranked plants. Contact allergy from the sap. One species, *P. cordatum*, which is often confused with *P. oxycardium*, the oxheart philodendron, is implicated in causing skin rash in nursery workers. Poisonous if eaten.

Phleum. 9 🗡

TIMOTHY. A common pasture grass for northern areas. Timothy is among the worst of all grasses for causing allergy. If possible, farmers using it for hay should mow the first crop early to prevent flowering. Early cuts of hay provide less tonnage but higher food value.

Phlomis fruticosa. 3

JERUSALEM SAGE. Tall, shrubby perennial with bright yellow flowers, hardy in all zones. Easy to grow and not fussy about soil. A member of the mint family.

Phlox. 3

Annuals and perennials, a few hardy to zone 3. Several different colors are available. Phlox grows best in full sun with plenty of water; the perennial varieties are long-lived once established.

Phoenix dactylifera. MALES 9 🗡, FEMALES 1 ✪

DATE PALM. The date palm of commerce is a tall, thin-trunked tree, cold-hardy to 10°F. Of the approximately fifteen other species of date palms, none is cold-hardy below 20°F. All members of this genus are separate-sexed, but no attempt has been made to sell them sexed, despite the fact that the trees are easy to propagate from root suckers, which produce young trees of the same sex as the parent. As with all separate-sexed trees, the males produce quantities of potent, airborne pollen. Canary Island date palms are very common street trees in California, Florida, and all along the Gulf Coast, creating a corridor of allergy when they bloom. The pollen of male Canary Island palms is occasionally used to pollinate female *P. dactylifera* but this results in smaller fruit.

PHOENIX TREE. See *Firmiana simplex*.

Phoradendron serotinum. MALES 6, FEMALES 1 ✪

AMERICAN MISTLETOE. A parasitic evergreen plant that grows on many species of trees. Most mistletoe is unisexual and males can cause pollen allergies. Mistletoe saps strength from the host trees and should be removed where possible. Mistletoe berries (from female plants) that are brought inside as holiday decorations pose little allergy threat; they are poisonous, however.

Phormium tenax. 3

NEW ZEALAND FLAX. Evergreen perennials for zones 7 to 10 that form tall clumps of broad grasslike bronze fronds marked with stripes. The red or yellow flowers, borne on tall, erect stalks, rise up out of the middle of these clumps; the entire plant may reach 12 feet. Although it looks like a grass plant, Phormium is related to the Agaves. Phormium is sometimes implicated in contact skin rash.

Photinia. 4

The deciduous *P. villosa* is hardy in zones 3 to 10. *P. × Fraseri* is a common evergreen shrub or small tree hardy in zones 9 to 10. Photinia flowers are usually white, occasionally pink, showy and, like the blossoms of the related pear, malodorous. When pruned hard, the new leaves grow back a bright red color, then slowly turn green as they mature. Despite its offensive smell, Photinia blossom is not a great contributor of allergenic pollen.

Phygelius capensis. 1 ✪

CAPE FUCHSIA. An easy-to-grow perennial for zones 7 to 10, with pendulous, red tubular flowers.

Phyla nodiflora. 2 ✪

LIPPIA. A drought-tolerant, low-growing perennial ground cover for zones 8 to 10, with small rose-colored flowers that attract bees. It does not compete well with weeds and becomes dormant in cold weather. It will tolerate desert conditions, but grows best with adequate water. Phyla is related to Verbena.

Phyllitis scolopendrium. 3

HART'S-TONGUE FERN. Long-lived hardy ferns for zones 5 to 10. They are popular potted plants, and will grow well in shady areas of their range.

PHYLLOSTACHYS. See *Bamboo*.

Physalis. 2 ✪

CHINESE LANTERN PLANT, GROUND CHERRY, STRAWBERRY TOMATO, TOMATILLO. Several species of annuals or frost-tender perennials, none of which causes allergy. The unripe fruits of some species, however, are poisonous.

PHYSIC NUT. See *Jatropha*.

Physocarpus. 4

NINEBARK. Easy-to-grow deciduous shrubs for full sun or partial shade, hardy in zones 2 to 10. The white flowers resemble those of Spiraea.

Physostegia virginiana. 3

FALSE DRAGONHEAD, OBEDIENCE PLANT. Hardy native perennial for all zones. Tall, upright plants bear tubular, rose-colored flowers on long spikes.

PHYTEUMA SCHEUCHZERI. See *Campanula*.

Phytolacca. 5 TO 8 DEPENDING ON SPECIES, 3 TO 8 DEPENDING ON SEX

POKE, POKE BERRY, POKE SALAD, POKEWEED. A group of herbs, shrubs, or treelike plants native to the tropics and to the southeastern United States. Many have poisonous roots and leaves, and the fruits are especially toxic. *P. americana*, usually called poke salad or pigeon berry, has leaves that are boiled and eaten in spring when the plants are small. The water must be changed several times to leach out the poisonous properties. Once the toxins are removed, the leaves are highly nutritious and are used much as collard greens. Mature poke plants have sap that is so dangerous that they should never be handled unless gloves are worn. Even small amounts of sap contacted through cuts or breaks in the skin can cause poisoning. The attractive red berries of poke have also proven fatal to children on numerous occasions. In addition, the pollen from male poke plants is both allergenic and poisonous. In Brazil, Uruguay, and Argentina, *P. dioica*, a tall (to 60 feet) evergreen separate-sexed tree, is used in landscaping, where the males do contribute to allergy. Several other species of Phytolacca, mostly herbs and flowers, are grown in China and Japan, but these are perfect-flowered and are not contributors to allergy.

Picea. 3

SPRUCE. Large evergreen, coniferous trees, hardy to zone 1, native to wide areas of the Northern Hemisphere, including North America, China, Japan, Tibet, and Scandinavia. Spruce grow best in cool summer, cold winter areas (and do not thrive in hot, dry climates) where soil is deep, well drained, moist, and acidic. They are related to pines, and like them, the pollen has a waxy coating that prevents it from irritating sensitive mucous membranes. As a result, spruce, like pine, is not an important tree in allergy even though it releases large amounts of pollen each year. Occasionally, some sensitive individuals may be allergic to the scent of spruce.

There are many species of Picea, ranging from ground covers to tall, handsome pyramid-shaped trees. The Colorado blue spruce (*P. pungens* 'Glauca') is a very popular slow-growing landscape tree. *P. abies*, the Norway spruce, is another common landscape plant that may reach 150 feet; it is also an important lumber tree.

PICKEREL WEED. See *Pontederia cordata*.

Pieris. 3

FETTERBUSH, LILY-OF-THE-VALLEY BUSH. Eight species of evergreen flowering ground covers, shrubs, or small trees, hardy in all zones. Some Pieris are native to Asia and others to the United States, but all grow best in partial shade in cool summer areas with well-drained, moist, acidic, peaty, or sandy soils. Pieris bears small, pink, drooping clusters of attractive buds, followed by white, pink, or occasionally red flowers. The leaves are glossy and handsome and the shrubs grow well alongside rhododendrons, which share their cultural requirements. All parts of the plant are highly poisonous if eaten.

PIGEON BERRY. See *Duranta*; *Phytolacca*.

PIGEON GRASS. See *Setaria*.

PIGEON PLUM. See *Coccoloba*.

PIGGY-BACK PLANT. See *Tolmiea menziesii*.

Pilea. MALES 5, FEMALES 1 ☻

ALUMINUM PLANT, ARTILLERY PLANT, CREEPING CHARLIE, PANAMIGA, PANAMIGO. A large group of frost-tender herbs often used as houseplants. The male flowers have limited allergy potential, so it is best to remove any blooms as they appear.

PILI NUT. See *Canarium ovatum*.

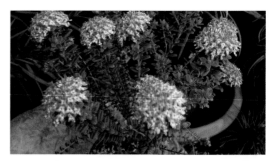

Pimelea coarctata, P. prostrata. 3

(*Pimelea ferruginea* pictured above.) Small evergreen shrub with fragrant white flowers that grows best in full sun with moist, acid, well-drained soil. *P. ferruginea* is a small, upright Australian subshrub with bright pink flowers for zones 9 to 10.

PIMPERNEL. See *Anagallis*.

Pimpinella anisum. 2 ☺

ANISE. Annual herb for all zones; easy to grow from seed in full sun with good moisture. The seeds and foliage are used to season foods.

Pinanga. 6

A group of more than 100 species of small- to medium-size attractive palms used mostly in tropical landscapes.

PINCUSHION FLOWER. See *Scabiosa.*

PINCUSHION TREE. See *Hakea.*

PINDO PALM. See *Butia capitata; Cocos australis.*

PINE. See *Pinus.*

PINE, WATER. See *Glyptostrobus lineatus.*

PINEAPPLE (ANANAS COMOSUS). See *Bromelia.*

PINEAPPLE FLOWER. See *Eucomis.*

PINEAPPLE GUAVA. See *Feijoa sellowiana.*

PINEAPPLE SAGE. See *Salvia.*

PINK BALL DOMBEYA. See *Dombeya.*

PINK CEDAR. See *Acrocarpus fraxinifolius.*

PINK IRONBARK. See *Eucalyptus.*

PINK POLKA-DOT PLANT. See *Hypoestes phyllostachya.*

PINK POWDER-PUFF BUSH. See *Calliandra.*

PINK. See *Dianthus.*

PINON, PINON NUT TREE. See *Pinus.*

Pinus. 4 (SEE EXCEPTION)

PINE, PINON, PINON NUT TREE. Evergreen coniferous trees and shrubs that are native to most temperate parts of the world, including Asia, Europe, and America. Some species are hardy into the coldest zones. In urban landscaping, large pine trees often overwhelm the area in which they are planted.

Pines shed enormous quantities of pollen, but because the pollen grains are waxy and not highly irritating to mucous membranes, their potential for allergy is rather low and, when it occurs, not usually severe. Allergic reactions to the scent of cut pine are reported but are also rare.

On the central coast of California most of the native Monterey pines have died off recently. The small, low-growing varieties such as the mugo pine, present even less allergy potential than larger types and are good choices for the allergy-free landscape.

Exception: One Pinus species, *P. contorta,* the lodgepole pine from Colorado, is known to cause asthma and has an OPALS ranking of 8. Use of lodgepole pine in landscaping should be discouraged.

Piper. MALES 6, FEMALES 1 ☺

PEPPER. A group of more than 1,000 different species of evergreen vines, shrubs, and small trees, many of which have high allergy potential from their odor, contact with their leaves and sap, and their pollen. Some species are separate-sexed plants, but all are tropical or subtropical, only grown in the United States in a few frost-free areas and in greenhouses. All male members of the Piper genus are high-allergy plants and should not be used in the allergy-free landscape.

P. betle, or betel, is a large shrubby vine, common in Asia and India. The leaves are chewed along with slaked lime and nuts from *Areca catechu* (the betel nut) as a stimulant.

P. kadsura is a climbing shrub from Asia, used in landscapes in Japan and Korea.

P. methysticum, kava-kava, is a large shrub or small tree, the roots of which are used to produce an herbal remedy for stress relief. The extract is also used in teas and mouth sprays as a calming agent.

P. nigrum, a large, woody vine, is the source of commercial pepper. Black pepper is made from the dried unripe fruits of the female vines. White pepper is made from ripe fruits.

Piqueria trinervia. 8

STEVIA. A small group of winter-blooming annuals and shrubs grown mostly in Mexico and Central America as florist crops for cut flowers. A high-allergy plant.

Pisonia. MALES 6, FEMALES 1 ☺

BIRD-CATCHER TREE, PARA-PARA. Houseplants, evergreen shrubs, or small trees in mildest parts of zone 10. From New Zealand and Australia, Pisonia bears tiny pink or white flowers.

Pistache. MALES 8, FEMALES 1 ☺

A group of deciduous and evergreen trees and shrubs from the southwestern United States, Mexico, the Mediterranean region, and the Canary Islands. All species are separate-sexed, and the male plants have very high potential for causing allergy and asthma. Pistache is in the Anacardiaceae (cashew) family of plants that includes poison ivy, poison oak, and poison sumac. Because of this close familial connection, it is probable that those with hypersensitivity to poison ivy or poison oak may eventually develop a severe allergy to either pistachio nuts, their pollen, or both.

P. atlantica, the Mount Atlas pistache, is a large, briefly deciduous separate-sexed tree for zones 8 to 10.

P

P. chinensis, the Chinese pistache tree, is a deciduous tree to 60 feet, prized for its orange and red autumn color in zones 8 to 10, and for the ornamental, glossy, half-red, half-blue-green fruit of the female trees. A popular street tree in California, the cultivar 'Keith Davey' is a male and should never be used. Some of these male street trees get to a huge size, and they look like they're smoking when the pollen is coming off of them.

P. vera is a small- to medium-size deciduous nut tree for hot summer areas of zones 8 to 10. Both sexes are needed to produce the edible nuts. Male *P. vera* trees are not as allergenic as those of *P. chinensis*. *P.* hybrid 'Red Push' is being sold as allergy-free, but from what I've seen so far, it is not; it looks to be a male plant.

Pisum sativum. 2 ✪
ENGLISH PEA, GARDEN PEA. Annual vines that produce edible peas and in some varieties, edible pods.

PITANGA. See *Eugenia*.

PITCHER PLANT. See *Sarracenia*.

Pithecellobium guadalupensis. MONOECIOUS 5, MALES 8, FEMALES 1 ✪
BLACKBEAD TREE. A tropical tree used in zone 10, especially in Florida. There are a few other species of this genus that are also of interest in allergy. *P. unguiscati*, cat's claw, is used in landscapes in south Florida, the West Indies, and Mexico. The male flowers of this species resemble those of Mimosa and are capable of releasing considerable allergenic airborne pollen. *P. flexicaule* is not separate-sexed, but has masses of exposed stamens and is suspected of causing allergies in some localities.

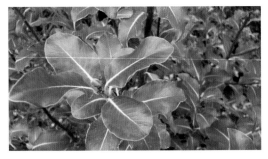

Pittosporum. BISEXUAL 4, MALES 7, FEMALES 1 ✪
CAPE PITTOSPORUM, KARO, KOHUHU, MOCK ORANGE, QUEENSLAND PITTOSPORUM, VICTORIAN BOX. (Pictured above.) Easy-to-grow, glossy-leafed evergreen shrubs and trees native to Australia, New Zealand, Japan, China, and South Africa, used as common landscape plants in zones 9 to 10. They are fairly drought-tolerant once established and not fussy about soil; they grow well in either sun or shade, but tend to legginess in deep shade. Pittosporums produce fragrant white flowers followed by rounded seedpods full of sticky seeds (their Latin name means "sticky seeds"), which may present a litter problem, especially with *P. undulatum*. The fragrance of some Pittosporum, especially *P. tobira*, can be intense, particularly on warm, still summer evenings, and this fragrance may be allergenic for odor-sensitive individuals.

There are at least two new allergy-free OPALS selected female cultivars of Pittosporum; see chapter 4.

Pityrogramma. 3
GOLDBACK FERN. A native of the West Coast from California to Alaska and used in landscapes in shady, dry spots. It becomes summer dormant and looks best during the winter.

PLANE TREE. See *Platanus*.

Planera aquatica. 10 ◈
PLANNER TREE, WATER ELM. A species of elm-related deciduous trees, native to swampy areas of the southeastern United States and hardy to zone 7. This is one of the few members of the elm family that produces separate male flowers, and as a result it is an especially heavy airborne pollinator.

PLANTAIN. See *Musa paradisiaca*.

PLANTAIN LILY. See *Hosta*.

Platanus. 8 (SEE EXCEPTION)
BUTTONBALL TREE, BUTTONWOOD, PLANE TREE, SYCAMORE. Big, fast-growing deciduous trees, some native, with attractive, peeling bark. Sycamore trees are used throughout the world and they cause some allergy everywhere they're cultivated. Several species grown from zones 3 to 10. The fuzzy leaves may cause contact rash in sensitive individuals. When they bloom in early spring, sycamores produce large amounts of airborne pollen, and allergy to sycamore is common. Sycamore leaves also often have a multitude of tiny sharp plant hairs on them, and these can become airborne and cause allergy, asthma, itching, and rash. Be careful when raking up the big leaves.

Exception: Existing sycamore trees that can't be removed can often be pollarded. Because almost all of the male pollen flowers are formed on old wood, pollarding each winter will eliminate almost all of the worst allergy potential. In London, England, many thousands of sycamore and London plane street trees are pollarded yearly to let in more light and to eliminate pollen. Annually pollarded sycamores can be considered to be fairly low-allergy trees.

Platycarya. 7
A deciduous Chinese tree, hardy in zones 6 to 10. The bark of these relatives of the walnut is used to make a black dye.

Platycerium. 3
STAGHORN FERN. Dry, shade-loving epiphytic fern that grows on trees or in hanging wire baskets in gardens in zones 9 to 10. Slow growing, it can get huge and quite beautiful with age.

Platycladus orientalis (Thuja orientalis; Biota orientalis). 7
BEVERLY HILLS ARBORVITAE, ORIENTAL ARBORVI-TAE. Evergreen coniferous shrubs, native to Korea and China, and hardy in zones 4 to 10. Extremely common landscape plants because of their tidy growth habits, these relatives of the cypress cause allergy.

Platycodon grandiflorus. 2 ✪
BALLOON FLOWER. An easy-to-grow perennial for full sun or partial shade in all zones. Its balloonlike blue or white flowers appear in summer on the upright plants.

Plectranthus. 1 ✪
SWEDISH IVY. Easy-to-grow houseplant related to Coleus.

Pleiogynium. MALES 7, FEMALES 1 ✪
BURDEKIN PLUM, HOG PLUM, QUEENSLAND HOG PLUM. Two species of separate-sexed trees from the Philippines, New Guinea, and Australia. Grown in California, Hawaii, and Florida, the hog plum is a large (to 60 feet) evergreen tree, the females of which produce small fruits popularly used in jellies and jams.

PLEIONE. See *Orchids.*

PLEROMA. See *Tibouchina.*

PLOVER EGGS. See *Adromischus.*

PLUM, FLOWERING. See *Prunus.*

PLUM, PATERSON. See *Lagunaria patersonii.*

PLUM YEW. See *Cephalotaxus.*

PLUMBAGO. See *Ceratostigma*; *Plumbago auriculata.*

Plumbago auriculata. 3
CAPE PLUMBAGO. Plumbago is a large group of more than 300 species, none of which is important in

allergy. The Cape plumbago is a large, sprawling shrub with sky-blue flowers, native to Ethiopia, and thrives on neglect in sunny areas of zone 10. Good bank cover plants. Very drought-tolerant. Direct contact with the leaves has been known to trigger skin rash and itch. Be careful when pruning. (See also *Ceratostigma.*)

PLUME CEDAR. See *Cryptomeria.*

Plumeria. 4
FRANGIPANI. Frost-tender evergreen and deciduous shrubs and small trees for sheltered locations of zone 10, or as greenhouse plants. Plumeria are easy to propagate from cuttings and make good container plants. Their extremely fragrant flowers may affect those with odor sensitivity. Flowers and leaves are poisonous. Sap can cause problems; do not get it in your eyes.

PLUMS, PRUNES. See *Prunus.*

Poa. GENUS 7, MALES 9 🌑, FEMALES 1 ✪
BLUEGRASS. *P. pratensis*, Kentucky bluegrass, is a popular lawn grass for northern areas, where it must be mowed often to keep it low and nonflowering. The common annual weed grass, *P. annua*, blooms at any height and also produces allergenic pollen.

Certain species of Poa make good pasture plants and in the future there should be some pollen-free selections. Hybrids between Kentucky and Texas bluegrass are often much less allergenic than either parent. Look for bluegrass plants and seed sold with an OPALS #1 tag, as some female selections are presently in the works. 'Bella' is a very interesting hybrid bluegrass clone; it stays short, grows in thick, produces very little pollen, is dark green, and is widely adapted. Plant 'Bella' from plugs.

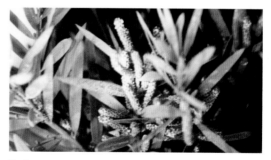

Podocarpus. MALES 10 🌑, FEMALES 1 ✪
FERN PINE, TOTARA, YEW PINE. (*Podocarpus*, male, pictured above.) A small group of separate-sexed coniferous evergreen shrubs or trees with leaves rather

than needles. The female trees produce small, round, fleshy covered seeds. *P. macrophyllus*, the yew pine, is a very common shrub in California and is hardy in zones 9 to 10. Several dwarf forms are sold for use as a ground cover or low hedges. 'Select Spreader' is a low-growing male cultivar that should be avoided for its allergy potential.

P. gracilior, the fern pine, is a medium- to large-size tree, occasionally well used to make a dense, large, tall hedge. *P. henkelii* is a handsome long-leafed shrub or small tree for zones 8 to 10, occasionally sold as long-leafed yellowwood. All species are separate-sexed.

Podocarpus are not related to pine but rather to yews (Taxus). Like their yew relatives, the leaves, stems, flowers, and pollen from Podocarpus are poisonous. The leaves, stems, bark, and pollen from Podocarpus are also cytotoxic, meaning, toxic to living cells. Male Podocarpus trees or shrubs growing next to bedroom windows represent a potentially very dangerous situation, as these plants bloom just as the nights warm up in spring and early summer. A chemotherapy drug is made from Podocarpus and used to treat leukemia. Heavy exposure to Podocarpus pollen can mimic chemotherapy treatments. *P. gracilior* has also been used as a source for the chemotherapy cancer drug Taxol (now sold as Paclitaxel).

The fruit on female trees is not poisonous, but it doesn't taste very good. Female trees that have no male trees within 100 feet will almost never make any fruit.

There are at least two very useful female cultivars, from several species, in the works now, and these will be sold with OPALS #1 ranked tags.

Podophyllum peltatum. 2 ✪
MAY APPLE, MAYAPPLE. A very hardy, small native perennial for shady areas, does well under deciduous trees. Small fruits are edible and used in jelly, but the leaves and roots of the may apple are poisonous.

POHUTUKAWA. See *Metrosideros*.

POINCIANA. See *Caesalpinia*.

POINSETTIA. See *Euphorbia*.

POINTED-LEAF MAPLE. See *Acer argutum*.

POISON BERRY. See *Solanum*.

POISON ELDER. See *Rhus*.

POISON IVY. See *Rhus*.

POISON OAK. See *Rhus toxicodendron*.

POKE, POKE BERRY, POKE SALAD, POKEWEED. See *Phytolacca*.

POKER PLANT. See *Kniphofia uvaria*.

POLECAT BUSH. See *Rhus*.

Polemonium. 2 ✪
JACOB'S LADDER. Hardy perennials best in cool summer areas in moist soil with good drainage. They bear stalks of blue or lavender flowers held erect above ferny foliage.

Polianthes tuberosa. 4
TUBEROSE. Tender tuberous perennial for the mildest areas of zone 10, Polianthes is used mostly as a potted plant. The powerfully fragrant, tubular white flowers are borne on tall spikes and may affect a few perfume-sensitive individuals.

POLKA-DOT PLANT. See *Hypoestes phyllostachya*.

Polyandrococos. 6
A palm tree from Brazil, with small, edible fruit, used in zones 9 to 10, especially in Florida.

POLYANTHUS. See *Primula*.

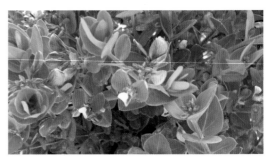

Polygala. 3
BIRD-ON-THE-WING, CANDYWEED, MILKWORT, SENECA SNAKEROOT, SWEET PEA SHRUB, VIOLET TREE, YELLOW BACHELOR'S BUTTON. (Pictured above.) Large group of evergreen perennials, shrubs, and small trees for light soils and partial shade in zones 7 to 12. Many species are frost-tender. The common name milkwort is derived from the belief that the plants could increase the flow of milk in cows.

Polygonatum. 2 ✪
SOLOMON'S SEAL. Tall perennials of the lily family, hardy in all zones. They grow in shady, moist areas, where they bear white or green-white bell-shaped flowers. Plants are poisonous.

Polygonum. **4 TO 6 DEPENDING ON SPECIES**
FLEECEFLOWER, KNOTWEED, SILVER LACE VINE,
SMARTWEED. Many species of worldwide distribution:
herbs, ground covers, vines, annuals, or perennials,
of varying hardiness. The Latin name means "many
joints," and refers to the many joints or nodes found
along the stems of these plants. Smartweed is a common weed that thrives in almost any moist area. Smartweed gets its name from the fact that the juice or sap
can "smart," or burn the skin. All Polygonum members
may cause skin rash from their caustic sap, and some
species may also cause airborne allergy. All parts of
plant are poisonous.

Polypodium. **INDIVIDUALLY RANKED**
The largest group of ferns, with more than 7,000 species worldwide.

Polypogon. **5**
BEARDGRASS, RABBIT'S FOOT GRASS. Small annual,
ornamental grass with large, fluffy heads. It often
naturalizes.

Polyscias. **1** ✪
MING ARALIA, PARSLEY PANAX. Tall, shrubby houseplants or small trees in tropical zone 10. Polyscias
grows best in partial shade.

Polystichum. **4**
HEDGE FERN, HOLLY FERN, SHIELD FERN, WESTERN
SWORD FERN. Large group of easy-to-grow landscape
ferns, some hardy to zones 4 to 5. All grow best in
shady spots in the garden.

POMEGRANATE. See *Punica granatum.*

POMPOM TREE. See *Dais cotinifolia.*

POND CYPRESS. See *Taxodium.*

PONDWEED, CAPE. See *Aponogeton distachyus.*

Pontederia cordata. **2** ✪
PICKEREL WEED. Pond plant for all zones; it bears tall
stalks of blue flowers.

PONYTAIL. See *Beaucarnea recurvata.*

POOR-MAN'S ORCHID. See *Schizanthus.*

POPLAR. See *Liriodendron*; *Populus.*

POPLAR, TULIP. See *Liriodendron.*

POPLAR, YELLOW. See *Liriodendron.*

POPOLO, YELLOW. See *Solanum.*

POPPY. See *Papaver.*

POPULUS GENUS

Populus. **MALES 8, FEMALES 1** ✪
ASPEN, COTTONWOOD, POPLAR. More than thirty
species of large, fast-growing, deciduous trees, members of the willow family, hardy in all zones and under
conditions ranging from arid deserts to wetlands,
depending on species. Almost all species of Populus are
separate-sexed; male trees often cause widespread and
severe allergy, and in many areas, poplar pollen is the
primary cause of springtime allergy. Female trees cause
no allergy but are often maligned for the "cotton," seeds
and fruit that they shed. Because they shed their seeds,
each with its parachute of highly visible "cotton," at the
same time that ragweeds, coyote bush, Chinese elm, and
other highly allergenic plants are shedding their pollen,
female poplars are unfairly blamed for the resulting
allergy. (Female trees often mature to larger, longer-
lived, rounder specimens than do male trees.) Trees
sold as cottonless cottonwoods or cottonless poplars are
males, and highly suspect in the allergy-free landscape.

The following named cultivars are all males and
should be avoided: 'Androscoggin', 'Cordeniensis',
'Majestic', 'Mojave Hybrid', 'N. E. 17', 'N. E. 308',
and 'Wheeler', as should *P. songarica* (*P. manchurica*).

P. x *berolinensis* 'Volunteer' is a female Russian
poplar, and *P. wilsoni* is a large female tree with
reddish twigs and leaves that are bluish above
and white below. Both are excellent choices for the
allergy-free landscape.

P. alba.
White poplar. The cultivar 'Nivea' is female; 'Pyramidalis'
is a male.

P. canadensis.
BLACK POPLAR. The cultivars 'Incrassata', 'Marilandica',
and 'Regenerata' are females and good choices for the
allergy-free landscape. 'Eugenei', 'Gelrica' or Dutch
poplar, 'Prairie Sky', and 'Robusta' are male and should
be avoided.

P. x *canadensis* (*P. deltoides* x *P. nigra*).
CAROLINA POPLAR. These are all male hybrids.

P. candicans (*P.* x *Jackii; P. balsamifera;
P. ontariensis*).
BALM-OF-GILEAD. These are female trees, and fine
choices for the allergy-free landscape. 'Candicans
Aurora' is a named female cultivar. 'Candicans Variegata'
is a beautiful female tree that is often used as a big
shrub. Cut to the ground each fall, it resprouts with
huge, variegated leaves, splashed with pink and white.

P

The cultivar 'Macrophylla' is a male and should not be used. The hybrid *P.* × *candicans* 'White' is a male.

P. × *canescens*.
The cultivar 'Tower' is a male tree; avoid use.

P. deltoides.
Among named cultivars, 'Carolin' and 'Siouxland' are males; 'Cordata' is a female.

P. fremontii.
'Zappetini' is a male.

P. × *Jackii*.
The named cultivar 'Generosa' can be either male or female; female trees are identified by their catkins, which are twice as long as the male's in this cultivar. Both 'Northwest' and 'Saskatchewan' are male.

P. lasiocarpa. 3
CHINESE NECKLACE POPLAR. A native of China, this is a rare example of a poplar that has bisexual flowers. It has very large leaves, and the pollen does not present much allergy potential.

P. nigra.
BLACK POPLAR. There are many named cultivars of black poplar, but unless the trees are sexed, it is best to avoid use. The Theves poplar 'Afghanica' is also called *P. thevestina*, *P. usbekistanica*, and *P. nigra* 'Ozbeki- stanica'. The Theves poplar is a tall, narrow tree, similar in appearance to Lombardy poplar (*P. nigra* 'Italica'), except that it is fuller and longer-lived. Theves poplar is female, as is the variety *P. nigra* 'Charkowiensis', which is a larger tree. 'Elegans' and 'Italica' are male. 'Noreaster' is one of the best, a sterile female.

P. nigra 'Italica'.
This is the tall, skinny, Lombardy poplar that grows so tall and fast but then dies off almost as quickly. Although this is the most widely planted poplar in the world, 'Italica' (or 'Lombardi') is always a male and should be avoided.

P. × *petrowskiana*.
'Waller' is a female.

P. × *pseudo-grandidentata*.
This is a weeping poplar, occasionally sold as *P. pendula*. It is a male.

P. simonii.
SIMON POPLAR. 'Fastigiata' and 'Pendula' are males.

P. tomentosa.
CHINESE WHITE POPLAR. Both sexes are sold; use only the female.

P. tremula.
EUROPEAN ASPEN. The varieties 'Erecta' and 'Pendula' are male.

P. tremuloides.
QUAKING ASPEN. 'Pendula' is a female.

PORCUPINE PALM. See *Rhapidophyllum hystrix*.

PORK-AND-BEANS. See *Sedum*.

PORT ORFORD CEDAR. See *Chamaecyparis*.

Portulaca grandiflora. 2 ✪
MOSS ROSE. An annual for hot, sunny spots. Bright roselike, little flowers in many colors cover these succulent bedding plants.

Portulacaria afra. 2 ✪
ELEPHANT'S FOOD, PURSLANE TREE. Tall succulent with many tiny, fleshy leaves borne on thick fleshy stalks. Easy to grow in sun or shade in protected areas of zones 9 to 10. Houseplant elsewhere, in good light.

POT MARIGOLD. See *Calendula officinalis*.

POTATO VINE, POTATO BUSH. See *Solanum*.

Potentilla. 3
CINQUEFOIL. Hardy evergreen and deciduous perennials and shrubs for all zones. Most Potentilla have bright yellow flowers but some are red, orange, or white. Several species are low-growing ground covers for partial shade with ample water.

POTHOS. See *Epipremnum aureum*.

POUND CAKE WEED. See *Parthenium hysterophorum*.

POVERTY GRASS. See *Corema*; *Hudsonia*.

PRAIRIE MIMOSA. See *Desmanthus*.

PRAIRIE TEA. See *Croton monanthogynus*.

Pratia angulata. 1 ✪
New Zealand perennial native used in desert areas of zones 7 to 10 as a ground cover, although it needs ample water. Pratia bears small white or blue flowers.

PRAYER PLANT. See *Maranta leuconeura*.

PREGNANT ONION. See *Ornithogalum*.

PRICKLEWEED. See *Desmanthus*.

PRICKLY ASH. See *Zanthoxylum*.

PRICKLY PEAR. See *Cactus*.

PRICKLY POPPY. See *Argemone*.

PRIDE-OF-BOLIVIA. See *Tipuana tipu.*

PRIDE OF CHINA. See *Melia.*

PRIDE OF INDIA. See *Melia.*

PRIDE OF MADEIRA. See *Echium fastuosum.*

PRIMROSE TREE. See *Lagunaria patersonii.*

Primula. 3 TO 6 DEPENDING ON SPECIES
AURICULA, COWSLIP, POLYANTHUS, PRIMROSE. Hardy
perennials often used as annuals. In hot areas primroses are best used as potted flowers, or in the garden
for winter color or as early spring annuals. Primroses
do not produce allergenic pollen, but some species,
especially *P. malacoides* and *P. obconica,* frequently are
the cause of severe skin rashes and lesions from simple
contact with the plants.

PRINCESS FLOWER. See *Tibouchina urvilleana.*

PRINCESS PALM. See *Dictyosperma.*

PRINCESS PINE. See *Lycopodium.*

PRIVET. See *Ligustrum; Phillyrea decora.*

PRIVET, SWAMP. See *Forestiera.*

Prosopis. 6 TO 7 DEPENDING ON SPECIES
MESQUITE, SCREW BEAN, TORNILLO. Twenty or more
species of summer-deciduous or evergreen thorny
shrubs or trees, native to desert areas of the southwestern United States and Mexico. With its fernlike foliage
and numerous pollen-shedding small yellow flowers,
mesquite is a major allergy plant in some areas.

Protea. 3
South African shrubs and trees, many with large,
unusual flowers, which are favored as centerpieces for
large flower arrangements. They are hardy only in zones
9 to 10.

Prunella. 2 ✪
HEAL-ALL, SELF-HEAL. Creeping perennial ground
cover with medicinal properties, for shade with ample
moisture.

PRUNUS GENUS

Prunus. INDIVIDUALLY RANKED
ALMOND, APRICOT, CHERRY, PEACH, PLUM, NECTAR-
INE. Prunus is a large group of more than 400 species of
deciduous shrubs and trees, mostly native to the Northern Hemisphere. Many species of Prunus are popular
and useful landscape shrubs and trees. Following are
some of the most common.

P. caroliniana. 6
CAROLINA LAUREL CHERRY. A native evergreen small
tree for zones 7 to 10.

P. ilicifolia. 5
HOLLYLEAF CHERRY. An evergreen ornamental shrub
or small tree for zones 8 to 10.

P. laurocerasus. 6
ENGLISH LAUREL, ZABEL LAUREL. An ornamental evergreen shrub, commonly used as a hedge in zones 7 to 9.

P. lusitanica. 5
PORTUGAL LAUREL. An evergreen ornamental shrub
with thick leathery leaves and white flowers. Hardy only
in warm winter areas.

P. lyonii. 6
CATALINA CHERRY. An ornamental flowering shrub for
zones 8 to 10.

P. maackii. 5
AMUR CHOKECHERRY. A cold-hardy, highly ornamental
cherry tree with incredibly beautiful bark, best in zones
4 to 7.

P. padus. 5
BIRD CHERRY, MAYBUSH, MAYDAY TREE. Tall ornamental cherry hardy to zone 4.

P. sargentii. 6
SARGENT CHERRY. A large tree, with small fruit that is
very attractive to birds.

P. serrula. 5
BIRCH BARK CHERRY. A large flowering tree with handsome leaves and bark, hardy to zone 4.

P. serrulata. DOUBLES 4, SINGLES 7
JAPANESE FLOWERING CHERRY. A popular and common flowering cherry, hardy to zone 4. Double-flowered
varieties are far less potent allergy trees.

P. virginiana. 5
CHOKECHERRY. Shrub or small tree, hardy even in zone
2. Chokecherry produces many dark red bitter fruits.
The leaves, stems, and unripe fruit of this species are
extremely poisonous, by far the most toxic of all Prunus
species.

The fruiting members of the Prunus genus (following) rarely present severe allergy problems, except for
almonds and sweet cherry, which are known to produce
copious amounts of highly irritant pollen. Normally
any Prunus species that is self-fertile, that does not
need a pollinator to set fruit, will be less allergenic.

P

P. armeniaca. 2 ✪

APRICOT. These are hardy in most zones, but do not fruit regularly in any but the mildest winter areas. Good trees often can be grown from seed, although they may take three or more years to fruit. They are especially beautiful when in bloom, and many have excellent fall color. Allergy to apricots is usually confined to those living in or near orchards; as the occasional yard tree, apricots are a very good choice for the allergy-free landscape. *P. glandulosa* is the flowering apricot.

P. avium, P. cerasus. 5 TO 7 DEPENDING ON CULTIVAR

CHERRY. Cherries are hardy, deciduous flowering trees that need a certain amount of winter cold to thrive. They will not grow well in zones 9 and 10. Sour cherry (*P. avium*) is hardier than sweet cherry (*P. cerasus*) and will grow as far north as zone 3. All varieties need good drainage to thrive. Pollen allergy is not uncommon. Those living in or near orchards are most at risk. As a rule, sour cherry is less allergenic than sweet cherry. Also, sweet cherry cultivars that are self-fertile, such as 'Stella', are considerably less allergenic. (Actually, with almost any kind of fruit trees, those that are self-fertile will pose much less potential for pollen allergy or asthma.) Flowering cherries (*P. lannesiana* or *P. siebolid*, see also *P. serrulata*) are commonly used as landscape and street trees and are a major source of pollen; double-flowered varieties release less pollen than single-flowered ones.

P. communis. 10 🖊

ALMOND. In allergy studies almonds frequently stand out as the cause of severe allergy. People living in or close to almond orchards are most likely to develop allergy, and although there is occasionally a cross-allergic reaction to eating almonds, this is less common. There is a small flowering shrub, the flowering almond, *Prunus triloba*, and it is considerably less allergenic than most other kinds of almond.

P. domestica, P. insititia. 3

PLUM. *P. cerasifera*, the purple-leaf plum, is a common landscape tree with several cultivars, notably 'Newport' and 'Krauter Vesuvius', that produce little pollen. *P. blireana*, another hardy red-leafed plum, is also a low pollen producer. The smaller, shrubby *P. cistena*, the dwarf red-leaf plum, is also not a high-risk tree but has a slightly higher potential for allergy. Ornamental

plum trees that actually make fruit are, as a rule, less allergenic than those that make none.

P. persica. 3 TO 4

NECTARINE, PEACH. Certain varieties of *P. persica* are hardy to zones 4 and 5, but most are not hardy past zone 6. The blossoms smell good, are pink and quite attractive; flowering varieties bloom very early and put on great shows. These flowering types have a greater allergy potential than do fruiting varieties. Nonetheless, allergy to peach or nectarine is uncommon, although the fuzz on peaches is sometimes the cause of rash or inhalant allergy. This allergy to peach fuzz is most common among those working in peach-packing operations.

In areas with foggy, cool nights, peach and nectarine are often afflicted with peach leaf curl, a fungal disease. They are best grown where spring and summer nights are warm and dry. Allergy ranking for fruiting peach and nectarine is 3; for flowering peach and nectarine, 4; and for double-flowered peach and nectarine, 3.

P. tomentosa. 4

NANKING CHERRY. Fruiting bush cherry with edible fruit; the most hardy of any semisweet-fruited cherries. Zones 3 to 7.

P. triloba. 4

FLOWERING ALMOND. Hardy to zone 3, *P. triloba* is considerably less allergenic than most other kinds of almond.

Pseudolarix kaempferi (Chrysolarix). 3

GOLDEN LARCH. A deciduous conifer with attractive foliage and good, bright yellow fall color. A native of China, it grows best in moist, acid soil in zones 6 to 8. Not an important allergy tree, despite its abundant pollen.

Pseudopanax. MALES 7, FEMALES 1 ✪

LANCEWOOD. Separate-sexed evergreen shrubs or small trees from New Zealand and Chile, grown in protected areas of zones 9 to 10. Female plants produce very small, one-seeded fruits.

Pseudophoenix. 5

CHERRY PALM. Four species of palm trees from the subtropics, used in zone 10.

Pseudotsuga. 3

BIG-CONE SPRUCE, DOUGLAS FIR. Five species of evergreen conifers, all large, tall trees, one native to Japan, the rest to the Pacific Northwest and hardy in zones 5 to 10. Although Pseudotsuga releases abundant pollen, none of the genus is an important allergy offender because the large pollen grains have a waxy coating that keeps them from being easily absorbed. Douglas fir, a giant tree, occasionally reaching a height of 300 feet, is perhaps the most important lumber tree in the world. Small Douglas firs are often used as Christmas trees and have the same aromatic smell as their close relatives, the pines. Douglas fir was named after David Douglas, a famous Scotch plant explorer who first discovered and named many species of the Pacific Coast. Douglas made three cross-continental trips across the U.S. searching for new plants before his untimely death in 1834, at the age of thirty-five, at the hands of inhabitants of the Sandwich Islands (Hawaii).

Pseudowintera. 5

WINTER'S BARK. Evergreen shrub or small tree, native of New Zealand and occasionally used in California.

Psidium. 3

GUAVA. Many species of mostly evergreen shrubs or small trees, often cultivated for the sweet yellow fruits with pink flesh. The hardiest of the true guavas is *P. littorale*, the small, reddish, strawberry guava, which grows in most areas of zone 9. *P. lucidum* is a similar plant but the small fruits are yellow. *P. guajava*, the common guava, is a zone 10 shrub that needs decent heat to produce sweet fruit. Although the pollen-bearing stamens are well exposed in Psidium flowers, and may present allergy problems if directly contacted, as a whole the genus does not pose much allergy potential. If *P. guajava* is planted in zone 9, it is suggested that it be planted on the south side of the house, directly under the overhang of the roof, if possible. This will provide it with a bit of frost protection. (See also *Feijoa*.)

Psoralea pinnata. 4

PURPLE GRAPE KOOL-AID SHRUB. This shrub has small purple-lilac flowers that up close smell almost exactly like grape Kool-Aid. Easy-to-grow shrub or small tree for zones 9 to 12. Not long-lived and needs annual pruning to cut out old dead growth. Reseeds and can be invasive in some areas. Stems are often sharp and sticky, and could pose some limited dermatitis risk.

Psylliostachys suworowii. 4

Annuals grown for their large leaves and spikes of pinkish lavender flowers, resembling statice, which are often used in dried flower arrangements.

Ptelea. MALES 7, FEMALES 1 ✪

HOP TREE, WAFER ASH. A deciduous shrub or small tree, related to and having flowers that smell like citrus. Hop tree is hardy to zone 3 if grown in a moist, shady spot. Separate-sexed; only the females produce the flat, hoplike seedpods.

Pteridium aquilinum. 5

BRACKEN FERN. A native fern, hardy in all zones, which may become invasive. The emerging fronds, called fiddleheads, are edible, although recent research indicates that they may contain a carcinogen. The spores may cause allergy.

Pteris. 5

BRAKE. Subtropical ferns, often grown as houseplants.

Pterocarpus. 3

ROSEWOOD, SANDALWOOD. Large group of tropical trees, with aromatic wood much prized for fine furniture.

Pterocarya. 6

WINGNUT TREE. A small group of deciduous trees related to walnut, grown for their attractive leaves and flowers. Various Pterocarya are hardy in zones 6 to 10, depending on species.

Pterostyrax. 4

EPAULETTE TREE, WISTERIA TREE. Deciduous trees from Asia, grown in zones 7 to 10. The long clusters of white flowers are followed by small, hairy seeds, which may be irritating to the skin. The flowers, however, present few pollen problems.

Ptychococcus. 7

A group of palm trees native from New Guinea to the Solomon Islands.

Ptychosperma. 7

ALEXANDER PALM, MACARTHUR PALM. A group of about thirty palm trees, many from Australia and occasionally used in zone 10. All can cause some allergy.

Pueraria lobata. 3

KUDZU. The vine that took over the South. An Asian native, kudzu has been planted in many southern areas as a pasture or hay crop because the feed value of the leaves is as good as alfalfa. Kudzu escaped cultivation, however, and has become a rampant, invasive weed throughout much of the South, often smothering native flora and buildings with its fast-growing vines. Highly invasive in southern areas.

PUERTO RICAN HAT PALM. See *Sabal*.

PUKA. See *Meryta sinclairii.*

Pulmonaria. 2 ✿

JERUSALEM SAGE, LUNGWORT. Perennials hardy in all zones, these shade-loving plants require ample moisture to bear their blue, purple, or red flowers.

Punica granatum. 2 ✿

POMEGRANATE. Deciduous shrubs or small trees, hardy to zone 7, but growing best in full sun, in hot summer areas of zones 8 to 9. Good heat is required to ripen sweet fruit. The large, orange flowers are followed by round fruits that require heat and adequate moisture to ripen fully. Although occasionally grown as an ornamental, pomegranates are good fruit trees, with the variety 'Wonderful' producing the largest fruit. Punica is easy to propagate from dormant cuttings.

PURPLE CONEFLOWER. See *Echinacea purpurea.*

PURPLE HEART. See *Setcreasea pallida.*

PURPLE LOOSESTRIFE. See *Lythrum.*

PURPLE MULLEIN. See *Verbascum.*

PURPLE OSIER. See *Salix.*

PURPLE RAGWORT. See *Senecio.*

PURPLE SAGE. See *Salvia.*

PURPLE VELVET PLANT. See *Gynura aurantiaca.*

PURPLE-LEAF PLUM. See *Prunus.*

PURPLELEAF ELDER. See *Sambucus.*

PURSLANE. See *Portulaca grandiflora.*

PURSLANE TREE. See *Portulacaria.*

PUSSY EARS. See *Calochortus tolmiei; Cyanotis.*

PUSSY TOES. See *Antennaria.*

PUSSY WILLOW. See *Salix.*

Putranjiva. 9 ◐

Small group of large trees native to India, Sri Lanka, and the former Borneo, all with great potential for allergy.

PUYA. See *Bromelia.*

PYCANTHEMUM MUTICUM. See *Mentha.*

Pycanthemum pilosum. 2 ✿

HAIRY MOUNTAIN MINT. Zones 4 to 8, a hardy, spreading native perennial with small white flowers that draw in huge numbers of pollinating wild bees, bumblebees, and small butterflies. Very little if any pollen and considerable nectar.

Pyracantha. 5

FIRETHORN. Several species of evergreen, thorny shrubs or small trees with small white flowers followed by round, reddish orange berries. The berries are poisonous but are eaten by some birds. Hardy in zones 7 to 10, Pyracantha is a common landscape shrub despite its long thorns and the fact that the malodorous flowers tend to attract flies. The odor may cause allergy in sensitive individuals. Pyracantha is closely related to hawthorn and cotoneaster, and may serve as a host for the bacterial disease fire blight.

Pyrethrum. 4

PAINTED DAISY. A daisy-flowered plant from which the botanical insecticide pyrethrum is derived. Those working in pyrethrum processing plants often become very allergic to the flowers and dust from the dried flowers. Pyrethrum is a common insecticide used in pet flea powders, and pet owners may exhibit allergy to this flower-based powder. Nonetheless, the common painted daisy in the garden poses little allergy risk. (See also *Chrysanthemum.*)

Pyrostegia venusta. 3

FLAME VINE. Big, fast-growing evergreen vine with long tubular orange flowers, for zone 10. Flame vine needs heat to grow well.

Pyrrosia lingua (Cyclophorus). 4

JAPANESE FELT FERN. Slow-growing, shade-loving small ferns for zones 9 to 10.

Pyrus. ORNAMENTALS 4, FRUITING VARIETIES 3

BRADFORD PEAR, PEAR. Deciduous fruit trees hardy to zone 4 but growing best in zones 7 to 9. Pear blossoms are attractive but malodorous, although the strong smell does not carry far in the air. The pollen is not usually a strong allergen. Among the many ornamental, flowering, nonfruiting pears grown, the most common and popular is the pyramidal Bradford pear. Asian pears, which have large, sweet fruit rounder than the common pear, are also prized for their good autumn color.

Pears often suffer from fire blight, a bacterial disease that can kill entire branches or even whole trees. Fire blight is spread through airborne spores and direct contact, so diseased branches should be burned, not composted. It is worst during cool, damp weather. Excessive growth encourages fire blight, so use of nitrogen fertilizers is not advised.

Allergy Index Scale: 1 is Best, 10 is Worst.
✪ for 1 and 2   ◗ for 9 and 10
No matter what the ranking, always read the full plant
description carefully and take note of any warnings.

QUACKGRASS. See *Agropyron*.

QUAILBUSH. See *Atriplex*.

QUAMOCLIT LOBATA. See *Mina lobata*.

QUAMOCLIT PENNATA. See *Ipomoea*.

QUEEN ANNE'S LACE. See *Daucus*.

QUEEN PALM. See *Arecastrum romanzoffianum*.

QUEEN'S TEARS. See *Billbergia*.

QUEEN'S WREATH. See *Antigonon*.

QUEENSLAND HOG PLUM. See *Pleiogynium*.

QUEENSLAND KAURI. See *Agathis robusta*.

QUEENSLAND LACEBARK. See *Brachychiton discolor*.

QUEENSLAND NUT. See *Macadamia*.

QUEENSLAND PITTOSPORUM. See *Pittosporum*.

QUEENSLAND POPLAR. See *Homalanthus populifolius*.

QUEENSLAND UMBRELLA TREE. See *Brassaia
actinophylla*.

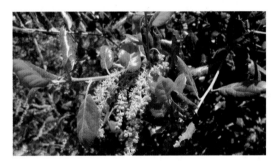

Quercus. **DECIDUOUS 8, EVERGREEN 9** ◗
OAK. (Pictured above.) With more than 400 species of
deciduous or evergreen hardy shrubs or trees worldwide, oaks are important timber and landscape plants
in much of the temperate world. All oaks make acorns,
the usually large, capped oak seeds. Acorns are eaten
by many wild animals and in the past were sometimes
used as food by native peoples.

Oaks are pollinated by the wind, and they produce
abundant pollen that provokes a great deal of allergy
in areas with many oaks. In some cities, planted
landscape oaks are the most common street trees
and these in turn contribute to frequent allergic
attacks; oak pollen can also trigger attacks of asthma.
The large deciduous trees usually flower while the
branches are still bare of leaves or as the new leaves
are budding out. The evergreen oaks often bloom later;
in California they are often at their peak around the

first of June. (In California there are so many kinds of oaks, both native and planted, all of them blooming at different times, that parts of the state have almost a perennial oak-pollen allergy season.)

Some oaks produce much more pollen than others, and an occasional oak tree does not ever bloom. It is hoped that in the future, nurserymen will seek out nonblooming oaks and graft them onto oak seedlings. A few rare individual oak trees, from numerous species, may never produce any male pollen flowers, and these could be considered to be allergy-free trees. However, no one yet sells these, alas.

The literature on oak allergy suggests that there are distinct differences in degree of severity between the allergy potential of the different species of oaks, but as yet, we are forced to group them into two, oversimplified groups, evergreen and deciduous. Some bright graduate student could do us all a wonderful service by sorting out the actual allergy potential of each species of oak, how much pollen each releases, and exactly how allergenic each kind of pollen is.

Allergy to oak pollen is such that if people are allergic to the pollen of red oak, for example, they will usually also be allergic to the pollen of white oak or any other oak. The actual degree of allergy from each species varies greatly and as yet is something of a mystery. Most oaks produce heavy pollen loads, but the evergreen or live oaks often produce the most pollen and produce it for a longer time. In California, *Q. agrifolia*, the coastal live oak, is a major allergy tree.

A large, spreading oak tree may well be the centerpiece of a landscape, and most people would be reluctant to remove it. If someone with allergies had a big oak, he or she would be wise to get skin-tested for oak pollen, and if positive, to undergo desensitizing shots for oak. For oaks that are not too large in height, it is hoped that the future will bring us some sort of nontoxic spray that could be used to knock down the huge amount of male flowers before they can release their pollen. Pollen from all types of oak is known to sometimes cause skin rashes from contact. Oak pollen is also high in tannic acid, and aerosol tannins have long been linked to a number of cancers.

Oaks can be pollarded, which will considerably reduce the amount of pollen produced. There are hundreds of natural oak hybrids, as most Quercus species will interbreed with others; it is likely that a few of these have produced male-sterile oak trees, but at this point in time, they have yet to be identified.

Quillaja saponaria. 4
SOAP BARK TREE. A tall evergreen tree from Chile, hardy in zones 8 to 10. Soap is made from the bark of some species.

QUINCE. See *Chaenomeles*.

QUINOA. See *Chenopodium*.

RABBIT'S FOOT GRASS. See *Polypogon*.

RABBIT'S PEA. See *Tephrosia*.

RAGWEED. See *Ambrosia*.

RAGWORT. See *Senecio*.

RAIN LILY. See *Zephyranthes*.

RAISIN TREE. See *Hovenia dulcis*.

RAMBUTAN. See *Nephelium lappaceum*.

RAMONA SAGE. See *Salvia*.

RAMONTCHI. See *Flacourtia*.

Ranunculus. 4
BUTTERCUPS, CROWFOOT, PERSIAN RANUNCULUS.
Colorful tuberous perennials usually grown as annuals, Ranunculus flowers (sometimes fully double) are held aloft on tall, wiry stems. They begin blooming in early spring and grow best in cool weather. *R. repens* is a true perennial, hardy in all zones, and useful as a ground cover for moist soils. As cut flowers, they pose some slight allergy potential. All parts of Ranunculus are quite poisonous if eaten.

RAPE. See *Brassica*.

Raqulia australis. 4
Low-growing, spreading perennial for zones 8 to 11. It requires full sun and good drainage to thrive.

RASPBERRY. See *Rubus*.

RATTAN PALM. See *Rhapis*.

RATTLEBOX. See *Crotalaria*.

RATTLESNAKE GRASS. See *Briza maxima*.

RED BAY. See *Persea borbonia*.

RED CEDAR. See *Juniperus*; *Thuja*.

RED CHOKEBERRY. See *Aronia arbutifolia*.

RED ELDER. See *Sambucus*.

RED ESCALLONIA. See *Escallonia*.

RED FIR. See *Abies*.

RED GUM. See *Eucalyptus*.

RED MAPLE. See *Acer rubrum*.

RED OSIER. See *Cornus*.

RED-APPLE ICEPLANT. See *Aptenia cordifolia*.

RED-BERRIED GREENBRIER. See *Smilax*.

RED-HOT POKER. See *Kniphofia uvaria*.

REDBIRD CACTUS. See *Pedilanthus tithymaloides*.

REDBUD. See *Cercis*.

REDONDO CREEPER. See *Lampranthus*.

REDTOP. See *Agrostis*.

REDWOOD. See *Sequoia sempervirens*.

REDWOOD, DAWN. See *Metasequoia glyptostroboides*.

REDWOOD, FORMOSAN. See *Taiwania cryptomerioides*.

REED, GIANT. See *Arundo donax*.

Rehmannia elata. 2 ✪
Tall, erect perennial for sun or shade in zones 9 to 12. The tubular multicolored flowers of Rehmannia persist over a long blooming period.

Reinwardtia indica. 4
YELLOW FLAX. Large shrublike perennial for zones 9 to 11. The bright yellow flowers bloom in late fall and early winter.

Reseda odorata. 3
MIGNONETTE. Fragrant, fast-growing warm-season annuals. The strongly fragrant blooms may present a challenge to the odor-sensitive if used as cut flowers.

RETINISPORA. See *Chamaecyparis*.

Rhamnus (*Cascara*). VARIES BY SPECIES, MALES 9 🗔, FEMALES 1 ✪
BEARBERRY, BUCKTHORN, CAROLINA BUCKTHORN, CASCARA SAGRADA, COFFEEBERRY, HOLLYLEAF RED-BERRY, INDIAN CHERRY. A large group of mostly decid-uous shrubs or small trees, native to the United States and Asia, especially to China and Japan; some are hardy to zone 3. In California, *R. californica*, the coffeeberry, is a commonly used native shrub, recently popular in the past wave of drought-tolerant native-based landscap-ing. All the Rhamnus species can cause allergy and this is well known and long documented.

Rhamnus flowers are small, numerous, and usually an off-white or greenish color; the pollen that they release triggers widespread and severe allergy. The inner bark of some species is boiled and used as a laxa-tive. The fresh leaves and the seeds of some species are poisonous if eaten.

Most species of Rhamnus are separate-sexed, and female plants produce no pollen; however, in certain moist climates seeding plants can become invasive.

R. purshiana (also *Cascara sagrada*), chitum, or "shit-um," is a hardy, deciduous native small tree or shrub from the Pacific Northwest. Hardy to zone 4, females make good landscape plants. The well-aged bark of this species is a powerful laxative.

Rhamnus frangula is sometimes listed under a separate genus, Frangula. This species looks very much like a typical buckthorn, but the flowers are somewhat different, and as a whole this group is less allergenic than the other species of Rhamnus. There is a new cultivar of *R. frangula*, 'Fine Line', that looks to be a female plant with low germination rates; thus it would be less allergenic and less likely to become invasive.

There are a couple of new cultivars of female Rham-nus that are now in the works; these eventually will be sold as pollen-free OPALS #1 selections.

Rhaphiolepis indica. 3
INDIA HAWTHORN. Several species of evergreen shrubs or small trees, some to 12 feet, common in zones 9 to 12. Rhaphiolepis grows in full sun or part shade, but flowers more profusely and holds its com-pact shape better in full sun. Although the attractive Rhaphiolepis is very common in urban landscapes, its overuse may eventually contribute to further allergy problems as urban biodiversity continues to decrease.

RHAPIDOPHORA AUREA. See *Epipremnum aureum*.

Rhapidophyllum hystrix. 5
BLUE PALMETTO, NEEDLE PALM, PORCUPINE PALM. Clumpy, short, native palms; the hardiest of all the palm species, they will grow in zone 7.

Rhapis. MALES 6, FEMALES 1 ✪
BAMBOO PALM, LADY PALM, MINIATURE FAN PALM, RATTAN PALM, SLENDER LADY PALM. Small palms often used as houseplants, or outside in zones 9 to 13. Native to China, Rhapis are separate-sexed, but are not yet sold sexed. The female plants produce small, one-seeded fleshy fruits.

Rheum. 4
RHUBARB. Rhubarb flowers cause limited allergy, but usually only in those living next to fields of Rheum. Nevertheless, these flowers are highly suspect given some of their allergenic cousins. A few rhubarb plants in the garden, however, pose little risk.

RHINO'S HORN. See *Agave attenuata*.

RHODES GRASS. See *Chloris*.

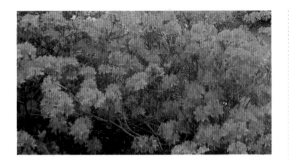

Rhododendron. AZALEA 3, RHODODENDRON 4
AZALEA, RHODODENDRON. (Pictured above.) A very large group of about 800 species of deciduous and evergreen shrubs or small trees. In general, azaleas are lower growing than rhododendrons, but all have colorful, extremely showy flowers, often in large, impressive clusters. They thrive in the partial shade of large deciduous trees, in deep, peaty, well-drained acid soils with a steady supply of moisture. Because they are completely unforgiving as far as drought is concerned, it is advisable to keep these plants deeply mulched at all times.

Rhododendron pollen is relatively heavy and not usually airborne; the male stamens are exposed, however, and direct contact with the pollen is possible. Tall plants should be used at the back of the garden, where the danger from dropping pollen is lessened. Tall rhododendrons should never be planted next to any bedroom windows. All parts of azalea and rhododendron, including the pollen, are poisonous.

Rhodosphaera rhodanthema. MALES 10 🍂, FEMALES 1 ✪
YELLOWWOOD. A separate-sexed Australian timber tree, to 40 feet. Female trees produce large one-seeded, nonedible fruits.

Rhoeo spathacea. 2 ✪
MOSES-IN-THE-CRADLE. A large-leafed plant with large white flowers that resemble small boats; for sheltered spots in zones 9 to 10.

Rhoicissus capensis. 2 ✪
EVERGREEN GRAPE. Rhoicissus is used as an attractive vine or ground cover in zones 9 to 10 and as a house-plant in cooler zones.

Rhopaloblaste. 4
A group of tropical palms.

Rhopalostylis. 5
FEATHER-DUSTER PALM, NIKAU PALM. A group of subtropical palms used in zones 9 to 10.

RHUBARB. See *Rheum.*

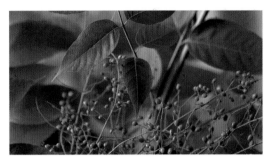

Rhus. MALES 8 TO 10 🍂, FEMALES 1 ✪ OR 3 DEPENDING ON SPECIES
AFRICAN SUMACH, CHINESE VARNISH TREE, FRAGRANT SUMAC, LAUREL SUMAC, LEMONADE BERRY, NUTGALL TREE, POISON ELDER, POISON IVY, POISON OAK, POLECAT BUSH, SMOOTH SUMAC, SUGAR BUSH, SUMAC, VINEGAR TREE, WILLOW SUMAC. (*Rhus verniciflua*, pictured above.) About 150 species of evergreen or deciduous shrubs and trees, from many regions. Most are separate-sexed, and the light, buoyant pollen produced by males of the species presents a distinctly serious allergy potential.

The most well known of the allergenic Rhus are poison sumac (*R. vernix*), poison ivy (*R. radicans*), and poison oak (*R. toxicodendron*), and cross-allergic reactions to the pollen of other Rhus species are a distinct possibility for those already hypersensitive to these three noxious weeds, vines, and shrubs.

Although several of the Rhus species are prized as landscape shrubs because of their ease of growth and their good fall color, few members of this genus are recommended for allergy-free landscapes because so many can present a host of allergy problems, from contact rashes to odor allergies.

In southern Italy, *R. coriaria*, tanner's sumac, is grown as a source of tannin for leather making. In Japan, *R. orientalis* is a vine with similar properties to our native poison ivy. In East Asia, Japan, and India, *R. succedanea*, the wax tree, is used to make both a commercial wax and a lacquer. Both the wax and the lacquer may cause allergy.

In Japan, the native *R. verniciflua*, or varnish tree, which is often described as "poisonous to touch," is used to make varnish or lacquer. It is occasionally

R

grown as an ornamental tree in the United States in zones 9 to 10, even though varnish or lacquer produced from the sap of this tree has been implicated as causing severe contact rash in individuals who handle furniture coated with this lacquer. Sometimes the contact triggering the rash is caused by varnished furniture where the varnish was applied a great many years ago.

R. integrifolia, a California native, has berries that are occasionally used as a substitute for lemons in lemonade but those who suffer allergy to any Rhus species should not drink this beverage. *R. ovata*, or sugar bush, is a large, drought-tolerant evergreen shrub native to the southwestern United States. Female plants (with red berries) are ranked 1, while males are ranked 6. Female plants of both *R. integrifolia* and *R. ovata* can make very decent low-allergy garden shrubs, and both are very drought-tolerant once established.

African sumac, *R. lancea*, zones 8 to 10, does well in hot desert areas. Female trees make small yellow-white berries but will form little if any fruit if there are no males nearby. I am in the process of propagating some female trees of this species, but it may be years before any female trees are available to nurseries.

R. aromatica, lemon sumac or fragrant sumac, is a low-growing, spreading native shrub that is suitable for difficult slopes and other poor soil sites as a ground cover. Look for a vigorous selection with great fall color called 'Grow-Lo Select', as it is a pollen-free female plant ranked 1.

Because Rhus species are separate-sexed, only the female plants have fruit. Because Rhus males produce allergenic pollen, in addition to all the other potential problems, the males should never be used. Last, it is important to realize that allergic response to Rhus species is almost always a delayed reaction. The actual allergy may not occur for hours, or even days, after the initial exposure.

RHYNCHOSPERMUM. See *Trachelospermum*.

RIBBON BUSH. See *Homalocladium platycladum*.

RIBBON CACTUS. See *Pedilanthus tithymaloides*.

RIBBONWOOD. See *Hoheria*.

Ribes. MALES 6, FEMALES 1 ✪
CATALINA PERFUME, CURRANT, GOOSEBERRY, TOSTA-BERRY. Very cold-hardy evergreen or deciduous shrubs grown in all zones, some for their fruit and others as landscape plants. There is a Ribes for almost any landscape situation ranging from shade to full sun,

and from dry to moist soils. Currants do not usually have thorns and gooseberries are usually prickly.

R. alpinum (alpine currant), *R. diacanthum*, *R. fasciculatum*, *R. orientale*, and *R. tenue* are all separate-sexed plants, although rarely sold sexed. There are several named cultivars of *R. alpinum*, and all of them are male plants. Hopefully, a female selection will be grown soon, as these are pollen-free and they also make attractive small red berries that wild birds like.

R. bracteosum, *R. glandulosum*, and *R. viburnifolium* all have malodorous flowers, leaves, or both, and should be avoided.

Both *R. nigrum*, black currant, and *R. sativum*, red currant, are grown for their fruit and neither poses an allergy problem. *R. uva-crispa*, the common, large-fruited gooseberry, is a prickly plant that also is fine for the allergy-free garden. *R. odoratum*, which has fragrant, yellow, complete flowers, also presents no allergy problem. Actually, separate-sexed or not, any Ribes that makes fruit is a low-allergy plant. Any that never do are suspect.

RICE. See *Oryza*.

RICE PAPER PLANT. See *Tetrapanax papyriferus*.

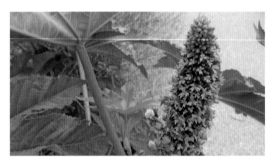

Ricinus communis. 10 ◐
CASTOR BEAN, CASTOR-OIL PLANT, PALMA CHRISTI, WONDER TREE. (Pictured above.) The castor bean is native to tropical Africa but has naturalized in the tropics, subtropics, and other warm regions around the world. A common large weedy shrub or small tree in zones 9 to 13, and used as an annual landscape foliage plant in all other zones, castor bean poses a severe allergy threat. Many acres of it were planted in the mid-western United States during World War II, and by the second season of this crop large numbers of allergies to castor bean appeared in people living close to these fields. Seed from these plantings escaped cultivation, and castor bean is a common and pernicious weed in

many areas. Allergy to Ricinus is common and severe and is a very potent trigger for asthma.

A member of the Euphorbia, or spurge, family, castor bean plants produce large amounts of very light, airborne pollen, and the watery sap causes skin rash, as can simple contact with the leaves, flowers, or seeds.

The odd-looking, mottled seeds, or "beans," of Ricinus contain a deadly poison called ricin. Ricin is so poisonous that terrorists use it, and a single small drop can kill an adult. Ricoleic acid, which is used in textile finishing and in the manufacture of some soaps, is also made from Ricinus, and cross-allergic reactions to these products are quite possible.

Those who are already allergic to castor bean may have cross-allergic reactions to latex rubber from *Hevea brasiliensis*, which is a related plant. In many parts of the South and in California castor bean has become an invasive plant. It is hard to kill, makes many seeds, and the seeds retain their viability for up to twenty years or more. On a grain-per-grain basis, it is entirely possible that there is no type of pollen that is as strongly allergenic as that of castor bean.

Ripidium ravennae. 9 🍂

HARDY PAMPAS GRASS, RAVENNA-GRASS. Older names include *Saccharum ravennae* and *Erianthus ravennae*. This very large, tall, ornamental grass is now being widely sold in colder climates as "hardy pampas grass," but it is not the same species as true pampas grass (*Cortaderia selloana*). Unlike the true pampas grass, this species is not separate-sexed and there are no female selections to be had. Considerable pollen, high-allergy potential.

RIVER WATTLE. See *Acacia*.

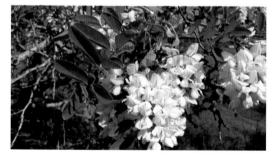

Robinia. 5

BLACK LOCUST, FALSE ACACIA, GUMMY ACACIA, LOCUST, SILVER CHAIN TREE, SMOOTH ROSE ACACIA, WHYA TREE. (Pictured above.) Robinia is a group of several species of large, fast-growing deciduous, often thorny, flowering trees of the legume family. All have very hard, durable wood and are well adapted to growing in hot, dry summer areas; some species are cold-hardy to zone 3. Because they cast a light, filtered shade, they are prized lawn trees. Some named cultivars are spineless. All Robinias have seeds, flowers, and leaves that are poisonous if eaten. (See also *Gleditsia triacanthos*; *Laburnum*.)

Rochea coccinea. 2 ✿

A tall, fleshy-leafed plant with bright red flowers that is grown as a greenhouse succulent or used outside in zones 10 to 13. It needs peaty, well-drained soil to thrive.

ROCK JASMINE. See *Androsace*.

ROCK MAPLE. See *Acer glabrum*.

ROCK PALM. See *Brahea edulis*.

ROCKBERRY. See *Empetrum*.

ROCKCRESS. See *Arabis*.

ROCKROSE. See *Cistus*.

ROCKY MOUNTAIN RED CEDAR. See *Juniperus scopulorum*.

Rodgersia. 2 ✿

Big bold perennials for zones 5 to 7, with large interesting leaves and flower spikes of many colors, including bright yellows or reds. Plants get 3 to 4 feet tall and as wide. Best in rich soil. Rodgersia are members of the Saxifrage family, a group not known for allergies. Native to Asia.

ROHDEA JAPONICA. See *Lilium*.

ROMAN CANDLE. See *Yucca*.

ROMAN LAUREL. See *Laurus nobilis*.

ROMAN WORMWOOD. See *Artemisia*.

Romneya coulteri. 4

MATILIJA POPPY. Very large perennial poppy for zones 9 to 11. Its gray-green leaves and huge white flowers can reach 8 feet. The Matilija poppy needs perfect drainage and is best grown on hillsides in sunny spots. All parts are poisonous.

Rondeletia. 3

Evergreen shrubs to 12 feet, for zones 10 to 13. Rondeletia bears long, tubular pink or yellow flowers in dense clusters.

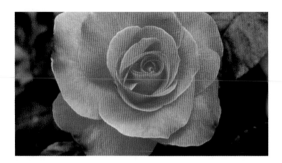

Rosa. VARIES BY VARIETY

ROSES. (*Rosa hybrida*, pictured above.) A large group of more than 100 species, hardy in all zones, according to species. Allergy to the fragrance of roses is more common than is allergy to the pollen, and any allergic response is usually low to moderate. Fully double roses release far less pollen than single-flowered varieties.

Roses grow best in full sun to partial shade and require fertile, well-drained soil and ample moisture to thrive. Many roses are easy to grow from dormant cuttings, which can often be rooted simply by using long cuttings, direct-stuck in a partially shaded spot. Roses are best purchased bare root in spring. Because they are susceptible to many diseases, including mildew, rust, and black spot, many garden roses are heavily sprayed. Both the spores of rose diseases and the chemicals used to control them may trigger allergic responses. Remove and replace disease-prone varieties with disease-resistant ones (a process rosarians refer to as "shovel-pruning").

When insects or diseases are a problem, a soapy water spray is usually enough to afford control. The botanical product neem is nontoxic and also controls both insects and disease.

The very best roses for an allergy-free garden are highly disease-resistant, have either light or absent fragrance, and are fully double. Good choices include 'Sally Holmes', a disease-resistant single that is a low-pollen producer; 'Iceberg', a semi-double white that releases almost no pollen (I've found that 'Iceberg' is also the best all-around white garden rose); 'New Day', a good yellow; 'Olympiad', a red; 'Gene Boerner', a superior pink; 'Singing in the Rain', a salmon-colored rose; and 'Touch of Class', a rosy coral hybrid tea that produces minimal amounts of pollen and has won many a blue ribbon. Miniature roses are also a good choice, because they release small amounts of pollen.

There is little point in trying to rank roses as a group, because of their incredible diversity. Very lightly scented or unscented roses with fully double blooms and many petals, combined with disease-resistance, would rank at 2. Multiflora roses with many highly fragrant, small flowers would rank as high as 5. Double roses with very high fragrance, such as 'Double Delight' or 'Fragrant Cloud', rank 4, unless they are cut and brought into the house. In that case, depending on the season, they could rank as high as 6, as roses are more fragrant in warm weather. Several old rose cultivars, the climbing 'Cecil Brunner', and the white- or yellow-flowered 'Rosa Banksia' roses (also a climber) are pretty close to being totally pollen-free. The 'Flower Carpet' series is also highly recommended, as they do not produce too much pollen, are self-fertile, and are not bothered by rust or mildew. Many of the 'David Austin' series are also good choices, being disease-resistant and low-pollen producing.

To reduce the amount of pollen released by your roses, consider not destroying earwigs, a common albeit minor pest of roses. Earwigs often eat only the pollen-producing stamens and rarely bother with the petals. Cucumber beetles also happily dine on rose pollen, but they also eat the leaves. (See image below.)

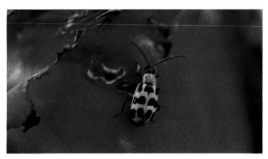

ROSARY PEA, ROSARY VINE. See *Abrus precatorius*; *Ceropegia woodii*.

Roscoea. 3

Perennial plants related to ginger. Hardy to zone 6.

ROSE ACACIA. See *Robinia*.

ROSE APPLE. See *Syzygium*.

ROSE MALLOW. See *Hibiscus*.

ROSE-OF-SHARON. See *Hibiscus syriacus*.

ROSEMARY. See *Rosmarinus officinalis*; *Ceratiola ericoides*.

ROSEWOOD. See *Pterocarpus*; *Tipuana tipu*; *Vauquelinia californica*.

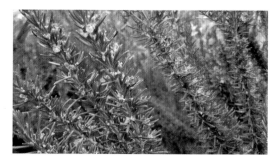

Rosmarinus officinalis. 3 TO 5 DEPENDING ON SELECTION

ROSEMARY. (Pictured above.) Evergreen erect or prostrate shrubby herbs for zones 8 to 13, with small, highly aromatic leaves and numerous small, sky-blue flowers. Rosemary is very drought-resistant and grows best in well-drained soil, in full sun. The fragrance is objectionable to many and allergenic to a few. In the future there may be some pollen-free selections of rosemary.

ROYAL BAY. See *Laurus nobilis*.

ROYAL FERN. See *Osmunda*.

ROYAL PALM. See *Roystonea regia*.

Roystonea regia. 7

CUBAN ROYAL PALM. A common allergy tree in Cuba.

RUBBER PLANT. See *Ficus elastica decora*.

RUBBER TREE. See *Ficus*; *Hevea brasiliensis*; *Parthenium*; *Sapium*.

Rubus. 3

BLACKBERRY, BOYSENBERRY, BRAMBLE, LOGANBERRY, RASPBERRY. Large group of prickly fruiting vines; one species is separate-sexed but most are perfect-flowered.

Rudbeckia. 5

BLACK-EYED SUSAN, GLORIOSA DAISY. Annuals, biennials, and perennials, hardy in all zones.

RUE. See *Ruta*.

Ruellia humilis. 3

WILD PETUNIA. Light purple petunia-like flowers on native perennials for full sun and dry soils in zones 4 to 10.

Rumex. 4 TO 8 DEPENDING ON SPECIES

DOCK, DOCK SORREL, SORREL, SPINACH. Large group of perennial herbs, some common weeds, others cultivated for their edible leaves and stalks, and others grown for their flowers, which are often used in dried flower arrangements. Numerous species of Rumex are important allergy plants and many of them cause some degree of allergy. Their use as dried flowers should be avoided.

R. hydrolapathum, R. hymenosepalus, R. patientia, and R. venosus present less allergy potential and are ranked at 4.

Rumohra adiantiformis (Aspidium). 3

LEATHERLEAF FERN. A moisture-loving fern for either part shade or full sun in zone 10.

RUNNING MOSS, RUNNING PINE. See *Lycopodium*.

Ruprechtia. MALES 7, FEMALES 1 ✪

BISCOCHITO. A group of separate-sexed tropical and subtropical shrubs and trees, native from Mexico to South America, and occasionally used in landscapes in Florida.

RUPTURE WORT. See *Herniaria*.

Ruscus. MALES 5, FEMALES 1 ✪

BOX HOLLY, BUTCHER'S BROOM, JEWISH MYRTLE. Evergreen shrublike plants for shady areas, native to the Mediterranean region and hardy in zones 8 to 11. These separate-sexed, slow-growing, evergreen plants are used as ground cover and as cut flowers.

RUSSIAN OLIVE. See *Elaeagnus angustifolia*.

Ruta. 4

RUE. Numerous species of strongly scented herbs. The odor may bother sensitive individuals. Contact skin rash is common.

RUTABAGA. See *Brassica*.

RYE. See *Secale cereale*.

RYEGRASS. See *Lolium*.

R

Sabal. 5

BERMUDA PALM, BUSH PALM, CABBAGE PALMETTO, DWARF PALM, HAT PALM, OAXACA PALMETTO, PALMETTO, PUERTO RICAN HAT PALM, SCRUB PALMETTO, SONORAN PALM, TEXAS PALM. A group of about twenty species of closely related small, fan-leafed palms, some to over 60 feet. This group of palms has complete flowers that are insect-pollinated but still produce some airborne pollen. The ratio of male parts to female is high and all stamens are fully exposed. Common in zones 8 to 13 and hardier than most palms, Sabal causes allergy only in those areas where it is extremely common. A few of these in a garden should pose little threat.

Saccharum. 4

SUGAR CANE. Tall grasses used in the production of cane sugar. Unlike many grasses, these are bisexual and do not cause as much allergy as might be supposed; also, sugar cane is almost always harvested before it flowers.

SAFFLOWER. See *Carthamus tinctorius.*

SAFFRON. See *Crocus.*

SAFFRON, FALSE. See *Carthamus tinctorius.*

SAGE. See *Salvia.*

SAGEBRUSH. See *Artemisia.*

Sageretia thea. 5

An occasionally thorny, evergreen, flowering shrub, native to China and hardy in zones 7 to 11. The small white flowers are followed by one-seeded purplish black fruits. A relative of Rhamnus or buckthorns, Sageretia causes less allergy.

Sagina subulata. 1 ✿

IRISH MOSS, SCOTCH MOSS. A low-growing, mosslike, spreading perennial hardy in all zones. Although difficult to establish, Sagina is useful as ground cover in partially shaded, moist areas.

SAGISI PALM. See *Heterospathe.*

SAGO CYCAS. See *Zamia.*

SAGO PALM. See *Cycas.*

SAGUARO CACTUS. See *Carnegiea gigantea.*

Saintpaulia ionantha. 1 ✿

AFRICAN VIOLET. Houseplants for filtered light. The handsome blue, lavender, white, or pink flowers are held above a rosette of fuzzy leaves. African violets are easy to propagate from leaf cuttings, rooted in water. The plants need acid-based potting soil and regular light feedings of complete fertilizer to thrive.

SALAL. See *Gaultheria.*

Salix. INDIVIDUALLY RANKED

OSIER, PUSSY WILLOW, SALLOW, WEEPING WILLOW, WILLOW. A large genus of mostly deciduous shrubs and trees, with more than 500 species worldwide. Various species are adapted to grow anywhere from desert washes to frozen tundra, and are native to every continent except Australia. The common willows and weeping willow are useful in damp spots where most trees fail to flourish. They grow quickly and may be used to form a quick-growing tall hedge. Low-growing willow shrubs are used as ground covers.

Because most willows are easily propagated from cuttings, a number of clones exist. Willows are often mentioned as potent allergen-producing plants, but because they are separate-sexed, the females of the species are excellent choices in the allergy-free landscape. Numerous willow species will be sold in the future with OPALS tags, and these will all be female trees—the safest bets.

S. acutifolia. 10 ✎
The cultivars 'Blue Streak' and 'Lady Aldenham' (despite her name!) are male trees.

S. aegyptiaca. 7
This species bears flowers of both sexes on the same tree; do not use.

S. alba. MALES 10 ✎, FEMALES 1 ✪
WHITE WILLOW. A group of common European trees. The cultivar 'Cardinalis' is a small, narrow, female tree. 'Chrysostela', 'Liempde', and 'Tristis' are male cultivars.

S. 'Americana'. 10 ✎
A male clone.

S. arbutifolia. 10 ✎
This is one of the worst willows for allergy; avoid its use.

S. 'Austree Hybrid'. 10 ✎
A new, fast-growing male clone marketed in Australia and California.

S. babylonica. MALES 10 ✎, FEMALES 1 ✪
CHINESE WEEPING WILLOW. In Asia, Europe, and the United States, female clones are available; in India, however, a male clone exists. 'Annularis', the ringleaf willow, is female.

S. calcodendron. 1 ✪
Grows to 40 feet; a female.

S. cantabrica. 1 ✪
A large shrub; a female.

S. caprea. MALES 6, FEMALES 1 ✪
GOAT WILLOW, SALLOW. 'Kilmarnock' is a male with scented flowers that cause less allergy than most male willows. 'Weeping Sally' is a female weeping pussy willow.

S. cinerea. MALES 6, FEMALES 1 ✪
'Variegata' is male; however, the flowers of this species are scented and it will cause less allergy than other Salix males.

S. daphnoides. MALES 10 ✎, FEMALES 1 ✪
The cultivars 'Aglaia' and 'Continental Purple' are male.

S. fragilis. MALES 10 ✎, FEMALES 1 ✪
BRITTLE WILLOW, CRACK WILLOW. 'Decipiens' is a male cultivar; 'Bedford Willow' is a female tree.

S. kinuiyanagi. MALES 10 ✎, FEMALES 1 ✪
The cultivar 'Kishu' is a small male tree; 'Kioryu' is a small female tree.

S. 'Maerd Brno'. 1 ✪
A small female tree.

S. matsudana. 1 ✪
S. matsudana 'Navajo' is a large female willow that grows well under desert conditions. S. matsudana 'Tortuosa', the corkscrew willow, is a female, however, S. pekinensis × S. alba is sometimes now also sold as 'Tortuosa' and it is a male tree. The variety known as S. babylonica 'Pekinensis' is female.

S. × pendulina. BISEXUAL 3, MALES 5, FEMALES 1 ✪
This is a rare species because sometimes it's bisexual. The cultivars 'Blanda' and 'Elegantissima' are female. 'Elegantissima' is similar in appearance to S. babylonica, the weeping willow, but is more cold-hardy. It is one of the best big weeping willows.

S. purpurea. MALES 10 ✎, FEMALES 1 ✪
PURPLE OSIER. The cultivar 'Eugene' is a male.

S. repens. MALES 6, FEMALES 1 ✪
The cultivar 'Boyd's Pendulous' is a male.

S. reticulata. MALES 6, FEMALES 1 ✪
This low-growing ground cover willow is a male.

S. × rubens. MALES 10 ✎, FEMALES 1 ✪
The cultivar 'Basfordiana' is male; 'Sanguinea' is a small female tree.

S. sachalinensis. MALES 10 ✎, FEMALES 1 ✪
The cultivar 'Sea' is a male tree.

S

S. × sepulcralis (S. × salamonii). **MALES 10** **, FEMALES 1** ✪
This is a female tree. A named variety, 'Chrysocoma', goes by many names: *S. alba* 'Aurea Pendula', 'Niobe', or 'Vitellina Pendula Nova'; *S. babylonica* 'Aurea'; the Niobe weeping willow; or the golden weeping willow. All are essentially the same tree and all are male.

S. × sericans. **10** ✎
A male hybrid.

S. triandra. **MALES 10** ✎**, FEMALES 1** ✪
'Black Maul' is a male cultivar.

S. × tsugaluensis. **1** ✪
WILLOW SHRUB. The cultivar 'Ginme' is a female with attractive reddish branchlets.

S. uva-ursi. **MALES 5, FEMALES 1** ✪
BEARBERRY. A very hardy (to zone 1), low-growing, spreading species used as a ground cover or bank cover. Not sold sexed; it would be a very useful plant if a female clone could be identified.

SALLOW. See *Salix*.

SALLY. See *Eucalyptus*.

Salpiglossis sinuata. **2** ✪
PAINTED TONGUE. An annual for warm sunny spots, it bears colorful flowers that resemble petunias. Salpiglossis makes good cut flowers.

SALT CEDAR. See *Tamarix*.

SALTBUSH. See *Atriplex*.

SALTGRASS. See *Distichlis*.

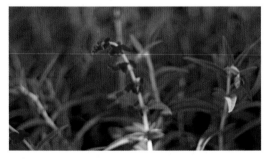

Salvia. **1** ✪ **TO 4 DEPENDING ON SPECIES AND CULTIVAR**
CREEPING SAGE, GREASEWOOD, MEXICAN BUSH SAGE, PINEAPPLE SAGE, PURPLE SAGE, RAMONA SAGE, SCARLET SAGE, VERVAIN. (Pictured above.) A large group of more than 700 species of mostly evergreen perennials, herbs, subshrubs, and shrubs, bearing small flowers of white, blue, lavender, purple, or bright red. Many Salvias thrive in hot, dry areas, while others do best in cool, moist situations. Some, like *Salvia azurea*, or blue sage, are hardy in zones 3 to 9, while many others, such as *S. leucantha*, or Mexican bush sage, do not grow outside of zones 8 to 13. Salvias are identifiable by their square stems. Many plants are called sage, and most sage are types of either Salvia or Artemisia. *S. officinalis* is true culinary sage. The Artemisias contribute greatly to allergy, but Salvias do not. Most Salvias thrive in full sun; in warm winter areas cut the plants back hard at least once a year, after a heavy bloom. There are a number of pollen-free selections, and with any luck some of these will be marketed before too long with OPALS tags.

Samanea saman. **6**
MONKEYPOD TREE, RAIN TREE. An evergreen tree with light green pinnate foliage, the pink flowers are very similar to those of *Albizzia julibrissin*. Zones 8 to 12.

SAMBUCUS GENUS

Sambucus. **INDIVIDUALLY RANKED**
BLACK ELDER, DANEWORT, DEVIL'S WOOD, ELDER-BERRY, PURPLELEAF ELDER, RED ELDER, STINKING ELDER, WALLWORT. Elders thrive in moist soil and par-tial shade. Where it is common, elderberry causes allergy, although certain species are worse than others. The sap of elderberry stems causes irritation to the skin, eyes, and nose in some. The plants are prized for their (usu-ally) edible fruits, although all fruit must be thoroughly cooked before eating. Eaten raw, the fruit is mildly toxic. Elder tea is made from the leaves, but should be used with caution because too much can cause illness. Stems, leaves, and unripe fruit are very poisonous.

The box elder, a variety of maple, is not related to Sambucus, nor is the swamp elder (Iva). Both box elder and swamp elder can be (depending on sex) potent allergy plants.

S. caerula. **6**
BLUE ELDER, STINKING ELDER. A tree, to 50 feet, this species gets one of its common names from its mal-odorous leaves.

S. canadensis. **4**
AMERICAN ELDER. A large shrub bearing black edible fruit, much loved by birds.

S. nigra. **5**
BLACK ELDERBERRY. A European elderberry grown for its sweet black fruit, which is used in jellies and wines.

S. pubens. 5
RED ELDER. Red elder is often found growing wild throughout the United States; the fruit is attractive but mildly poisonous.

SAN JOSE HESPER PALM. See *Brahea*.

SAND VERBENA. See *Abronia*.

SANDALWOOD. See *Pterocarpus*.

SANDBOX TREE. See *Hura*.

SANDHILL SAGE. See *Artemisia*.

SANDWORT. See *Arenaria*.

Sanguinaria canadensis. 3
BLOODROOT. A hardy perennial with large leaves and white-pink flowers, for moist, shady areas of zones 2 to 7. The thick, fleshy roots exude a blood-red sap when cut.

Sanguisorba menziesii. 2 ✪
RED BURNET. A native perennial plant in Alaska, hardy to zone 2, useful in landscaping, with attractive flower spikes and handsome leaves. Easy to grow and will do well in containers; prefers moist soils.

Sansevieria trifasciata. 1 ✪
BOWSTRING HEMP, MOTHER-IN-LAW'S TONGUE, SNAKE PLANT. A common houseplant with stiffly erect, long, narrow leaves with light margins. Sansevieria thrives on neglect, needing little in the way of fertilizer, light, or water. As houseplants these should occasionally be washed clean of dust.

SANTA LUCIA FIR. See *Abies*.

Santalum. 6
SANDALWOOD. Several species of evergreen shrubs and trees from India to Australia to Hawaii with aromatic wood. Santalum is the sandalwood oil source. Zones 10 to 13.

Santolina. 5
GRAY SANTOLINA, GREEN SANTOLINA, LAVENDER COTTON. A shrubby perennial for full sun in zones 7 to 10. Santolina bears small, daisylike yellow flowers; the bruised leaves release a pungent odor.

Sanvitalia procumbens. 4
CREEPING ZINNIA. A native annual of Mexico for sunny areas.

Sapindus. MALES 8, FEMALES 3
CHINESE SOAPBERRY, SOAPBERRY, WILD CHINA TREE. A dozen species of shrubs and trees, some native, some Asian, for zones 8 to 12 and commonly used in Florida and California. Some species of Sapindus are separate-sexed, but all cause allergy. All parts of the Sapindus tree are poisonous if eaten, and contact with leaves or, especially, sap, can cause contact dermatitis. The female trees bear small yellow-orange fruits that are occasionally used to make soap. Do not use soap made from Sapindus berries.

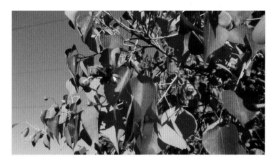

Sapium. MALES 10 ✎, FEMALES 4
CHINESE TALLOW TREE. (*Sapium*, female, pictured above.) The Japanese native *S. japonica* is hardy only in zones 8 to 10; *S. sebiferum*, the Chinese tallow tree, is hardy in zones 4 to 10. As members of the Euphorbia family, Sapiums share in its diverse allergenic properties. Some of the genera are separate-sexed, but all have a distinctly high allergy potential. The sap of all Sapium is poisonous and may cause skin rash; the pollen is also toxic and the cause of allergy. Contact with the leaves of some species may cause rash.

Sapodilla. 3
A large group of tropical and subtropical trees and shrubs with milky latex sap that is used to make, among other things, chewing gum.

Saponaria. 3
CHINA TREE, SOAPWORT. A group of low-growing, mat-forming perennials and annuals, hardy in any zone. The small flowers are usually pink.

SAPOTE, WHITE. See *Casimiroa edulis*.

SAPPHIRE BERRY. See *Symplocos*.

Sarcobatus. 7
GREASEWOOD. A spiny, deciduous shrub native to the western United States. The hard yellow wood is much used as quick-kindling firewood. Plants are monoecious and pollen is allergenic.

Sarcococca. 5
SWEET BOX, SWEET SARCOCOCCA. Evergreen shrubs
of the boxwood family, native to China and commonly
used as shrubs for shady areas in zones 8 to 10. The
pollen has some, although slight, allergenic potential.
The scent of its flowers may cause allergy in perfume-
sensitive individuals.

Sarracenia. 3
PITCHER PLANT. Odd insect-catching perennials native
to the United States. One species, *S. purpurea*, is a bog
plant and is hardy to zone 3.

SARSAPARILLA, WILD. See *Schisandra*; *Smilax*.

Sassafras. MALES 7, FEMALES 1 ☺
Three species of large deciduous trees, one native to the
southeastern United States and two native to China.
The bark is used to make an aromatic oil and a tea.
Sassafras is separate-sexed; the females are identifiable
by their small dark fruits.

SATINWOOD. See *Zanthoxylum*.

**Satureja (Micromeria). 1 ☺ TO 3 DEPENDING ON
CULTIVAR**
CALAMINT, SUMMER SAVORY, WINTER SAVORY, YERBA
BUENA. Annual and perennial herbs of the mint family,
Satureja are winter hardy in all zones. The fragrant
leaves are used for tea. (See *Mentha*, for cautions.)

SAUROMATUM. See *Lilium*.

SAVIN. See *Juniperus*.

SAVORY. See *Satureja*.

SAWLEAF ZELKOVA. See *Zelkova*.

Saxifraga. 3
BERGENIA, SAXIFRAGE. A group of more than 300 species of small perennials, often grown for their attractive foliage. Some species are used as houseplants and
others as garden plants, thriving in partial shade with
average moisture.

Scabiosa. 3
MOURNING BRIDE, PINCUSHION FLOWER. Annuals and
perennials with many small, pom-pom-shaped, pastel
flowers; most interesting for the tall stamens, held
well above the petals, and resembling pins stuck into a
pincushion. Thriving in full sun, Scabiosa are slightly
fragrant and highly attractive to butterflies. They make
a long-lasting cut flower if placed in water immediately after cutting. Because of the highly exposed,
pollen-producing stamens, avoid directly inhaling the
fragrance of Scabiosa flowers.

Scaevola. 3
BEACH NAUPKA. Spreading, drought-resistant, shrubby
perennials covered with mauve flowers, for zone 10.

SCARLET GILIA. See *Ipomopsis*.

SCARLET MAPLE. See *Acer rubrum*.

SCARLET SAGE. See *Salvia*.

SCARLET WISTERIA TREE. See *Sesbania tripetii*.

Scheelea. 7
A group of about forty species of large, slow-growing,
thick-trunked tropical palm trees, used as landscape
trees in zones 9 to 10.

SCHEFFLERA. See *Brassaia actinophylla*.

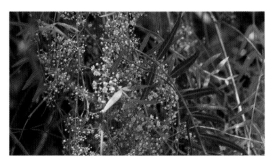

Schinus. MALES 10 🍃, FEMALES 3
PEPPER TREE. (Pictured above.) Twenty-eight species
of separate-sexed South American evergreen trees. All
members of Schinus are heavy flowering and the males
produce abundant pollen, much of which becomes
airborne. Schinus is a member of the Anacardiaceae
family, with many noxious close relatives like poison
ivy, poison sumac, and poison oak; people with sensitivity to these plants are at increased risk of allergy
from Schinus pollen.

Although these trees are called pepper trees and have
a peppery odor, they are not true pepper plants; true
black and white peppers come from *Piper nigrum*, which
is not related to Schinus. The red Schinus berries, called
"peppercorns" by many, are sometimes combined with
the black and white seeds of true pepper to produce a
colorful mixture. Schinus seeds, however, are not edible
and may cause allergy in those using this combination.

Because the plants are separate-sexed, the female
trees do not produce pollen, automatically making them
far superior to the males. Nonetheless, all Schinus
trees may cause skin rashes, eye inflammations, facial
swellings, and odor allergies. The pollen, in addition to
causing respiratory allergy, can also trigger asthma or

skin irritation. Allergies caused by Schinus are usually delayed, and identifying the cause of the reaction may be difficult.

S. molle, called the California pepper tree, Australian pepper, Peruvian pepper tree, or pirul, is a common street tree in zones 9 to 13, and especially so in California, where many mistakenly believe it to be a native species. *S. terebinthifolius*, the Brazilian pepper tree, or Christmas berry tree, is another widely used species, especially in Hawaii, Florida, and California. *S. terebinthifolius* in Florida has become a highly invasive species and now grows wild in most areas. *Terebinthifolius* means "turpentine scented" in Latin, and the crushed leaves emit a powerful, pungent odor when crushed. Of all the members of the genus, this is the most highly allergenic. The leaves are poisonous if eaten, the pollen is allergenic, mere contact with the leaves will cause rash for some, and when the plants are pruned or clipped, the volatile organic compounds (VOCs) released cause irritation to the eyes and/or respiratory tract. The trees are not normally sold sexed; a named cultivar of *S. molle*, 'Shamel,' is a male.

S. latifolius, a popular landscaping plant in its native Chile, is a small tree with white flowers followed by small lavender fruits. *S. polygamous*, a spiny, narrow tree, also from Chile, is commonly used in California. *S. lentiscifolius* is a Brazilian native, commonly used as a landscape shrub because of its white flowers and pink fruits. *S. longifolius* is a small tree used in Argentina.

Schippia. 1 ⊘
A tall (to 30 feet) slim-trunked palm tree from Belize.

Schisandra. MALES 5, FEMALES 1 ⊘
BAY STAR VINE, MAGNOLIA VINE, WILD SARSAPARILLA. Separate-sexed vining shrubs, some hardy in zones 5 to 13. One species is native to the United States and the others are from China. The female vines bear red berries when fertilized.

Schizanthus. 2 ⊘
BUTTERFLY FLOWER, POOR-MAN'S ORCHID. Easy-to-grow annuals for partial shade. They bear small colorful flowers, resembling orchids, on tall, drooping stems.

SCHIZOCENTRON. See *Heterocentron*.

Schizophragma hydrangeoides. 6
JAPANESE HYDRANGEA VINE. Shade plant for moist soils in zones 4 to 8, climber, masses of white flowers. Do not plant this where it will grow close to any bedroom windows. Will grow up masonry walls.

SCHIZOSTYLIS. See *Lilium*.

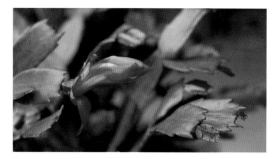

Schlumbergera. 2 ⊘
CHRISTMAS CACTUS, CRAB CACTUS. (Pictured above.) Houseplants or outside in zones 10 to 13, in partial shade. Schlumbergera need regular watering and frequent feeding to thrive.

Sciadopitys. 7
UMBRELLA PINE. A slow-growing Japanese native evergreen tree, to 100 feet. The umbrella pine grows best in shaded, moist soil. It is unrelated to pines.

Scilla. 3
BLUEBELLS, SQUILL. Easy-to-grow, blue-flowered perennials from bulbs; some species of Scilla are hardy in all zones. Scilla is quite poisonous, and some gardeners claim that if gophers eat it, they die. (See also *Endymion*.)

Scindapsus pictus. 3
Vining houseplants that resemble Pothos, but need a sunny window to thrive. The sap may cause rash.

Scirpus. 5
LOW BULRUSH. A tall reedy plant for wetlands or to edge ponds.

SCOTCH BROOM. See *Cytisus*.

SCOTCH HEATHER. See *Calluna*.

SCOTCH MOSS. See *Sagina subulata*.

SCREW BEAN. See *Prosopis*.

SCREW PINE. See *Pandanus*.

SCRUB PALMETTO. See *Sabal*.

Scutellaria alpina. 2 ⊘
ALPINE SKULLCAP. Native perennials in the mint family, hardy in zones 5 to 10, easy to grow, likes moisture but is drought-tolerant. Cultivars with either blue, pink, lavender, white, or yellow flowers. Good pollinator plants with little pollen but much nectar.

SEA ASH. See *Zanthoxylum*.

S

SEA BUCKTHORN. See *Hippophae*.

SEA FIG. See *Carpobrotus*.

SEA GRAPE. See *Coccoloba*.

SEA HOLLY. See *Eryngium*.

SEA LAVENDER. See *Limonium*.

SEA PINK. See *Armeria*.

SEA POPPY. See *Glaucium*.

SEA URCHIN. See *Hakea*.

SEASIDE DAISY. See *Erigeron*.

Secale cereale. NOT YET RANKED
RYE. A cool-season grain crop, unrelated to ryegrass (Lolium), which is a common, allergenic lawn grass. There are five species of Secale, both annuals and perennials. Rye is not a major allergy plant because the pollen is heavy and does not travel far.

SEDGE. See *Carex*; *Cyperus*.

Sedum. 2 ☻
DONKEY TAIL, PORK-AND-BEANS, STONECROP. A large group of about 600 species of succulent perennials, hardy in zones 3 to 13, depending on species. Sedum flowers may be yellow, red, orange, or lavender. They are easy plants to grow, doing best in full sun but tolerant of light shade. They are easily propagated from cuttings.

Selenicereus. 1 ☻
MOON CACTUS, NIGHT-BLOOMING CEREUS. Tall, night-blooming cactus.

SELF-HEAL. See *Prunella*.

Semecarpus. MALES 10 ☙, FEMALES 8
MARKING-NUT TREE, VARNISH TREE. About forty species of tropical and subtropical trees, the sap of which is used to make a black dye used for ink. Both the dye and the ink have allergenic properties, and the leaves of Semecarpus can cause very severe contact skin rash. Semecarpus is dioecious, but because of the extreme potential for dermatitis, neither sex is recommended.

Semele androgyna. 5
CLIMBING BUTCHER'S VINE. A climbing, evergreen native of the Canary Islands, Semele is used as a greenhouse plant and is occasionally mistaken as a relative of asparagus, to which it is unrelated.

SEMINOLE BREAD. See *Zamia*.

Sempervivum. 1 ☻
HENS-AND-CHICKS, HOUSELEEK. Easy-to-grow, drought-tolerant creeping succulents for sunny spots

in zones 7 to 13, and as houseplants in sunny rooms elsewhere.

SENECA SNAKEROOT. See *Polygala*.

Senecio (Jacobaea; Kleinea; Kleinia repens).
4 TO 10 ☙ DEPENDING ON SPECIES
CALIFORNIA GERANIUM, CANDLE PLANT, CINERARIA, DUSTY MILLER, FLAME VINE, GERMAN IVY, GOLDEN RAGWORT, HOT-DOG CACTUS, INCHWORM, KENYA IVY, LEOPARD'S BANE, NATAL IVY, PARLOR IVY, PURPLE RAGWORT, SPEARHEAD, STRING OF BEADS, TANSY RAGWORT, TAPE WORM, VELVET GROUNDSEL, WATER IVY, WAX VINE. A very large genus of nearly 3,000 species of annuals, biennials, perennials, vines, and shrubs, with worldwide distribution. Forming a group of plants whose uses range from flower garden herbs to landscape plants to weeds, most are implicated in causing some degree of allergy.

Because of the close relationship between Senecio and ragweed, Senecio pollen is a cause of airborne allergy and, in areas where they are numerous, may be the primary cause of summer and fall allergies. Most Senecio species bear small yellow flowers but a few, like the *S. cineraria*, bear larger, more colorful flowers that do not release nearly as much pollen as the small-flowered species. With many members of the genus, there is a distinct chance of contact skin rash from the leaves and flowers. The flowers and leaves of most Senecio are poisonous if eaten.

SENNA. See *Cassia*.

SENSITIVE PLANT. See *Mimosa pudica*.

SENTRY PALM. See *Howea*.

Sequoia sempervirens. 5
COAST REDWOOD. One of the tallest trees in the world, hardy in zones 8 to 10. There are many cultivars of redwood, including a few dwarf or weeping varieties. Sequoia pollen causes some allergy, although it is neither common nor usually severe. The large forms of redwood should not be used as landscape plants because they soon outgrow their surroundings. The allergy potential from the dwarf forms is slight.

Sequoiadendron giganteum. 5
BIG TREE, GIANT SEQUOIA. A giant redwood that grows inland on the western slopes of the Sierra Nevada. Hardier than the coast redwood, it thrives in zones 4 to 10. It has the largest trunk diameter of any tree in the world. Sequoiadendron is generally unsuitable as a landscape tree, because of its immense mature size.

SERVICE BERRY. See *Amelanchier laevis*.

Sesbania tripetii. 3
SCARLET WISTERIA TREE. Fast-growing deciduous shrub or small tree for sunny areas of zones 8 to 12. Sesbania is occasionally grown in large pots. Can be very invasive.

Setaria. 7
BRISTLEGRASS, FOXTAIL MILLET, PIGEON GRASS. European grasses used in warm zones of the United States.

Setcreasea pallida. 2 ✪
PURPLE HEART. An easy-to-grow perennial for shady areas of zones 10 to 13, or as a houseplant elsewhere. The leaves, stems, and flowers are purple.

SHADBLOW, SHADBUSH. See *Amelanchier*.

SHAGBARK HICKORY. See *Carya ovata*.

SHAMROCK. See *Oxalis*.

SHARPBERRY TREE. See *Phillyrea decora*.

SHASTA DAISY. See *Chrysanthemum*.

SHE-OAK. See *Casuarina*.

SHEEP BUR. See *Acaena*.

Shepherdia. MALES 6, FEMALES 1 ✪
BUFFALO BERRY, SOAPBERRY. Three species of separate-sexed deciduous shrubs or small trees, hardy to zone 2. Adapted to dry, cold, rocky soils, female buffalo berry plants produce small edible fruits that are used for jelly. If one male plant is used with two or more female plants, the potential for allergy is slight.

SHIBATAEA. See *Bamboo*.

SHIMPAKU. See *Juniperus chinensis*.

SHISO. See *Perilla frutescens*.

SHOOTING STAR. See *Dodecatheon*.

SHORE BAY. See *Persea borbonia*.

Shortia. 2 ✪
FRINGE BELLS, FRINGED GALAX, OCONEE BELLS. Attractive small evergreen plants for shady areas in zones 3 to 8.

SHRIMP PLANT. See *Justicia*.

SIBERIAN PEASHRUB. See *Caragana arborescens*.

Sibiraea. 7
Several species of deciduous shrubs from Asia, used in zones 5 to 8.

SIERRA LAUREL. See *Leucothoe*.

SIERRA MAPLE. See *Acer glabrum*.

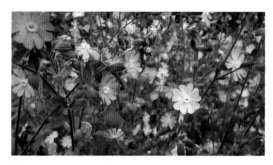

Silene. 1 ✪ TO 5 DEPENDING ON SPECIES, SEX, OR CULTIVAR
CAMPION, CATCHFLY, COCKLE, CUSHION PINK, EVENING LYCHNIS, INDIAN PINK, MORNING COCKLE, MOSS CAMPION. (Pictured above.) Tall, easy-to-grow annuals and perennials, for all zones; some species are adapted to dry areas and others to wet locations. Some Silene are separate-sexed, but as yet are not sold sexed. Male Silenes do shed considerable pollen.

SILK TASSEL. See *Garrya*.

SILK TREE. See *Grevillea*; *Albizia julibrissin*.

SILKY CAMELLIA. See *Stewartia*.

Silphium. 5
COMPASS PLANT. A small group of tall, hardy, flowering perennials, excellent for sunny spots in the back of flower borders. As a cut flower it has some distinct allergy potential.

SILVER CHAIN TREE. See *Robinia*.

SILVER FIR. See *Abies*.

SILVER LACE VINE. See *Polygonum*.

SILVER LINDEN. See *Tilia*.

SILVER MAPLE. See *Acer saccharinum*.

SILVER PALM. See *Coccothrinax*.

SILVER TREE. See *Leucodendron*.

SILVER WATTLE. See *Acacia*.

SILVERBELL TREE. See *Halesia*.

SILVERBERRY. See *Eleagnus commutata*.

Silybum. 5
HOLY THISTLE, ST. MARY'S THISTLE. Tall perennials often naturalized as weeds. Possibly invasive.

Simarouba. MALES 8, FEMALES 1 ✪
ACEITUNO, BITTERWOOD, PARADISE TREE. Large tropical evergreen trees, often separate-sexed, for zones 10 to 13.

Simmondsia. MALES 7, FEMALES 1 ✪
GOATNUT, JOJOBA. Two dozen species of separate-sexed, evergreen shrubs, adapted to desert conditions and very drought-tolerant. Simmondsia is often raised for its seeds, from which jojoba oil, a high-quality oil used as a substitute for whale oil, is pressed.

Sinningia. 2 ✪
Many species from Mexico to Brazil. Perennials or shrubs, none is hardy outside of zones 9 to 13. *S. speciosa* is the florist's gloxinia, a plant that is beautiful when purchased, but one that never seems to thrive in the garden.

Sinofranchetia chinensis. MALES 6, FEMALES 1 ✪
A tall, separate-sexed vining shrub native to China.

Sinowilsonia henryi. 7
A small deciduous, monoecious flowering tree from China.

Siphokentia. 5
Several species of palms from Molucca Islands, frost-tender, used in zone 10.

Sisyrinchium. 1 ✪
BLUE-EYED GRASS. Easy-to-grow, spreading perennials with grassy foliage and small blue flowers. Related to iris.

Skimmia japonica. MALES 5, FEMALES 1 ✪
A red-flowered, attractive evergreen shrub from Japan, hardy to zone 8. These are sold sexed by Monrovia Nursery, in Southern California. Female plants make very cute, bright red berries. One male plant will pollinate half a dozen females. Best in a shady spot, deeply mulched, in acidic soils, Skimmia is not drought-tolerant.

SKUNK CABBAGE. See *Veratrum*.

SKUNKBUSH. See *Rhus*.

SKY FLOWER. See *Duranta*; *Thunbergia*.

SLENDER LADY PALM. See *Rhapis*.

SLIPPER PLANT. See *Pedilanthus tithymaloides*.

SMARTWEED. See *Polygonum*.

Smilacina. 3
FALSE SOLOMON'S SEAL. A shade-loving woodland perennial for zones 3 to 9.

Smilax. MALES 4, FEMALES 1 ✪
CARRION FLOWER, JACOB'S LADDER, RED-BERRIED GREENBRIER, WILD SARSAPARILLA. Separate-sexed vines, many species native to the southern United States. Some species may form small shrubs under the right conditions. Insect-pollinated.

SMOKE BUSH. See *Cotinus*.

SMOKE TREE. See *Cotinus*; *Dalea spinosa*.

SMOOTH ROSE ACACIA. See *Robinia*.

SMOOTH SUMAC. See *Rhus*.

SNAIL VINE. See *Vigna*.

SNAIL'S TRAIL. See *Acanthus mollis*.

SNAILSEED. See *Coccoloba*; *Cocculus laurifolius*.

SNAKE LILY. See *Dichelostemma*.

SNAKE PLANT. See *Sansevieria trifasciata*.

SNAKEROOT. See *Cimicifuga*; *Eupatorium*.

SNAPDRAGON. See *Antirrhinum majus*.

SNAPDRAGON, FALSE. See *Chaenorrhinum*.

SNEEZEWEED. See *Helenium autumnale*.

SNOW-IN-SUMMER. See *Cerastium tomentosum*.

SNOW-ON-THE-MOUNTAIN. See *Euphorbia*.

SNOWBALL BUSH. See *Viburnum*.

SNOWBELL TREE. See *Styrax*.

SNOWBERRY. See *Symphoricarpos*.

SNOWDROP TREE. See *Halesia*; *Styrax*.

SNOWDROPS. See *Galanthus*.

SNOWFLAKE. See *Leucojum*.

SNOWFLAKE TREE. See *Trevesia*.

SOAP BARK TREE. See *Quillaja saponaria*.

SOAP TREE. See *Yucca*.

SOAPBERRY. See *Sapindus*; *Shepherdia*.

SOAPWELL. See *Yucca*.

SOAPWORT. See *Saponaria*.

SOCIETY GARLIC. See *Tulbaghia violacea*.

SODA APPLE. See *Solanum*.

Solandra maxima. 3
CUP-OF-GOLD VINE. Large-flowered, night-fragrant evergreen vine for warmest parts of zone 10 to 13. Solandra thrives in the humidity of coastal areas; its heavy vines, lacking tendrils, need support. Poisonous.

Solanum. INDIVIDUALLY RANKED

APPLE OF SODOM, DEADLY NIGHTSHADE, EGGPLANT, JERUSALEM CHERRY, LOVE APPLE, LULO, NIGHTSHADE, POISON BERRY, POTATO TREE, POTATO VINE, SODA APPLE, WHITE POTATO, YELLOW POPOLO. Solanum is a very large genus of more than 1,500 species, including potatoes; eggplants; pepino; many domesticated flowers, shrubs, and vines; a few trees; and numerous weeds and wildflowers. In most species, the leaves, flowers, and berries are poisonous.

In medieval times young women put drops of juice of nightshade in their eyes to enlarge the pupils and make them brilliant (a beauty practice that often resulted in blindness). The Latin name for nightshade, *belladonna* (pretty lady), reflects this practice.

Allergy to potatoes and eggplants is fairly rare, as is allergy to Solanum pollen. More likely, however, are poisonings caused by ingesting the attractive orange or yellow fruits of various Solanum species, especially those of Jerusalem cherry, *S. pseudocapsicum*. A few species of Solanum produce edible fruits, notably the garden huckleberry and eggplant. One species, wonderberry, is used as a sugar substitute.

Soleirolia soleirolii. 3

ANGEL'S TEARS, BABY'S TEARS. A small-leafed evergreen ground cover in zones 9 to 10; it becomes winter dormant in zones 6 to 8. Baby's tears grows best in shade and requires ample water to thrive. In sunnier areas, it is more compact.

Solidago. 6

GOLDENROD. A tall, bright yellow, beautiful fall-flowering perennial, hardy in all zones but most common in the eastern and midwestern U.S. Much has been written about goldenrod and allergy, with many claiming that because it blooms at the same time as most ragweeds, it is unfairly blamed for allergy. Goldenrod, however, is related to ragweed and can cause allergy, albeit far less than its more potent cousin. Solidago pollen is heavier and less likely to become airborne than ragweed pollen. Thirty percent of those who suffer from ragweed allergy are also allergic to goldenrod pollen. Limit plantings to a few, and keep them away from the house. Goldenrod may cause contact skin rash. Goldenrod is amphiphilous, pollinated by both insects and the wind.

Solidaster (x Solidaster). 2 ✪

A very attractive sterile hybrid of Aster and Solidago (goldenrod). Propagated from cuttings, viable seeds are not produced.

Sollya heterophylla. 3

AUSTRALIAN BLUEBELL CREEPER. Evergreen vine or shrub for zones 9 to 10. The bluebell creeper needs excellent drainage to thrive; when in bloom, it is covered with small, bell-shaped bright blue flowers. A Pittosporum relative.

SOLOMON'S SEAL. See *Polygonatum*.

SONORAN PALM. See *Sabal*.

Sophora. 6

A large group of deciduous, leguminous trees. The largest is *S. japonica*, the Chinese scholar or Japanese pagoda tree, which bears small yellow-white flowers followed by small beanlike pods. The seeds are poisonous if eaten in quantity; in very small doses, the seeds can cause hallucinations and a deep, comalike sleep, lasting for up to three days.

S. secundiflora, the Mexican or Texas mountain laurel or mescal bean tree, is well adapted to hot, dry areas, where it can grow to 50 feet. It bears long lavender flowers. Its seeds are extremely poisonous—to a small child, a single seed may be fatal. Possible negative cross-reactions with other existing legume (soy, peanut) allergies.

Sorbaria sorbifolia. 4

FALSE SPIRAEA. A large, deciduous shrub for zones 3 to 9 that bears clusters of small white flowers. False spiraea blooms on new wood only.

Sorbus. 4

MOUNTAIN ASH. A group of about eighty species of deciduous trees and large shrubs producing small, edible fruits, hardy to zone 3. Mountain ash has leaves resembling true ash, but it is a member of the rose family. They are beautiful trees when in full bloom and are also attractive when heavy with small red or orange fruit, which is used to make the sweetener sorbital. The pollen of Sorbus may cause limited allergy. Important food source for songbirds in northern areas.

Sorghum. 6 TO 10 ◐

GRAIN SORGHUM, GYP CORN, JOHNSON GRASS, MILO, SUDANGRASS. Grain sorghum causes limited allergy, but the weed *S. halepense*, or Johnson grass, is a major allergy plant. The species planted for grain crops are considerably less allergenic than those for forage grass. Some species may be invasive.

SORREL. See *Oxalis*; *Rumex*.

SORREL TREE. See *Oxydendrum*.

SOUR GUM. See *Nyssa*.

S

SOUR WEED. See *Oxalis*.

SOURWOOD. See *Oxydendrum*.

SOUTH AMERICAN LILY. See *Alstroemeria*.

SOUTHERNWOOD. See *Artemisia*.

SPANISH BAYONET. See *Yucca*.

SPANISH BROOM. See *Genista*; *Spartium junceum*.

SPANISH CEDAR. See *Cedrela*.

SPANISH FIR. See *Abies*.

SPANISH FLAG. See *Mina lobata*.

SPANISH LIME. See *Melicoccus*.

SPANISH SHAWL. See *Heterocentron elegans*.

SPANISH TEA. See *Chenopodium*.

Sparaxis. 2 ✪
Perennial corms for zones 9 to 13.

Sparmannia africana. 6
AFRICAN LINDEN. An evergreen tree for zones 9 to 13, or grown as a houseplant elsewhere.

Spartina. 7
CORDGRASS, MARSH GRASS. Native grass that grows in southern coastal tidewater regions.

Spartium junceum. 7
SPANISH BROOM. A large evergreen shrub for dry, sunny areas of zones 8 to 13. Under optimum conditions, it can become invasive and spread to large areas and is then a source of local allergy. All parts of these plants, including the seeds, are poisonous.

Spathiphyllum. 2 ✪
Houseplants prized for their large dark green leaves and unusual, large, long-lasting white flowers.

SPEAR LILY. See *Doryanthes palmeri*.

SPEARHEAD. See *Senecio*.

SPEEDWELL. See *Veronica*.

Sphaeropteris. 5
TREE FERNS. More than 100 species of very large, tall, treelike ferns, some hardy in zone 10 in shady locations. Although strikingly beautiful, tree ferns drop spores that trigger allergic reactions, so placement is important; do not plant next to doors or windows that will be opened. The stems have many tiny, sharp hairs that can cause rash.

SPICEBERRY. See *Ardisia*.

SPICEBUSH. See *Calycanthus*; *Lindera*.

SPIDER FLOWER. See *Cleome spinosa*.

SPIDER LILY. See *Crinum*; *Hymenocallis*.

SPIDER PLANT. See *Chlorophytum comosum*.

SPIDERWORT. See *Tradescantia*.

Spigelia marilandica. 2 ✪
INDIAN PINK. Great shade perennial plants for almost any soil in shade to partial sun. Bright green leaves and large numbers of striking red flowers with yellow star centers that attract hummingbirds. Will grow in dry shaded areas and spread. Native to the southeastern states of the U.S. Hardy to zone 5.

SPIKED CABBAGE TREE. See *Cussonia spicata*.

SPINACH. See *Rumex*; *Spinacia*.

SPINACH, WILD. See *Chenopodium*.

Spinacia. MALES 5, FEMALES 2 ✪
SPINACH. A popular cool-weather garden vegetable plant, spinach is separate-sexed and related to other species that cause a great deal of allergy. In recent years, spinach has had its reputation as a highly nutritious leafy green tarnished because of the allergenic properties of the leaves.

SPINDLE TREE. See *Euonymus*.

SPINY-CLUB PALM. See *Bactris*.

Spiraea. 5
BRIDAL WREATH. Many species of mostly deciduous shrubs of the Northern Hemisphere, most bearing heavy panicles of small, bright white flowers. Allergy to Spiraea is not common, but may be severe when it does occur. It is best planted far from doors and windows.

Spiranthes cernua. 1 ✪
NODDING LADIES' TRESSES. A very nice perennial native orchid with fragrant white flowers in spikes. Native to the eastern U.S. and Canada, hardy to zone 2. Plants are from 6 to 20 inches tall and for orchids are fairly easy to grow in moist soil.

SPLIT-LEAF PHILODENDRON. See *Monstera*.

SPOON FLOWER. See *Dasylirion*.

SPREKELIA. See *Lilium*.

SPRING BEAUTY. See *Claytonia*.

SPRING STAR FLOWER. See *Ipheion uniflorum*.

SPRUCE. See *Picea*.

SPURGE. See *Euphorbia*.

SPURGE LAUREL. See *Daphne adorata*.

SPURGE NETTLE. See *Cnidoscolus*.

SQUAWBERRY. See *Viburnum*.

SQUAWBUSH. See *Rhus*.

SQUIRREL CORN. See *Dicentra*.

ST. AUGUSTINE GRASS. See *Stenotaphrum secundatum*.

ST. JOHN'S BREAD. See *Ceratonia siliqua*.

ST. JOHN'S WORT. See *Hypericum*.

ST. MARY'S THISTLE. See *Silybum*.

Stachys byzantina. 3
LAMB'S EAR. Small perennials grown for their soft, fuzzy gray leaves; for sun or shade in zones 3 to 11. They bear inconspicuous purple flowers on erect stalks.

Stachyurus. 2 ✿
A group of shade-loving deciduous shrubs from China, hardy in zones 7 to 10, but growing best in zones 7 to 8. Stachyurus is prized for its bright green leaves, drooping clusters of little yellow flowers, and good fall color.

STAGHORN FERN. See *Platycerium*.

Stapelia. 2 ✿
CARRION FLOWER, STARFISH FLOWER. Unusual succulents with large, malodorous star-shaped flowers. They are popular in zones 9 to 13, and are occasionally used as potted plants.

Staphylea. 3
BLADDERNUT. Attractive shrubs or small trees, native to North America, for zones 5 to 9.

STAR APPLE. See *Chrysophyllum cainito*.

STAR BUSH. See *Turraea obtusifolia*.

STAR JASMINE. See *Trachelospermum*.

STAR LILY. See *Zigadenus*.

STAR OF BETHLEHEM. See *Campanula*; *Ornithogalum*.

STARFISH FLOWER. See *Stapelia*.

STAR FLOWER, SPRING. See *Ipheion uniflorum*.

STATICE. See *Limonium*.

Stauntonia. MALES 7, FEMALES 1 ✿
Several dioecious species of evergreen, woody climbing vines from Japan and China, and hardy to zone 8. Stauntonia bears fragrant white or pink flowers and thrives in moist, shady spots with rich soil. Female plants make blue fruits.

STEER'S HEAD. See *Dicentra*.

Stenocarpus sinuatus. 4
FIREWHEEL TREE. An evergreen tree for zones 10 to 13, adopted by the Rotary Club as its mascot plant. Slow growing and slow to come into bloom, the bright red, round flower clusters cover the plant. Young plants have beautiful foliage and are occasionally used as houseplants.

STENOLOBIUM. See *Tecoma*.

Stenotaphrum secundatum. 4
ST. AUGUSTINE GRASS. A broad-leafed, coarse, perennial lawn grass for zones 9 to 13. If it escapes cultivation to unmowed areas, it will grow tall, flower, and cause allergy. In the well-tended lawn, however, St. Augustine grass rarely grows tall enough to bloom and produce pollen.

Stephanandra incise. 5
A hardy, attractive, deciduous subshrub from Asia. Best in zones 4 to 7, with very attractive leaves and masses of tiny white flowers. Rose family.

Stephanotis. 7
MADAGASCAR JASMINE, WAX FLOWER VINE. An evergreen flowering vine for the very mildest coastal areas of zone 10, or grown as a houseplant or greenhouse plant elsewhere. The waxy white flowers are very fragrant, and may affect those with odor sensitivities. Stephanotis grows best with roots in shade and tops in sun. Recent reports from Holland documented asthma outbreaks among nursery workers exposed to the sap of the wax flower vine. The bright white flowers are often used in wedding bouquets and brides would be well advised to handle these flowers with extra care. Skin rash and itch from the sap is also a distinct possibility.

STERCULIA. See *Brachychiton*.

Sternbergia lutea. 2 ✿
Small flowering plants from bulbs, hardy in all zones. Similar to crocus.

Stevia. 3 TO 9 ✿ DEPENDING ON SEX AND SPECIES
A large group of more than 200 species of perennial herbs and shrubs native to the tropics of North and South America and India. *S. serrata* is common in zones 8 to 10 and in Mexico. *S. rebaudiana* is used to make a strong natural sweetener. Another plant called stevia is *Piqueria trinervia*. Some Stevia are dioecious but none is sold sexed. All species have propensity for allergy, especially for those individuals who are already allergic to ragweed (to which Stevia are related). Allergic reactions from the sweetener have been quite common.

Stewartia. 3
MOUNTAIN CAMELLIA, SILKY CAMELLIA, STUARTIA.
Attractive deciduous shrubs or small trees bearing
large, showy flowers and with good fall color. They are
hardy to zones 4 or 5, but grow best in zones 5 to 8.
Stewartia thrives only in cool, moist, well-drained acid
soil, in partial shade. Several of the larger, less hardy
species are Asian natives; *S. ovata* is native to the mountains of North Carolina and Tennessee. Choice shrubs
for allergy-free gardens.

STICKY MONKEY FLOWER. See *Mimulus.*

Stigmaphyllon. 2 ✪
AMAZON VINE, BRAZILIAN GOLDEN VINE, BUTTER-
FLY VINE, GOLDEN CREEPER, ORCHID VINE. Vigorous
evergreen vines, native to tropical America and bearing
bright yellow, orchidlike flowers, for zones 10 to 13.

STINK TREE. See *Ailanthus.*

STINKING CEDAR, STINKING YEW. See *Torreya.*

STINKING ELDER. See *Sambucus.*

STOCK. See *Matthiola.*

Stokesia laevis. 5
STOKES ASTER. Perennials bearing blue, purple, or
white flowers, hardy in all zones.

STONE COTTON TREE. See *Eucommia ulmoides.*

STONECRESS. See *Aethionema.*

STONECROP. See *Sedum.*

STONEFACE. See *Lithops.*

STONEWOOD. See *Ostrya.*

STORAX. See *Styrax.*

Stranvaesia. 4
Evergreen shrubs or small trees, native to Asia, and
hardy in zones 8 to 10. The small white flowers appear
in June and are followed by clusters of bright red berry-
like fruits, occasionally used for Christmas decorations.
Plants are closely related to Photinia species.

STRAWBERRY. See *Fragaria.*

STRAWBERRY GERANIUM. See *Saxifraga.*

STRAWBERRY GROUND COVER. See *Waldsteinia
fragarioides.*

STRAWBERRY TOMATO. See *Physalis.*

STRAWBERRY TREE. See *Arbutus.*

STRAWFLOWER. See *Helichrysum.*

STREAM ORCHID. See *Epipactis gigantea.*

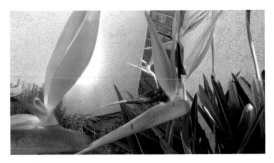

Strelitzia. 1 ✪
BIRD-OF-PARADISE. (Pictured above.) *S. regina,* the
bird-of-paradise, is the official flower of the city of Los
Angeles, despite the fact that it is native to South Africa
and the tropics. The long-stemmed orange and blue
flowers are popular in floral arrangements.

    S. nicolai, the giant bird-of-paradise, grows much
larger and taller, resembling a banana tree. The flowers
are very large and more unusual than beautiful. These
treelike plants are often used with good effect in indoor
shopping mall landscaping.

    The birds-of-paradise are not known to cause
allergy, and the design of their flowers keeps pollen
inside. Because it produces no airborne pollen and
lacks the insect needed to pollinate it, bird-of-paradise
rarely sets seed in the United States. The flowers can be
hand-pollinated and the resulting seeds are large, hard,
and black, with a small fuzzy orange tuft. Easy to grow
from seed or divisions. Sun or shade in zones 10 to 13,
houseplants for sunny windows in other areas.

Streptocarpus. 2 ✪
CAPE PRIMROSE. Perennials for the mildest parts of
zone 10 and houseplants elsewhere. Streptocarpus
grows best in cool, moist, partial shade outdoors, and
inside requires cultural conditions similar to those for
African violets, to which they are related.

Streptosolen jamesonii. 2 ✪
FIREBUSH, MARMALADE BUSH, ORANGE BROWALLIA.
An attractive evergreen (sometimes) vining subshrub
for zones 9 to 13, or popular as a greenhouse plant in
other zones. Streptosolen bears bright, orange-red flowers in large clusters. It needs full sun and good drainage
with ample water to thrive. Not long-lived.

STRING OF BEADS. See *Senecio.*

STRIPED MAPLE. See *Acer pensylvanicum.*

STUARTIA. See *Stewartia.*

Styrax. 4
FRAGRANT SNOWBELL, JAPANESE SNOWBELL, SNOWBELL TREE, SNOWDROP TREE, STORAX. A group of about 100 species of deciduous and evergreen shrubs and trees, some Asian and others native to the United States. Some species of Styrax are hardy to zone 3. The small attractive flowers are usually white, lightly scented, and appear in early summer. Although the pollen is innocuous, the sap of some Styrax species may cause rash.

SUCCULENTS. LISTED INDIVIDUALLY
In general, most succulents pose little allergy potential.

SUDANGRASS. See *Sorghum.*

SUGAR BUSH. See *Rhus ovata.*

SUGAR CANE. See *Saccharum.*

SUGAR MAPLE. See *Acer saccharum.*

SUGARBERRY. See *Celtis.*

SUMAC. See *Rhus.*

SUMMER CYPRESS. See *Kochia.*

SUMMER HOLLY. See *Comarostaphylis diversifolia.*

SUMMER HYACINTH. See *Galtonia candicans.*

SUMMER SAVORY. See *Satureja.*

SUMMERBERRY. See *Viburnum.*

SUNFLOWER. See *Helianthus.*

SUNROSE. See *Halimium; Helianthemum nummularium.*

SURINAM CHERRY. See *Eugenia.*

SWAMP BAY. See *Persea borbonia.*

SWAMP CANDLEBERRY. See *Myrica.*

SWAMP CYPRESS. See *Cyrilla racemosa; Glyptostrobus lineatus.*

SWAMP GUM. See *Nyssa.*

SWAMP HAW. See *Viburnum.*

SWAMP PRIVET. See *Forestiera.*

SWAN RIVER DAISY. See *Brachycome iberidifolia.*

SWAN RIVER PEA SHRUB. See *Brachysema lanceolatum.*

SWEDISH IVY. See *Plectranthus.*

SWEET ALYSSUM. See *Lobularia maritima.*

SWEET BAY. See *Laurus nobilis; Magnolia.*

SWEET BOX. See *Sarcococca.*

SWEET BRUSH. See *Cercocarpus.*

SWEET CICELY. See *Myrrhis odorata.*

SWEET CLOVER. See *Melilotus.*

SWEET FERN. See *Comptonia peregrina.*

SWEET GALE. See *Myrica.*

SWEET GUM. See *Liquidambar.*

SWEET HAKEA. See *Hakea.*

SWEET LAUREL. See *Laurus nobilis.*

SWEET MARJORAM. See *Origanum majorana.*

SWEET OLIVE. See *Osmanthus.*

SWEET PEA. See *Lathyrus.*

SWEET PEA SHRUB. See *Polygala.*

SWEET PEPPERBUSH. See *Clethra alnifolia.*

SWEET POTATO. See *Dioscorea.*

SWEET ROCKET. See *Hesperis matronalis.*

SWEET SULTAN. See *Centaurea.*

SWEET VERNAL GRASS. See *Anthoxanthum.*

SWEET WILLIAM. See *Dianthus.*

SWEET WOODRUFF. See *Galium odoratum.*

SWEETBERRY. See *Viburnum.*

SWEETLEAF. See *Symplocos.*

SWEETSHADE. See *Hymenosporum flavum.*

SWEETSPIRE. See *Itea ilicifolia.*

Swietenia. 3
MAHOGANY. Six species of large evergreen tropical or zone 10 to 13 trees, occasionally used as street trees.

SWISS CHARD. See *Beta vulgaris.*

SWISS CHEESE PLANT. See *Monstera.*

SWORD FERN. See *Nephrolepis; Fern.*

Syagrus. 6
COCOS PALM, LICURI PALM, OURICURI PALM. A group of palms from South America, occasionally used in the United States in zones 9 to 13. Some species of Syagrus are used for palm oil.

SYCAMORE. See *Platanus.*

SYCAMORE MAPLE. See *Acer pseudoplatanus.*

Sycopsis. 6
Six species of monoecious evergreen shrubs or trees from China, the Himalayas, and the Philippines, with showy male flowers.

S

Symphoricarpos. 3

CORALBERRY, INDIAN CURRANT, SNOWBERRY, WAX-BERRY, WOLFBERRY. Deciduous shrubs native to the United States and China, used for their ornamental red fruits and attractive foliage. Easy to grow, some of the hardier species will grow to zone 3. Snowberry thrives in sun or shade, in almost any kind of soil.

SYMPHYANDRA ZANZEGUR. See *Campanula*.

Symphytum officinale. 3

COMFREY. Hardy perennial herb for all zones. Traditionally, comfrey was grown as a medicinal herb and a nutritious pot green or forage crop, but modern research indicates that the leaves contain a low-level poison.

Symplocos. 4

SAPPHIRE BERRY, SWEETLEAF. A large group of trees and shrubs from Eurasia, the Americas, and Australia. *S. paniculata*, the sapphire berry, grows to 40 feet and is hardy to zone 5.

Synadenium grantii. 10 ◕

AFRICAN MILKBUSH. A large Euphorbia relative with numerous highly allergenic properties, including blindness from the sap and severe skin rash; all parts of the plant are very poisonous. These are planted sometimes in zones 10 to 13, and are also sold as houseplants, which is a very bad idea.

Syneilesis aconitifolia. 3

SHREDDED UMBRELLA PLANT. A handsome hardy perennial with large interesting leaves, growing to 2 feet wide and 18 inches tall, in shaded areas in zones 4 to 8. Small, white, daisylike flowers on spikes above the foliage.

Syngonium podophyllum. 2 ✿

AFRICAN EVERGREEN, ARROWHEAD VINE. Occasionally sold as *Nephthytis afzelii*. A common and popular, easy-to-grow houseplant that resembles Philodendron. Because they produce separate male flowers, Syngonium may cause allergy, but as houseplants they rarely flower.

Synsepalum dulcificum. 2 ✿

MIRACULOUS FRUIT, WONDERBERRY. A tall shrub (to 12 feet), native to West Africa. Grows in zone 10 only. It bears white flowers, followed by small, succulent, oblong red fruits. After chewing the fruit, sour foods taste sweet. At one time showing promise as an artificial sweetener, miraculous fruit has been abandoned as a commercial venture. A member of the Sapote family.

SYRIAN BEAD TREE. See *Melia*.

Syringa. 5 TO 6 DEPENDING ON SPECIES AND CULTIVAR

LILAC. Deciduous shrubs or small trees, hardy to zone 3. *S. vulgaris*, the common lilac, is a tall shrub bearing clusters of highly fragrant flowers in early spring. The intensely sweet fragrance may produce allergic reactions in those with odor sensitivities. As a member of the olive family, lilac has allergenic pollen, but because it is rarely airborne, it does not present much allergy potential. Lilacs should be planted away from doors and windows. Some of the smaller varieties have beautiful flowers that have less fragrance, and they pose less allergy potential. Lilac flowers cut and brought inside may trigger allergies for those with already existing allergies to privet or olive pollen.

Syzygium. 5 TO 6 DEPENDING ON SPECIES

AUSTRALIAN BUSH CHERRY, EUGENIA, JAMBU, JAVA APPLE, JAVA PLUM, LILLY-PILLY TREE, MALABAR PLUM, MALAY APPLE, ROSE APPLE, WAX APPLE. More than 400 species worldwide of evergreen shrubs and trees, some quite large, for zones 9 to 10.

Some species are raised for their edible plumlike fruits and one, *S. aromaticum*, is the source of cloves. Syzygium belong to the myrtle family, and those who are allergic to Eucalyptus should avoid them. Although the genus has not been well studied for allergy potential, the flowers are numerous, produced over a very long period, and have exposed, pollen-producing stamens, all of which suggest good potential for allergy.

The most commonly used species in the United States (zones 9 to 10) is *S. paniculatum*, the Australian bush cherry, often sold as *Eugenia myrtifolia*. This is usually seen as a landscape shrub or hedge plant, although when left unsheared it quickly grows into a large tree. Easy to grow in any soil and somewhat drought-tolerant when established, bush cherry must be kept closely sheared to prevent flowering. Its small purple fruits, thought by many to be poisonous, are edible but certainly not especially delicious. Eugenia would make a good hedge plant except that a large number of the plants will likely get infected with tiny psyllid insects that disfigure the leaves. The psyllids are themselves allergenic. Chemical control of these insects is difficult, and not worth the effort. There are far better choices for tall hedges; see chapter 4.

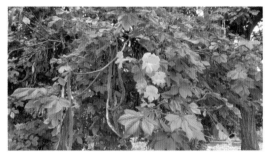

Tabebuia. 5

TRUMPET VINE TREE. (*Tabebuia chrysotricha*, pictured
above.) Large evergreen flowering trees from the
tropics and subtropics, occasionally used in zones 9
to 10. Two species, *T. avellanedae* and *T. chrysotricha*
(the golden trumpet tree), are hardier than others of
this genus. In the United States, these trees rarely get
taller than 25 feet, but in the tropics they may grow to
100 feet. They are closely related to the hardy catalpa
tree, which is known to cause allergy. Because these
three trees have many similarities, use Tabebuia as
a landscape tree with discretion. Tabebuia pollen is
heavy and does not fall far from the tree; plant these
trees away from the house.

Taenidia intergerrima. 5

YELLOW PIMPERNEL. Hardy perennial for shade or sun
in poor soils, good on slopes, drought-tolerant, and
visited by a great number of wild bees and butterflies.
Carrot family. Do not bring inside as a cut flower or use
in flower bouquets, as they may shed more pollen if
brought indoors.

Tagetes. 3 TO 6 DEPENDING ON SPECIES

MARIGOLD. Very common annual flowers, usually yellow, gold, or orange. They are frost-tender, easy and fast
from seed, and grow best in full sun. Marigolds are clas-
sified as either French or dwarf marigolds (*T. patula*),
or African or tall marigolds (*T. erecta*), despite the fact
that marigolds are native to neither Africa nor France,
but to Mexico and Central America. One species,
T. signata (Mexican marigold), is known to cause severe
skin rash and should not be used. *T. lemmonii* is native
to Arizona and makes a good garden subshrub, but
contact with the leaves and flowers is known to trigger
itch and rash.

The fragrance of marigold is offensive to some and
may cause allergy for a few perfume-sensitive individuals, if used as cut flowers. Although allergy to marigolds
is not common, the plants are related to ragweeds
and share some similarities. Fully double varieties
hide their pollen deep within the flower and generally

present less of an allergy potential than single-flowered varieties. The pollen is long-spined and light, and may become airborne, yet most allergy from marigolds is from direct contact with the open flowers.

Taiwania cryptomerioides. 7
FORMOSAN REDWOOD, TAIWAN CEDAR. An evergreen coniferous tree discovered in 1904 in the mountains of Taiwan. A rare tree in the United States, Taiwania closely resembles the Japanese cedar (*Cryptomeria japonica*), but is more closely related to bald cypress. Because both of these species are well-documented allergy producers, it can be assumed that Taiwania is also a potential allergen.

TALA PALM. See *Borassus*.

TALL FESCUE. See *Fescue elatior*.

TALL OATGRASS. See *Arrhenatherum elatius*.

TALLHEDGE BUCKTHORN. See *Rhamnus*.

TALLOW TREE. See *Sapium*.

TAM. See *Juniperus sabina*.

TAMARACK. See *Larix*.

TAMARIND-OF-THE-INDIES. See *Vangueria*.

Tamarindus indica. 2 ✪
TAMARIND. A large evergreen tree from the tropics, also grown in south Florida for its fine shape, attractive foliage, and sweet fruit, which is very popular in Mexico and Latin America. Tamarind is entirely insect-pollinated and is not known to cause allergy.

Tamarix. MOST SPECIES 7 (SEE EXCEPTION)
SALT CEDAR, TAMARISK. Deciduous trees native to the deserts of Arizona and California, and also native to parts of Africa and the Mediterranean. They are used in landscaping in the western desert and in many coastal areas. Tamarisk trees occasionally become summer dormant and regrow their leaves as the weather cools. Extremely drought-resistant, Tamarisk have tiny leaves, green stems, and many tiny pinkish flowers. They are the cause of some allergy, especially in Arizona and California, where they have an extended blooming period.

Exception: At least one species, *T. dioica*, is separate-sexed. This small tree, native to India, Pakistan, Afghanistan, and Iran, but also cultivated in the United States, causes more allergy than other Tamarix species. It has an allergy ranking of 9 for the male plants and an allergy ranking of 1 for the female plants. All species of tamarisk have invasive potential.

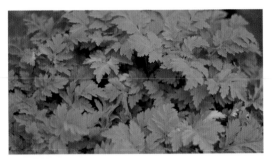

Tanacetum. 5
TANSY. (Pictured above.) A common, tall perennial with about fifty species native to the Northern Hemisphere. The leaves and flowers are highly aromatic and may cause allergy in perfume-sensitive individuals. Tansy also releases some airborne pollen and is the cause of allergy in areas where it is most common. The smaller, golden-leafed cultivars now sold as bedding plants are less allergenic. All parts of tansy are poisonous if eaten in quantity.

Tanakaea. MALES 6, FEMALES 1 ✪
A separate-sexed evergreen herb used in landscapes in China and Japan. The male plants produce airborne pollen.

TANBARK OAK. See *Lithocarpus densiflorus*.

TANGERINE. See *Citrus*.

TANNER'S SUMAC. See *Rhus*.

TANNER'S TREE. See *Coriaria japonica*.

TANSY. See *Tanacetum*.

TANSY RAGWORT. See *Senecio*.

TAPE GRASS. See *Vallisneria*.

TAPE WORM. See *Senecio*.

Taraxacum officinale. 5
DANDELION. A common European weed that has naturalized over much of the Northern Hemisphere. Dandelion sheds airborne pollen and causes limited allergy, but the weed-killing lawn chemicals (also includes so-called "weed and feed" fertilizers) applied to eradicate it cause more allergy. These chemicals can cause not only allergy, but also leukemia in dogs and cats using the lawn. Avoid these chemicals. Dandelions can be held in check by applying high-nitrogen lawn fertilizer frequently, mowing regularly, and if necessary, pricking them out with a knife or a dandelion digger.

TARO. See *Colocasia esculenta*.

TARRAGON. See *Artemisia*.

TASMANIAN TREE FERN. See *Dicksonia*.

TATARIAN MAPLE. See *Acer tataricum*.

Taxodium. 8

BALD CYPRESS, MONTEZUMA CYPRESS, POND CYPRESS, TAIWAN CEDAR. Two species of coniferous trees hardy in zones 7 to 11. Bald cypress, which grows in swamps and shallow lakes of the southern United States, produces a buttressed lower trunk. Montezuma cypress is a tree of the Pacific Coast, growing southward into Mexico. Both species are well-known allergens and both produce copious amounts of airborne pollen, which is the cause of local wintertime allergy. Occasionally used in landscapes in wet situations, Taxodium is best left in the swamps. These are sometimes used as very interesting bonsai plants, and as such, these should not bloom and thus pose little allergy potential.

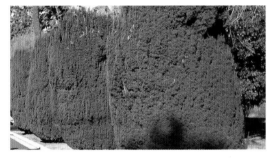

Taxus. MALES 10 🗡, FEMALES 1 ⊙

YEW. (*Taxus*, male, pictured above.) Eight species of evergreen coniferous trees and shrubs, all native to the Northern Hemisphere. Several species are native to the United States and some are imported from Japan and China. Most Taxus are separate-sexed. Young female Taxus species often make fine foundation shrubs, adding a luxurious look to the landscape. If there are male plants present, the female plants will often form red berries. (All parts of the plant except the berries are poisonous; the seeds inside the berries are poisonous.)

Taxus are slow growing, very long-lived, and shade-tolerant, and they thrive only in moist, acid soils. The bark of *T. brevifolia*, the western yew, used to be the main source of the anticancer drug Taxol. Although there is some disagreement about the prevalence of allergy from Taxus, yew pollen is very similar to the

well-known allergenic juniper pollen, and likely shares its allergenic potential. Plant female yews only.

The greatest health hazard from yews is low-dose poisoning from the cytotoxic pollen from nearby male plants. The pollen is as toxic as the leaves, but no one would eat the leaves because they don't taste good. Pollen, however, can all too easily be inhaled without one's knowing it. The greatest danger comes from male yews that are planted directly underneath or right next to bedroom windows. Male yews will bloom and produce abundant pollen in the spring, as the weather is warming up (and at the same time people would want to leave their bedroom windows open). A window screen is no protection at all from these minute pollen grains. In the nursery trade in northern climates a disproportionately large number of older nursery workers develop "the shakes," and it is thought by some that this comes from handling large numbers of potted male yews while they are in bloom. The greatest number of yews sold in the trade are sold during springtime, and this is when they are blooming. Nursery workers have told me that sometimes after loading trucks with hundreds of 1- and 5-gallon male yews they have ended up literally covered with this pollen.

T. baccata is the English yew. 'Fastigiata' is an upright, variegated female. *T. brevifolia* is the Pacific or western yew. It is not sold sexed; look for the red berries that indicate a female plant. *T. cuspidata* is the Japanese yew, which is hardier than the English yew, to zone 3. Again, look for berries.

T. × *media* is a hybrid cross between the Japanese and English yews, and nearly as hardy as Japanese yew. 'Anthony Wayne' is a tall, vigorous female, despite its masculine name, as are 'Hicksii', 'Kelseyi', 'Pyramidalis', and 'Sentinalis'. To be perfectly assured of getting only female yew plants, either buy ones that already have berries on them or look for ones with an OPALS female tag on them. (Note: In spring the berries on females will still be small, and they will still be green.)

The prevalence of male or female yews in landscapes often varies considerably by city. Often a large popular nursery sold large numbers of one clone, and these are the ones you'll find growing in those areas. For example, in Washington, D.C., in the area in and around the White House, almost all the yews I saw there were male clones.

Besides triggering allergies, pollen from male yews can cause irritation of the eyes, nose, and throat; can trigger skin rash, aching joints, itch, headaches, and lethargy; and yew pollen is also a trigger for asthma.

TEA. See *Camellia*; *Thea sinensis*.

TEA TREE. See *Leptospermum*.

TEABERRY. See *Gaultheria*; *Viburnum*.

TEAK. See *Tectona grandis*.

Tecoma (Stenolobium). 3
A group of trumpet vine species for zones 9 to 12 that needs heat, sun, rich soil, and ample water to thrive.

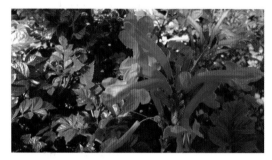

Tecomaria capensis. 3
CAPE HONEYSUCKLE. (Pictured above.) A shrub or vine native to South Africa and common in zones 9 to 13. It grows best in full sun or partial shade, and can be clipped to form a hedge. Tecomaria's orange tubular flowers are attractive to hummingbirds. There is a yellow-flowering variety that needs more light and heat to thrive. Tecomaria is unrelated to common or Japanese honeysuckle (Lonicera).

Tectona grandis. 3
TEAK. A very large (to 150 feet) deciduous tree native to India and Myanmar, and occasionally grown in zones 10 to 13. A fine landscape plant and an important timber tree. Sawdust from teak wood is a known allergen and often causes rash and itch.

TEDDY BEARS. See *Cyanotis*.

Tellima grandiflora. 2 ✿
FRINGE CUP. Unusual perennial with spotted leaves and tall spikes of reddish flowers, hardy in zones 6 to 10. It thrives in the partial shade beneath large deciduous trees.

TENDER MAPLE. See *Acer rubescens*.

Tephrosia. 4
CAT GUT, FISH POISON PEA, RABBIT'S PEA. A group of more than 300 species of the legume or pea family from the tropics and subtropics, some used in zones 5 to 13. Several species produce poisonous seeds that are used

by native fishermen to kill fish and are also used to produce the organic insecticide rotenone.

Ternstroemia gymnanthera. 2 ✿
A group of about eighty species of evergreen shrubs and trees from Japan and India, used in landscapes in the United States in zones 7 to 11. Related to the Camellia, they require well-drained, moist, acid soil to thrive. Ternstroemia grows in sun or shade, but the leaves are reddish in full sun.

Tetraclinis. 9 ◐
ARAR TREE. A small coniferous evergreen tree from the dry areas of the Mediterranean regions, grown in zones 10 to 13. The arar tree closely resembles its relatives, the cypresses, and like them also causes allergy.

Tetragonia. GENUS 4, MALES 6, FEMALES 1 ✿
Fifty species of herbs or small shrubs from Australia, New Zealand, Africa, Asia, and South America. *T. tetragonioides*, or New Zealand spinach, is grown as a perennial vegetable. These are occasionally separate-sexed plants but the allergy potential is small.

Tetrapanax papyriferus. 6
CHINESE RICE PAPER PLANT. A tall, very large-leafed evergreen shrub for sun or shade in zones 8 to 13. It bears white flowers that are not implicated in allergy, but the leaves are coated in fine hairs that cause skin rash and serious irritation.

Tetrastigma. MALES 6, FEMALES 1 ✿
JAVAN GRAPE. About ninety species of separate-sexed evergreen vines, natives of Southeast Asia and the Philippines, for zones 9 to 13. *T. voinieranum*, chestnut vine, lizard plant, or lizard vine, is used in landscaping in California and Florida. There is scant evidence of allergy from the pollen-producing males, but because Tetrastigma is not sold sexed, it is wise to avoid its use.

Teucrium. 2 ✿
GERMANDER. Small shrublike plants for hot, dry situations in all zones. The white flowers are attractive to bees.

TEXAS BLUEBELL. See *Eustoma grandiflorum*.

TEXAS BUCKEYE. See *Ungnadia*.

TEXAS MOUNTAIN LAUREL. See *Sophora*.

TEXAS PALM. See *Sabal*.

TEXAS RANGER. See *Leucophyllum frutescens*.

TEXAS UMBRELLA TREE. See *Melia*.

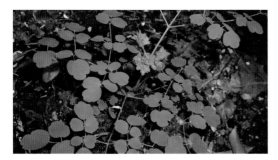

Thalictrum. MALES 9 🥀, FEMALES 1 ✪
BUTTERCUPS, LAVENDER MIST, MEADOW RUE.
(Pictured above.) Perennials for all zones, but grow best in zones 2 to 8; they are common plants in the high latitudes of the Northern Hemisphere. Meadow rue usually grows 2 to 3 feet tall, but one species, *T. diptero-carpum*, Chinese meadow rue, may grow to 6 feet. The yellow, violet, lavender, purple, or white flowers are often used in floral arrangements. Thalictrum are heavy producers of airborne pollen that causes allergy during their extended bloom period—March through August. One species in particular, *T. rochebrunianum*, is now widely sold in nurseries, almost always as a male clone. This plant has beautiful flowers but they are all male and exceptionally allergenic. At the present time there are no female cultivars of any species of Thalictrum. *T. aquilegifolium* and *T. occidentale* are also sold in nurseries. Seedlings of these species will have both male and female plants; special selections will always be male.

THATCH PALM. See *Thrinax.*

Thea sinensis. 2 ✪
TEA. An evergreen shrub or tree, similar in many ways to its close relative, the Camellia. Tea is grown in India, Ceylon, Japan, Indonesia, Pakistan, Russia, Brazil, Chile, and Peru. Unpruned, a tea tree can grow to 50 feet, but commercial plantation shrubs are usually kept clipped to about 6 feet. Like Camellia, Thea causes little or no allergy.

Theobroma cacao. 2 ✪
CACAO TREE. An evergreen tree, to 25 feet, from Central and South America, the seeds of which are used to produce cocoa and chocolate.

Theophrasta. MALES 6, FEMALES 1 ✪
About sixty species of evergreen shrubs and trees from Hawaii and tropical America, many of them separate-sexed. In Florida, a Mexican native shrub

called Jacquinia is used in landscaping. Most of the Theophrasta family has not been ranked yet, but may well contain numerous allergy plants. Jacquinia looks to be a functionally dioecious shrub with separate-sexed flowers on each plant, but it does not look like a prolific pollen producer.

Thevetia. 5
BE-STILL PLANT, LUCKY TREE, YELLOW OLEANDER. A fast-growing small tree or shrub from tropical America and Mexico, used in landscapes in zones 9 to 13. Its common name of be-still plant derives from the fact that its long green leaves tremble in the slightest breeze. Thevetia tolerates a little light frost but does best in hot, frost-free areas. The sap has allergy potential. All parts of the plant are extremely poisonous.

THORN APPLE. See *Datura.*

THREAD PALM. See *Washingtonia.*

THREADLEAF FALSE ARALIA. See *Dizygotheca.*

THRIFT. See *Armeria.*

Thrinax. 2 ✪
FLORIDA THATCH PALM, KEY PALM, PALMETTO THATCH, THATCH PALM. Several species of medium-size fan palms, native to Mexico, Honduras, the West Indies, and Florida. All are insect-pollinated and do not cause much allergy. Zones 10 to 13.

Thuja. 8
ARBORVITAE, THUYA, WESTERN RED CEDAR, WHITE CEDAR. Five species of evergreen coniferous trees native to North America and eastern Asia. Many of these trees are used as either trees or shrubs in all plant zones in the United States. Many cultivars of Thuja are sold as arborvitae. Popular shrub forms of Thuja are sold as either "globe" or "pyramid" types. All species of Thuja release large amounts of airborne pollen over an extended period of time; those allergic to cypress or juniper have a good chance of cross-allergic reaction to arborvitae. Sawdust from western red cedar is known to trigger dermatitis in woodworkers. Wood shavings from this plant may well be allergenic for small animals such as mice, rats, and hamsters.

Thujopsis dolabrata. 9 🥀
BATTLE AX CEDAR, DEERHORN CEDAR, FALSE ARBOR-VITAE, HIBA ARBORVITAE, HIBA CEDAR. A large ever-green, coniferous tree native to Japan and growing to 100 feet in its native land. In the United States in zones 7 to 11, the many named cultivars of Thujopsis are used as landscape plants.

T

Thunbergia. 2 ✿
BLACK-EYED SUSAN VINE, ORANGE CLOCK VINE, SKY FLOWER. Perennial vines for sunny areas of zones 9 to 13, and hanging basket annual plants elsewhere.

THUYA. See *Thuja*.

THYMOPHYLLA. See *Dyssodia tenuiloba*.

Thymus. 3
THYME. Perennial ground covers, small shrubs, or culinary herb for sunny areas of zones 4 to 10. The fragrance may rarely affect perfume-sensitive individuals. Some thyme may be all-female plants, but there will be no all-male individuals.

TI. See *Cordyline*.

Tiarella. 3
FOAMFLOWERS. Interesting native perennials with spikes of white or pink flowers, hardy in zones 3 to 8. Many hybrid cultivars, with numerous interesting colored large leaves. Good woodland plants for shady areas; flowers attract butterflies. Saxifrage relatives.

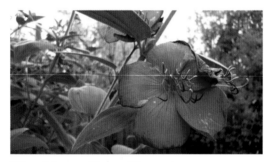

Tibouchina urvilleana (Pleroma). 2 ✿
GLORY BUSH, PRINCESS FLOWER. (Pictured above.) A tall, loosely limbed, evergreen shrub with large, very soft, velvety leaves and large attractive purple flowers, hardy in the mildest areas of zones 9 to 10, and as a green houseplant elsewhere. Native to Brazil, Tibouchina is actually a large genus of plants with more than 300 species, the best known of which is *T. urvilleana*, the princess flower. Fast growing under the right conditions, Tibouchina does best with its roots in shade and its top in the sun, in mulched, well-drained, slightly acidic soil with adequate water.

TICKSEED. See *Coreopsis*.

TIDYTIPS. See *Layia platyglossa*.

Tigridia. 3
TIGER FLOWER. The brilliant orange, trumpet-shaped flowers, flecked with black, are held aloft on stiff, erect stems. Tigridia bulbs are hardy in zones 8 to 10.

Tilia. 6
BASSWOOD, CRIMEAN LINDEN, FEMALE LINDEN, LIME TREE, LINDEN, LITTLELEAF LINDEN, MALE LINDEN, MONGOLIAN LINDEN, SILVER LINDEN, WHISTLEWOOD, WHITE LINDEN, WHITTLEWOOD. A group of about thirty species of fast-growing, spreading, deciduous trees, native to most of the Northern Hemisphere and popular as street trees and valuable lumber trees. They thrive only in areas of adequate moisture.

Despite some of their common names, no linden is actually either a male- or a female-only tree. They produce many small white flowers; although honeybees visit these flowers often, the trees are imperfectly insect-pollinated, and a good deal of pollen becomes airborne. Tilia pollen, although often allergenic, is fairly heavy and does not easily travel far from the tree. Exposure to linden pollen is often caused by trees growing in the allergy sufferer's own yard or workplace (proximity pollinosis).

TILLANDSIA. See *Bromelia*.

TIMOTHY. See *Phleum*.

Tipuana tipu. 3
PRIDE-OF-BOLIVIA, ROSEWOOD TREE, TIPU TREE. An evergreen or deciduous tree native to South America, and used in the United States in zones 9 to 11 as an ornamental. Tipuana is hardy to about 20°F. It bears clusters of apricot-colored pealike flowers in spring, and has long leaves divided into eleven or twelve leaflets.

Tithonia rotundifolia. 5
MEXICAN SUNFLOWER. Tall perennial with large, bright orange flowers, used as an annual in sunny areas of most zones.

TITI. See *Cyrilla racemosa*; *Oxydendrum*.

TOADFLAX. See *Linaria*.

TOBACCO, FLOWERING. See *Nicotiana*.

TOBIRA. See *Pittosporum*.

TODDY PALM. See *Borassus*.

Tolmiea menziesii. 1 ✿
PIGGY-BACK PLANT. Native to California's Coastal Range, the piggy-back plant is popular in gardens in zones 8 to 13 and as a houseplant elsewhere. It is tolerant of wet soil, grows well in the shade, and causes little or no allergy.

TOMATILLO. See *Physalis*.

TOMATO. See *Lycopersicon lycopersicum*.

TOONA TREE. See *Cedrela toona*.

TOOTHACHE TREE. See *Zanthoxylum*.

TORCH LILY. See *Kniphofia uvaria*.

TORCHWOOD FAMILY. See *Burseraceae*.

Torenia. 3
BLUEWINGS, WISHBONE FLOWER, WISHBONE PLANT. About forty species of annuals and perennials, most used as summer annuals. The colorful flowers resemble those of gloxinias.

TORNILLO. See *Prosopis*.

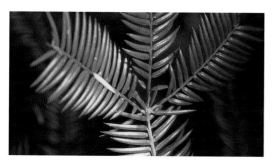

Torreya. MALES 7, FEMALES 1 ☉
CALIFORNIA NUTMEG, FLORIDA TORREYA, JAPA-NESE NUTMEG TREE, NUTMEG TREE, STINKING CEDAR, STINKING YEW. (Pictured above.) Six species of evergreen coniferous trees native to California's cool canyons, Georgia, Florida, China, and Japan, and used in zones 6 to 11. The very slow-growing Japanese nutmeg female tree produces edible seeds; it thrives only in moist, shady situations. Torreya is related to yews (Taxus) and like the yews some species of Torreya are separate-sexed. Because they are not sold sexed, it is best to avoid their use. Leaves are poisonous and the pollen may be also.

TOTARA. See *Podocarpus*.

TOUCH-ME-NOT. See *Impatiens*.

TOWER OF JEWELS. See *Echium fastuosum*.

TOYON. See *Heteromeles arbutifolia*.

Trachelospermum (Rhynchospermum). 5
CONFEDERATE JASMINE, STAR JASMINE. A group of about a dozen species of shrubby, vining evergreen plants with bright, star-shaped, highly fragrant white flowers. These very popular landscape plants are often used as ground covers in sun or shade, in zones 8 to 13. Star jasmine's milky sap can occasionally cause rash, and the heavy fragrance is allergenic to those who are perfume-sensitive. The fragrance is most intense on still, warm summer nights and it should not be planted under bedroom windows. Unrelated to true jasmine (Jasminum). Those who cannot tolerate the heavy fragrance of Jasminum may not be as affected by Trach-elospermum. Plants in full sun appear to be much more fragrant than those growing in the shade.

Trachycarpus. MALES 7, FEMALES 1 ☉
WINDMILL PALM. Several species of small- to medium-size palm trees native to the Himalayan region of Asia. One species in particular, *T. fortunei*, the Chinese windmill or hemp palm, is among the hardiest of all palms, down to 7°F or 8°F. Used in landscaping in zones 8 to 13, windmill palm is also commonly grown in all zones as a houseplant. Landscapers in zones 8 to 9 like these palms because of their ability to tolerate cold; in warm areas the trees grow quickly to 40 feet tall, but in colder, more borderline hardy areas they grow much more slowly.

Separate-sexed, they are not sold sexed. The females produce fruits that resemble large blueberries. The male trees produce allergenic pollen. It has been errone-ously stated that fan-leafed palms cause no allergy because they are perfect-flowered and pollinated only by insects. The windmill palm is not the only exception to the rule.

Trachymene coerulea (Didiscus). 4
BLUE LACE FLOWER. Two-foot-tall annuals with clus-ters of lacy blue flowers on long stems; they grow best in cool weather.

Tradescantia (Zebrina). 4
CHAIN PLANT, SPIDERWORT, WANDERING JEW. Common houseplants or ground covers for shady areas with ample water in zones 9 to 13. Wandering Jew has handsome multicolored leaves. It occasionally causes allergies—especially red, runny eyes—in dogs and cats. In humans, allergy is uncommon.

TRAILING ARBUTUS. See *Epigaea repens*.

TRANSVAAL DAISY. See *Gerbera jamesonii*.

Treculia. MALES 9 ◗, FEMALES 1 ☉
A dozen species of shrubs and trees from tropical Africa; one species, *T. africana*, the African bread tree, is grown in the United States in the mildest areas of zone 10 and in zones 11 to 13. Separate-sexed plants related

to mulberry, the female trees produce huge, seed-filled fruits (to 30 pounds) with many seeds. The male plants have high allergy potential; the females, almost none.

TREE FERN. See *Blechnum*; *Cibotium*; *Dicksonia*; *Sphaeropteris*.

TREE FERN, TASMANIAN. See *Dicksonia*.

TREE MALLOW. See *Lavatera*.

TREE-OF-HEAVEN. See *Ailanthus*.

TREE-OF-SADNESS. See *Nyctanthes*.

TREFOIL. See *Lotus*.

Trema. 9 ◐

About twenty species of trees or shrubs from the tropics and subtropics of both hemispheres. They are related to elm, and some of these species have separate, male-only flowers, which undoubtedly produce considerable pollen. Unfortunately, not much is yet known about individual species, so it is necessary to rank them all as a single group.

Trevesia. 5

SNOWFLAKE TREE. Houseplants grown for their large, snowflake-shaped leaves, held aloft on prickly, long stalks.

TRICHOSPORUM. See *Aeschynanthus*.

Trichostema lanatum. 3

WOOLLY BLUE CURLS. An evergreen shrub native to California's Coastal Range, in zones 9 to 10; it is extremely drought-tolerant.

TRICUSPIDARIA. See *Crinodendron*.

Tricyrtis formosana. 2 ✿

TOAD LILY. Easy-to-grow perennial for part shade in zones 4 to 8. Blooming late summer into the fall.

TRIDENT MAPLE. See *Acer buergeranum*.

Trifolium. 3

CLOVER. Allergy to fresh, growing clover is uncommon, but adverse reaction to dried clover hay is extensive and often severe. The cause of the reaction is not the clover itself, but the mold spores that form when hay is baled while still wet. Dairy farmers, working in enclosed areas with this hay, are frequent sufferers of this allergy, known as "farmer's lung."

Triglochin. 6

ARROW GRASS. A perennial grasslike plant common to marshy areas of much of the world and used as a landscape plant around ponds and small pools.

Trigonella. 2 ✿

FENUGREEK. An annual grown for its aromatic seeds, which have both medicinal and culinary uses.

Trillium. 2 ✿

WAKE ROBIN. Hardy perennials for moist, shady areas in even the coldest zones. They bear attractive, three-lobed white flowers in early spring.

TRINIDAD FLAME BUSH. See *Calliandra tweedii*.

TRIPLET LILY. See *Triteleia*.

Tripleurospermum. 5

BRIDAL ROBE, TURFING DAISY. A group of spreading, ground cover perennials from Asia, Europe, Syria, and Lebanon, now naturalized in the eastern United States. They bear small, daisylike flowers.

Tripogandra multiflora. 5

BRIDAL VEIL. A houseplant very similar to wandering Jew, except that the leaves are much smaller and it produces numerous small, white flowers. It is often sold as *Tradescantia multiflora*.

Tripsacum. 6 TO 9 ◐ DEPENDING ON SPECIES

GAMMA GRASS. A common pasture or forage crop. Some Mexican species are separate-sexed.

Tristania conferta. 5

BRISBANE BOX. An Australian evergreen tree with large leaves and interesting, molting bark, for zones 9 to 13. It is a popular landscape tree in Florida and California. Brisbane box is related to Eucalyptus and sheds some pollen, but little is yet known about its allergy potential. Brisbane box leaves do not have the strong smell characteristic of Eucalyptus foliage. It is, however, like Eucalyptus, a very high VOC-emitting tree.

Triteleia. 3

BRODIAEA, GRASS NUT, ITHURIEL'S SPEAR, TRIPLET LILY. Native to California, *T. laxa*, Ithuriel's spear, is grown from corms and bears large, trumpet-shaped blue flowers.

Trithrinax. 3

Small and medium-size, spiny-trunked palm trees from South America, used in the United States in zones 9 to 11.

Triticum. 6

WHEAT. Wheat is a type of grass and as such there are occasional cross-allergic reactions to its pollen, although the pollen usually does not travel far in the air. Because of this cross-allergic potential, many allergists suggest that people suffering from grass pollen allergies refrain from eating foods made from wheat during peak grass pollen months. This avoidance technique often works quite well. Allergy to hay made from wheat is also common.

TRITOMA. See *Kniphofia uvaria*.

Tritonia (Montbretia). 3
FLAME FREESIA. Grown from corms in zones 9 to 13, Tritonia bears bright orange flowers on tall spikes.

Trollius. 3
GLOBE FLOWER. Large-flowered orange, yellow, or gold perennials, hardy to zone 3. Globe flowers are long-lasting cut flowers.

Tropaeolum. 3
CANARY BIRD FLOWER, NASTURTIUM. Two species of Tropaeolum are commonly used in landscaping. *T. majus*, the common garden nasturtium, is a perennial that is used as a fast-growing annual. The large, round leaves and bright yellow or orange flowers are edible and piquant, and are occasionally added to salads. *T. peregrinum*, the climbing nasturtium, can reach 12 feet. It is yellow-flowered. Some individuals may be sensitive to its fragrance.

TRUMPET CREEPER. See *Campsis*.

TRUMPET VINE. See *Bignonia*; *Campsis*; *Distictis*; *Tecoma*.

TRUMPET VINE TREE. See *Tabebuia*.

TRUMPET VINE, YELLOW. See *Anemopaegma chamberlaynii*; *Macfadyena unguis-cati*.

Tsuga. 3
HEMLOCK, HEMLOCK SPRUCE. A group of ten species of tall evergreen coniferous trees, native to Canada, the United States, and Japan. The Canada hemlock is the most hardy, to zone 2, but the other species are all hardy to at least zone 6. Hemlocks are beautiful trees and can be used to good effect as clipped hedges or as bonsai specimens. They grow best in moist, acid soil and do not do well in full sun or in spots with no protection from strong winds. Tsuga does not tolerate hot, dry conditions. Members of the pine family, Tsuga shed abundant pollen, but because it has a waxy coating it is not irritating to mucous membranes.

TUBEROSE. See *Polianthes tuberosa*.

TUCKEROO. See *Cupaniopsis anacardiodes*.

Tulbaghia violacea. 5
SOCIETY GARLIC. A long-lived perennial with onionlike leaves and small lavender flowers. It has naturalized in some areas. The pollen is nonallergenic. Some find the smell of the crushed leaves or the plants themselves to be objectionable; it may cause allergy in odor-sensitive individuals.

TULIP POPLAR, TULIP TREE. See *Liriodendron*.

TULIP POPPY, MEXICAN. See *Hunnemannia*.

Tulipa. DOUBLES 1 ✪, SINGLES 3
TULIP. A popular spring-blooming flower, grown from bulbs in all zones. Tulip pollen is rarely allergenic, but "tulip rash," caused by handling the bulbs, is not unusual and often severe. There are now many double forms of tulips, and many of these lack any pollen parts; these double tulips are also very long lasting as cut flowers.

TUNG OIL TREE. See *Aleurites fordii*.

TUPELO. See *Nyssa*.

Tupidanthus. 2 ✪
Tall plants that resemble schefflera, for zone 10 or as houseplants elsewhere.

TURFING DAISY. See *Tripleurospermum*.

TURKEY CORN. See *Dicentra*.

TURKEY MULLEIN. See *Eremocarpus setigerus*; *Verbascum*.

TURNIP. See *Brassica*.

Turraea obtusifolia. 2 ✪
STAR BUSH. An evergreen shrub with large, bright white, star-shaped flowers that thrives in light shade in the mildest parts of zone 10. It needs regular deep irrigation.

Tussilago. 5
COLTSFOOT. A common wildflower sometimes grown as a perennial for its very early spring bloom of yellow flowers. It may become invasive and is hard to eradicate where established. Coltsfoot is used medicinally as a cough remedy.

TWINBERRY. See *Lonicera*.

TWINFLOWER. See *Linnaea borealis*.

TWINSPUR. See *Diascia*.

Typha. 6
CATTAIL. A common wetland plant.

Ugni molinae (Myrtus ugni).   2 ✿

CHILEAN GUAVA. An evergreen shrub from Chile, hardy in zones 9 to 13. This handsome shrub has dark green leaves with a slight bronzy tint, rosy white flowers, and small, fragrant, delicious dark purple fruit. Ugni grows best in slightly acid soil with ample water. Easy to grow from cuttings.

Ulmus.   5 TO 9 ◣ DEPENDING ON SPECIES

ELM. A group of eighteen deciduous or partially evergreen trees, native to the United States, Mexico, Europe, and Asia. All the elms are bisexual, having both male and female parts in the same flowers (despite reports that elms possess both unisexual and bisexual flowers). Many plants with bisexual flowers do not release much airborne pollen, but with elms this is not the case; they release significant amounts of pollen into the air. Part of the confusion about the elm flowering systems is probably caused by the fact that some close relatives—Aphananthe, Hemiptelea, Holoptelea, Planera, Trema, and Zelkova—produce unisexual (one-sex) flowers.

All elms produce allergenic pollen. Most deciduous elms produce their pollen in early spring, just before or at the same time as new leaves are appearing. An exception to this is *U. crassifolia*, the cedar elm, which blooms in the fall. It is ranked at 8 on the allergy-potential scale. The Chinese elm (*U. parvifolia*), which can be found growing throughout zones 6 to 10, is often evergreen in the warmest winter areas. Chinese elm releases its pollen from late summer into early winter. It is ranked at 9.

There are also at least three cultivars of elm that never bloom, making them fine allergy-free landscape trees: *U. americana* 'Ascendens', a large columnar tree; *U. glabra* 'Horizontalis', a weeping selection of Scotch elm; and *U. minor* 'Gracilis', a cultivar of the European smoothleaf elm. All three of these nonflowering elms are grown by cuttings or are budded onto seedling elm rootstock. They are ranked as excellent (1) for the allergy-free landscape.

Because Dutch elm disease (DED) has killed off millions of elm trees worldwide, the prevalence of elm allergy has dropped considerably. In areas where elms have been replaced by disease-resistant look-alikes like the Chinese elm, however, the replacements may be more potent allergenic trees than the vanished elms. In fact, a strong argument can be made that the huge rise in urban allergy is directly linked to the millions of monoecious and dioecious male trees that were used to replace so many of the dead elms.

It should also be noted that some of the newer DED-resistant American elm trees are triploid hybrids, and some of these produce very little pollen. Not yet ranked by cultivar.

U. pumilia, the Siberian elm, blooms in early spring and produces large amounts of allergenic pollen; it is ranked 9.

Umbellularia californica. 6
BAY LAUREL, CALIFORNIA BAY, CALIFORNIA LAUREL, MYRTLE, OREGON MYRTLE, PEPPERWOOD. A very large, spreading broadleaf evergreen tree, native to California and Oregon and hardy in zones 8 to 10. The leaves of this tree are occasionally used in cooking, in a similar fashion to its relative, *Laurus nobilis*, the bay laurel or sweet bay tree. However, unlike the pleasant odor of crushed *Laurus nobilis* leaves, the leaves of Umbellularia when crushed are malodorous. Inhaling this odor can cause immediate and severe (although not long-lasting) headache. The fallen leaves also have this smell and odor-sensitive individuals should avoid them. The Umbellularia is perfect-flowered, but it also produces numerous tiny white flowers with exposed stamens and plentiful pollen.

UMBRELLA PALM. See *Hedyscepe canterburyana*.

UMBRELLA PINE. See *Sciadopitys*.

UMBRELLA PLANT. See *Cyperus*.

UMBRELLA TREE. See *Brassaia actinophylla*; *Melia*.

UMBRELLA TREE, QUEENSLAND. See *Brassaia actinophylla*.

UMKOKOLO. See *Dovyalis hebecarpa*.

Ungnadia. 5
FALSE BUCKEYE, MEXICAN BUCKEYE, TEXAS BUCKEYE. A small, shrubby deciduous tree native to Texas, New Mexico, and Mexico, and used in landscaping in zones 7 to 12. The 1-inch fragrant white flowers appear before the leaves, in early spring.

Ursinia. 4
A group of daisy-flowered annuals, perennials, and shrubs from South Africa, some used in all zones in the United States as ornamentals. Many are strong-smelling, and the pollen of a few species may cause limited allergy.

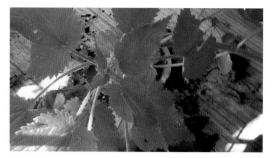

Urtica. MALES 9 ✎, FEMALES 5
NETTLES. (Pictured above.) A large family of noxious weeds and allergy plants. *U. piluifera*, the Roman nettle, is a tall annual grown in greenhouses as an ornamental flower. It, like many others in this family, can cause allergy. Stinging nettles cause immediate contact rash. The male plants produce abundant airborne pollen and have long been implicated in allergy studies. It should be noted that nettles are separate-sexed and only male plants produce the pollen. Nonetheless, few people would want either sex of these stinging plants in their garden.

When nettle leaves are collected (carefully, and with gloves!) they can be steamed or boiled and are nutritious and tasty, although for some (including me), cooked nettles make them sleepy. Nettles have long been a natural medicine for the prostate gland of men; nettle leaves or roots from male plants are more potent for this purpose.

Uvularia grandiflora. 3
BELLWORT. A hardy native perennial for shady gardens with moist soil, bellwort flowers are drooping, yellow, and quite attractive, especially in wildland gardens. Lily family.

U

Allergy Index Scale: 1 is Best, 10 is Worst.
✿ for 1 and 2   ❧ for 9 and 10
No matter what the ranking, always read the full plant description carefully and take note of any warnings.

Vaccinium. 2 ✿

BILBERRY, BLUEBERRY, CRANBERRY, CROWBERRY, FOXBERRY, HUCKLEBERRY. A genus of evergreen and deciduous shrubs, all with edible fruit, some hardy to zone 2. Vaccinium is an intriguing group of fruiting plants, most with small, bell-shaped white flowers that flourish only in very well-drained, moist, acid soil. They grow best when well mulched. Blueberries tolerate some shade but will not take drought. Bilberry is said to be good for improving eyesight, and the juice of wild blueberries has long been an effective remedy for quickly curing diarrhea. Cranberries and their juice are recognized as beneficial for curing or preventing bladder infections, and slowing or stopping gum disease. Vaccinium fruits and juices may also be useful in relieving severe lower back pain caused by liver disorder.

VALERIAN. See *Valeriana.*

VALERIAN, RED. See *Centranthus ruber.*

Valeriana. 2 ✿ TO 4 DEPENDING ON SPECIES

GARDEN HELIOTROPE, VALERIAN. Many species of ornamental and medicinal annuals and perennials, native to every continent except Australia and grown in all zones. The most commonly cultivated is *V. officinalis,*

garden valerian, which has tall stems (to 4 feet) and clusters of tiny white, pink, red, or lavender flowers. The plants self-seed readily. The fragrant flowers may bother perfume-sensitive individuals. In *V. officinalis,* pollen is not a problem, but with some other species of this large group it is possible.

Vallisneria. MALES 7, FEMALES 1 ✿

EEL GRASS, TAPE GRASS, WATER CELERY, WILD CELERY. A small group of separate-sexed plants used in landscaping ponds and small pools. The males produce airborne pollen suspected of causing allergy.

VALLOTA. See *Hippeastrum.*

VAN HOUTTAN PALM. See *Nephrosperma.*

Vancouveria. 3

INSIDE-OUT FLOWER. Deciduous and evergreen perennials native from California to Vancouver, Canada, and grown as a ground cover in shady areas of zones 7 to 9. They bear yellow, white, or white-and-lavender flowers.

VANDA. See *Orchids.*

Vangueria. 5

TAMARIND-OF-THE-INDIES. A group of shrubs and trees from the tropics, some with edible seeds or edible seedpods.

VARIEGATED BOX ELDER. See *Acer negundo* 'Variegatum'.

VARNISH TREE. See *Firmiana simplex; Koelreuteria paniculata; Rhus; Semecarpus.*

VASE PLANT. See *Billbergia.*

Vauquelinia californica. **5**
ARIZONA ROSEWOOD. Drought-tolerant, evergreen shrub or small tree used in desert landscapes of zones 8 to 9. It bears masses of single white flowers that resemble tiny roses. There is little allergy data on this native species, but those with allergies would be wise to keep their noses out of these flowers!

Veitchia. **6**
CHRISTMAS PALM, MANILA PALM. A group of about twenty species of palm trees from the Fiji Islands, Vanuata, and the Philippines. Highly ornamental, these are widely used in tropical landscapes in zones 11 to 13, and in zone 10, especially in Florida.

VELVET GRASS. *See Holcus.*

VELVET GROUNDSEL. *See Senecio.*

VELVET PLANT. *See Gynura aurantiaca.*

Venidium. **4**
CAPE DAISY, NAMAQUALAND DAISY. A small group of perennial flowers from South Africa. The cape daisy bears bright orange flowers and grows to 2 to 3 feet. It thrives in full sun.

Veratrum. **8**
CORN LILY, EUROPEAN WHITE HELLEBORE, FALSE HELLEBORE, INDIAN POKE, ITCHWEED, SKUNK CABBAGE. A genus of about forty-five species of perennial herbs native to North America, Europe, and Asia. Veratrum are usually wildflowers or weeds, but some species are used in the perennial garden. Veratrum thrive only in moist ground.

The false hellebores are an unusual group whose flowers may be white, green, brown, maroon, or purple, always borne in loose clusters on the ends of the stems. All parts are considered highly poisonous; sheep ingesting Veratrum give birth to lambs with fatal deformities. Even so, Veratrum species are used to make various forms of insecticides and are used also as medicinal plants. Avoid both products! Veratrum also causes skin rash, and is suspected of causing pollen-induced allergy.

Verbascum. **2 ✪ TO 5 DEPENDING ON SPECIES AND CULTIVAR**
FLANNEL PLANT, MOTH MULLEIN, MULLEIN, PURPLE MULLEIN, TURKEY MULLEIN. A large genus of several hundred or more of mostly hardy biennial herbs, native to Asia and Europe, but now common in most of the United States. Several species are used in flower gardens. Some species have leaves with a very disagreeable odor. There are now a great number of newer Verbascum

hybrids, some of them interspecific crosses, and all of these have very low allergy potential.

Verbena. **3**
BLUE VERVAIN, GARDEN VERBENA, VERVAIN, WHITE VERVAIN. A genus of about 200 species, annuals and perennials, some low growing and others tall and almost shrublike. *V. hybrida* is the common Verbena sold in most nurseries, and is grown as a short-lived perennial or ground cover in zones 9 to 11, and as an annual in other zones. Verbenas are heat-loving plants needing full sun and fast-draining soil for best results. Grown well, they flower profusely. Verbena is occasionally implicated in causing skin rash, and the scent of a few species, especially when planted en masse, can be unpleasant to some.

Verbesina. **4**
BUTTER DAISY, CROWN-BEARD, WINGSTEM, YELLOW IRONWEED. A group of North and South American herbs, shrubs, and a few trees, rarely used in zones 5 to 10.

VERNAL GRASS. *See Anthoxanthum.*

Vernonia. **4**
IRONWEED. A very large group of herbs, shrubs, trees, and vines with almost worldwide distribution. Few are used in landscaping in the United States.

Veronica. **2 ✪**
BROOKLIME, SPEEDWELL. About 250 species of annuals and perennials from the North Temperate Zone, widely used in landscaping. (A New Zealand shrub called both Veronica and Hebe, and commonly used in most of California, is now placed in the genus Hebe.) Most garden Veronicas are hardy, summer-flowering perennials, bearing white, rose, pink, or blue flowers on erect spikes. Veronicas grow best in full sun and need ample watering. Several prostrate varieties are used as ground covers.

Veronicastrum virginicum. **5**
CULVER'S ROOT. An easy-to-grow, tall, native perennial hardy to zone 2 and widely adapted to much of the eastern U.S. and Canada. Does well with full sun in northern areas but best with partial shade in southern states. White or pink flowers on tall spikes. A few of these in the garden ought to be of little problem, but don't use the flowers as cut flowers, as they may shed more pollen if brought indoors.

Verschaffeltia splendida. **6**
A tall palm tree used in Florida.

VERVAIN. *See Salvia; Verbena.*

Viburnum. DECIDUOUS 3, EVERGREEN 5, STERILE CULTIVARS 1 ✪
ARROWWOOD, COWBERRY, CRANBERRY, CRAN-BERRY BUSH, FRAGRANT SNOWBALL, GROUSEBERRY, GUELDER ROSE, HAW, LAURUSTINUS, LEATHERLEAF, MOOSEBERRY, NANNYBERRY, SNOWBALL BUSH, SQUAWBERRY, SUMMERBERRY, SWAMP HAW, SWEET-BERRY, TEABERRY, WAYFARING TREE, WHITTEN TREE. Deciduous or evergreen shrubs or small trees, native to America, Asia, and Europe and hardy in all zones, depending on species. Viburnums are important long-lived landscape plants and are often used as foundation shrubs, hedges, solitary flowering shrubs, topiary, and small trees; relatives of honeysuckles. Most allergy occurs from close, direct inhaling of the pollen of the small, white, lightly fragrant flowers.

In California, *V. tinus*, the laurustinus or evergreen viburnum, is commonly seen as a small tree or flowering hedge. *V. tinus* needs good air circulation and mildews in humid climates, or when planted too close to a building.

V. opulus, the cranberry bush or snowball, is very popular in zones 3 to 10. Deciduous and hardy, it bears huge round clusters of small white flowers. Usually grown as a shrub, it makes a handsome little multi-trunked tree. In some cultivars, the flowers are followed by bright red edible berries. *Viburnum opulus sterilis* is pollen-free and ranks 1.

A very similar species, *V. carlcephalum*, produces more fragrant flowers and sets no fruit. *V. plicatum* 'Sterilis' is also similar and bears sterile flowers. (Sterility means that pollen may be present, but the flowers don't set seed. However, in most cases of sterility, either no allergic pollen is shed, or the amount produced is considerably reduced.)

Allergy to Viburnum pollen is uncommon; the pollen is heavy and rarely becomes airborne. Perfume-sensitive individuals may be affected by the scent of Viburnum flowers when in full bloom, and bees find them particularly attractive. Those with bee-sting allergies should limit the use of Viburnums. Evergreen species of Viburnum are often infested with aphids, scale, and spider mites, and these small insects may be potent allergens in themselves.

Vicia faba. NOT YET RANKED
FABA BEANS, FAVA BEANS. Large, robust, upright-growing annual broad beans. When some people eat faba beans they develop a condition called favism, which makes them quite sick, or in some cases can be deadly. This reaction is most common in people from the Mediterranean area, Greeks, Italians, and Jews. Among people of African descent, 15 percent also cannot tolerate faba beans. The pollen of faba bean flowers can also set off favism in susceptible people. Faba is not allergy ranked, but should be used with some caution.

VICTORIAN BOX. See *Pittosporum*.

Vigna. 2 ✪
SNAIL VINE. A perennial vine for zones 9 to 10. Snail vine and its flowers resemble those of a large bean vine. It dies back in winter and resprouts in spring.

Villebrunea. MALES 8, FEMALES 2 ✪, DECIDUOUS 3
A small group of shrubs and vining trees from Taiwan and Japan. *V. pedunculosa,* is used as a small landscape tree. Some of the species in this genus are separate-sexed and, as relatives of the nettles, all male plants present distinct allergy potential.

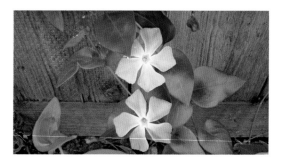

Vinca. 2 ✪
MYRTLE, PERIWINKLE. (*Vinca major*, pictured above.) *V. minor* is a small-leafed, slow-growing, prostrate vine, hardy to zone 3, where it is used as a ground cover. *V. major* is a fast-growing, large-leafed version, not as hardy. Both vines bear five-petaled purple-blue flowers and have attractive dark, leathery leaves. Variegated forms of both species are available. Vinca grows well in full sun to full shade, but becomes tall and less compact in deep shade. Drought-tolerant once established, it performs better when provided with adequate water. Because the flowers have almost no exposed pollen, Vinca makes a very good substitute for more allergenic Algerian or English ivy. The plant known as *V. rosea*, or annual periwinkle, is a fine, sun-loving annual flower properly named *Catharanthus roseus*. Vinca sap may cause allergic skin rash, and although this is uncommon, use care when shearing the vines.

VINE MAPLE. See *Acer circinatum*.

VINEGAR TREE. See *Rhus*.

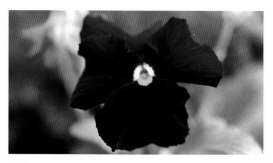

Viola. 1 ✪

JOHNNY-JUMP-UP, PANSY, VIOLA, VIOLET. (Pictured above.) Common, cold-hardy, small perennials, usually grown as annuals and performing best in cool weather, Violas are planted in all zones. In zones 6 to 10, they grow well in spring, fall, and winter. In colder regions, Violas are best in spring. They flourish in full sun to partial shade and require ample water to thrive. The garden violas bear medium-size flowers. Those with very small flowers are known as Johnny-jump-ups. Those bearing the largest and most colorful flowers are called pansy. Long-lived and occasionally fragrant violets, *V. odorata*, are true perennials; this species is also quite poisonous. All Violas reseed with abandon and may (on rare occasion) become an invasive weed.

Violas produce very little pollen and are entirely insect-pollinated. Perfume-sensitive individuals may have adverse reaction to the scent of fragrant violets, but this too, is rare.

VIOLET TREE. See *Polygala*.

VIOLET TRUMPET VINE. See *Clytostoma callistegioides*.

VIRGINIA BLUEBELLS. See *Mertensia*.

VIRGINIA CREEPER. See *Parthenocissus*.

VIRGINIAN STOCK. See *Malcolmia maritima*.

VISCARIA. See *Lychnis*.

Viscum cruciatum. MALES 6, FEMALES 2 ✪

EUROPEAN MISTLETOE. A dioecious (separate-sexed) species; sprigs of berry-covered female plants are used as Christmas decoration. These berries themselves do not cause allergy, although all parts of the plant are poisonous. The common American mistletoe is *Phoradendron serotinum*. It is rarely a good idea to leave mistletoe growing in a tree if it can be knocked down. Most mistletoe is dioecious.

Vitex. 4

CHASTE TREE, HEMP TREE, MONK'S-PEPPER TREE. A large group of more than 200 deciduous or evergreen shrubs or trees from the tropics and subtropics, hardy in zones 4 to 10. Some species have contact-allergy potential. The two most commonly seen Vitex are *V. agnus-castus*, the chaste tree, and the less hardy *V. lucens*, or New Zealand chaste tree, both of which bear spikes of blue or lavender flowers. They are used as large flowering shrubs or multi-trunked small trees. *V. negundo* is a large shrub with clusters of blue flowers and is hardy to zone 4. Chaste tree needs good summer heat to produce the best flowers and has become invasive and naturalized in some warm southern states. Products from Vitex all have very high estrogenic potential.

Vitis. SELF-FERTILE 3, MALES 6, FEMALES 1 ✪

GRAPE. All grape flowers release pollen, but it is not a common allergen. More common is skin rash on those pruning or harvesting grapes: the undersides of the leaves are covered with fine hairs that may cause irritation, although not a classic allergic response. Dander from the small insects, especially aphids, that are common pests of grapes may cause inhalant allergy.

The muscadine grape is an exception, in that it is separate-sexed and males produce airborne pollen, which has been implicated as causing allergy. If muscadine grapes are to be grown (only in zones 9 to 10), there are self-fertile cultivars that can be used to pollinate the all-female vines. Do not use any all-male plants, as they can cause allergy, and are not needed. 'Arlene', 'Black Beauty', 'Janet', 'Pam', 'Scuppernong', 'Supreme', and 'Sweet Jenny' are all excellent all-female muscadine cultivars. Any of them can be pollinated with self-fertile varieties such as 'Dixie Red', 'Fry', 'Ison', or 'Pineapple'.

Most commonly sold grape vines are either self-fertile or they are female plants that set parthenocarpic (seedless) fruit. Grapes are easy to grow and root easily from foot-long pencil-thick dormant cuttings taken in winter. 'Concord' is a self-fertile vine hardy in zones 5 to 10.

Vittadinia australis. 5

A bushy subshrub used in Australia and New Zealand, the Vittadinia bears daisylike white flowers on a low-growing fuzzy-leafed plant.

Vonitra. 6

Several species of slender palms from Madagascar, used to produce fiber.

VRIESEA. See *Bromelia*.

V

WAFER ASH. See *Ptelea*.

WAFFLE PLANT. See *Hemigraphis*.

WAKE ROBIN. See *Trillium*.

Waldsteinia fragarioides. 1 TO 2 ⊕

BARREN STRAWBERRY, STRAWBERRY GROUND COVER.
Not related to strawberries (see *Fragaria*), this small,
prostrate creeper for zones 6 to 10 bears five-petaled
yellow flowers that resemble those of strawberry but
produces small, inedible fruits. A spreading perennial
native to the eastern U.S., it is a useful ground cover
plant for shady areas in zones 4 to 8, but will also grow
in full sun.

Wallaceodendron celebicum. 6

A large and large-leafed tree from Celebes, used in
tropical landscapes. Growing to 125 feet, this tree produces numerous flowers with petals that are brown on
the outside and white, yellow, and green inside.

WALLFLOWER. See *Cheiranthus cheiri*; *Erysimum*.

Wallichia. 2 ⊕

Six species of small monocarpic palms that bloom once
and die. They are used in zones 9 to 13. Because they
flower only once, these plants produce copious amounts
of pollen when blooming; they are, however, insect-
pollinated and present little allergy threat. Some palms
called Wallichia are actually Arenga.

WALLWORT. See *Sambucus*.

WALNUT. See *Juglans*.

WAND FLOWER. See *Galax urceolata*.

WANDERING JEW. See *Callisia*; *Tradescantia*;
Tripogandra multiflora.

WARMINSTER BROOM. See *Cytisus*.

Warszewiczella. 2 ⊕

A few species of trees from the tropics, occasionally
seen in greenhouse collections in the United States.

WASHINGTON THORN. See *Crataegus*.

Washingtonia. 3

WASHINGTON PALM. Two species native to dry areas of
Mexico, California, and Arizona. *W. filifera*, the desert
palm, California fan palm, or petticoat palm, is a thick-
trunked, very stout palm tree that can eventually reach
80 feet. It is native to desert streams and springs, and is
hardy to 18°F.

 W. robusta, the Mexican fan or thread palm, is a
very tall tree with a slender trunk. It is the most common palm tree in California. It is hardy to about 20°F.
Luckily for the many people living with these tall fan
palms towering overhead, both species are entirely
insect-pollinated and shed very little pollen. In almost

all urban areas where these palms are common, the trees are used yearly as nesting sites for orioles, kestrels, and barn owls. These trees should never be pruned (de-thatched) during the nesting months of January to July, as all of these birds are important native species.

WATER CELERY. See *Vallisneria*.

WATER ELM. See *Planera aquatica*.

WATER HAWTHORN. See *Aponogeton distachyus*.

WATER HYACINTH. See *Eichhornia crassipes*.

WATER IVY. See *Senecio*.

WATER LILY. See *Aponogeton distachyus*; *Nelumbo*; *Nymphaea*.

WATER PINE. See *Glyptostrobus lineatus*.

WATERCRESS. See *Tropaeolum*.

WATERMELON PEPEROMIA. See *Peperomia*.

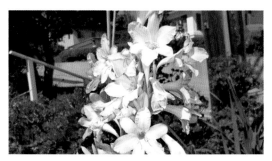

Watsonia. 2 ⊕
BUGLE LILY, WATSONIA LILY. (Pictured above.) Easy to grow, planted with corms, for zones 4 to 12, these tall, colorful plants often naturalize. Highly recommended. In coldest areas it may be necessary to dig and store corms in the fall and then replant them in the spring. Long-lasting flowers.

WATTLE. See *Acacia*.

WAX APPLE. See *Syzygium*.

WAX MYRTLE. See *Myrica*.

WAX PALM. See *Ceroxylon*.

WAX PLANT. See *Hoya*.

WAX VINE. See *Senecio*.

WAXBERRY. See *Symphoricarpos*.

WAXFLOWER. See *Chamelaucium uncinatum*; *Hoya*; *Stephanotis*.

WAYFARING TREE. See *Viburnum*.

WEDDEL PALM. See *Microcoelum*.

Wedelia triloba. 3
Tender ground cover perennial bearing small yellow flowers, for zone 10.

WEEPING WILLOW. See *Salix*.

Weigela. 3
Deciduous shrubs that are widely used in zones 3 to 8, with many named cultivars. Because they flower on new wood, hard pruning after bloom encourages next season's blossoms. There are about a dozen different species of Weigela, usually bearing pink, purple, or carmine-colored flowers. All need ample water to thrive, but are otherwise easy to grow. Not often implicated in allergy, they are related to honeysuckle and those with allergy to honeysuckle should avoid inhaling the fragrance of Weigela.

Weinmannia. MALES 7, FEMALES 1 ⊕
A large genus of evergreen shrubs and trees from Africa and the Southern Hemisphere; several species are used around the world in landscapes for their large glossy leaves and pink or white flowers. Many species of Weinmannia are separate-sexed, and the group as a whole is closely related to several other important allergy plants. Zones 10 to 13.

Welwitschia mirabilis. NOT YET RANKED
A separate-sexed perennial from the deserts of Africa, occasionally found in the United States as a curiosity.

WEST INDIAN CEDAR. See *Cedrela*.

WEST INDIAN CHERRY. See *Malpighia glabra*.

WEST INDIAN SATINWOOD. See *Zanthoxylum*.

WESTERN JUNE GRASS. See *Koeleria*.

Westringia. 2 ⊕
A small group of shrubby Australian plants, similar in many ways to perennial Salvia. They are popular in zones 9 to 11, especially in California, where they are grown for their brown-spotted white flowers.

WHEAT. See *Triticum*.

WHEATGRASS. See *Agropyron*.

Whipplea modesta. 4
YERBA DE SALVA. A trailing subshrub or ground cover for zones 7 to 10, Whipplea grows best in cool, shady woods where it bears clusters of white flowers.

WHISTLEWOOD. See *Tilia*.

WHITE BLADDER FLOWER. See *Araujia*.

WHITE CAMAS. See *Zigadenus*.

WHITE CEDAR. See *Cedrus*; *Chamaecyparis*; *Juniperus*; *Thuja*.

WHITE FORSYTHIA. See *Abeliophyllum distichum*.

WHITE MULBERRY. See *Morus alba*.

WHITE PEPPER. See *Piper*.

WHITE VERVAIN. See *Verbena*.

WHITETHORN. See *Acacia*.

Whitfieldia. 2 ✪

A small group of tropical African shrubs used in zones 10 to 13 for their white or red flowers.

WHITTEN TREE. See *Viburnum*.

WHITTLEWOOD. See *Tilia*.

WHYA TREE. See *Robinia*.

Widdringtonia. MONOECIOUS 8 TO 9 🌑, DIOECIOUS MALES 10 🌑, DIOECIOUS FEMALES 2 ✪

AFRICAN CYPRESS, BERG CYPRESS, CLANWILLIAM CEDAR, MLANJE CEDAR, WILLOWMORE CEDAR. Evergreen, coniferous trees, some of which reach great height, native to Africa and Madagascar and used in the United States only in the mildest areas of zone 10 and 11. Some of the species are separate-sexed and, as close relatives of allergenic cypress, they are a potent allergy threat.

WILD BUCKWHEAT. See *Eriogonum*.

WILD CARROT. See *Daucus*.

WILD CELERY. See *Vallisneria*.

WILD CHINA TREE. See *Sapindus*.

WILD CINNAMON. See *Canella*.

WILD GINGER. See *Asarum*.

WILD HELIOTROPE. See *Phacelia distans*.

WILD HYACINTH. See *Dichelostemma*.

WILD INDIGO. See *Baptisia australis*.

WILD LILAC. See *Ceanothus*.

WILD LIME. See *Zanthoxylum*.

WILD MUSTARD. See *Brassica*.

WILD OLIVE. See *Nyssa*.

WILD RICE. See *Zizania*.

WILD RYE. See *Elymus canadensis*.

WILD SPINACH. See *Chenopodium*.

WILD STRAWBERRY. See *Fragaria*.

WILGA. See *Geijera parviflora*.

WILLOW. See *Salix*.

WILLOW SUMACH. See *Rhus*.

WINDFLOWER. See *Anemone*.

WINDMILL PALM. See *Trachycarpus*.

WINE PALM. See *Borassus*; *Caryota*.

WINGNUT TREE. See *Pterocarya*.

WINGSTEM. See *Verbesina*.

WINTER ACONITE See *Eranthis hyemalis*.

WINTER CREEPER. See *Euonymus*.

WINTER DAPHNE. See *Daphne odorata*.

WINTER HAZEL. See *Corylopsis*.

WINTER SAVORY. See *Satureja*.

Winteraceae. NOT YET RANKED

BARK FAMILY. A group of about eight genera and seventy species, mostly native to the Southern Hemisphere. They are related to Magnolias but have separate male flowers that produce airborne pollen. Only two kinds are used as ornamentals in the United States, Drimys and Pseudowintera.

WINTERBLOOM. See *Hamamelis*.

WINTERGREEN. See *Gaultheria*.

WINTER'S BARK. See *Drimys winteri*; *Pseudowintera*.

WINTERSWEET. See *Chimonanthus praecox*.

WIRE VINE. See *Muehlenbeckia complexa*.

WISHBONE FLOWER, WISHBONE PLANT. See *Torenia*.

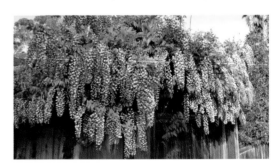

Wisteria. 4

(*Wisteria sinensis*, pictured above.) Less than a dozen species of woody vines native to Asia and the eastern United States. Two species, *W. floribunda* and *W. sinensis*, are commonly used worldwide. *W. floribunda*, the Japanese wisteria, is hardy in zones 4 to 10, long-lived, heavy-flowering, and may grow far up into trees or onto houses. Its fragrant flowers are white, purple, or lavender and are borne in long drooping clusters. The cultivar 'Plena' has fully double, deep blue-violet flowers. 'Plena' releases almost no pollen and is a fine choice for the allergy-free garden.

W. sinensis, the Chinese wisteria, has shorter, faintly fragrant, purple flower clusters that open all at once, making them very showy in bloom. 'Alba' is a highly fragrant white cultivar. Hardiness is similar to *W. floribunda*.

W. macrostachya is a native species, found in wet areas of the southeast, west to Arkansas. It has foot-long clusters of lilac-blue flowers and its pods are smooth. Another native is *W. frutescens*, also from the southeast, west to Texas; it produces 5-inch-long lilac-colored flower clusters.

All species produce long pods filled with poisonous seeds that eject forcefully when ripe, often with a bang like a small firecracker. Frequently, as one pod explodes, others quickly join in; it sometimes sounds like the yard has just come under gunfire! Wisteria is difficult to propagate from cuttings (as are most members of Leguminosae or pea family), but it is easy from seed and good selections can be budded or grafted. Vines often take many years to bloom and occasionally, if the soil is too rich in nitrogen, the vines grow rampant but never bloom. Graft incompatibility is fairly common, and if the top of a grafted plant dies off suddenly, the rootstock will still sprout, grow, and eventually flower.

Generally speaking, wisteria is not much of an allergy concern, but, because it is a large-flowering legume, and because cross-reactive responses are not uncommon with legume (peanut, soy) allergy, this should be considered if someone in a household has any kind of peanut allergy. Dogs that eat the big, hard seeds may also become sick.

WISTERIA TREE. *See Pterostyrax; Sesbania tripetii.*

WITCH HAZEL. *See Hamamelis.*

WOLFBERRY. *See Symphoricarpos.*

Wollemia nobilis. 4
WOLLEMIA PINE. Zones 9 to 11 evergreen conifer trees with large male and female cones on same tree.

WONDER TREE. *See Idesia polycarpa; Ricinus communis.*

WONDERBERRY. *See Synsepalum dulcificum.*

WONGA-WONGA VINE. *See Pandorea.*

WOOD FERN. *See Dryopteris.*

WOOD SORREL. *See Oxalis.*

WOODBINE. *See Lonicera; Parthenocissus.*

Woodfordia. 5
Two species of shrubs from Africa, Madagascar, and Asia, occasionally used in Florida. *W. fruticosa*, a large shrub, is the most common; it bears clusters of red flowers. Zones 10 to 13.

WOODRUFF. *See Galium odoratum.*

Woodwardia fimbriata. 5
GIANT CHAIN FERN. Easy-to-grow, very large fern for zones 7 to 12.

WOOLLY BLUE CURLS. *See Trichostema lanatum.*

WOOLY SENNA. *See Cassia.*

WORMSEED. *See Chenopodium.*

WORMWOOD. *See Artemisia.*

Wrightia. 6
Fifteen species of trees and shrubs from the tropics of the Old World, with poisonous seeds and a sap that causes contact allergy.

Wyethia. 4
A small genus of a dozen species of herbs native to the western United States and occasionally used as perennial plants for their yellow flowers.

Allergy Index Scale: 1 is Best, 10 is Worst.
✿ for 1 and 2   ❧ for 9 and 10
No matter what the ranking, always read the full plant description carefully and take note of any warnings.

Xantheranthemum. 1 ✿

A perennial herb from Peru, grown as a houseplant or greenhouse plant for its attractive dark green leaves with veins that are yellow above and purple below.

Xanthoceras. 6

Two species of shrubs or small trees from China, hardy in zones 6 to 11. They resemble horse chestnut or buckeye (Aesculus). The seeds are poisonous.

Xanthorrhoea. 4

BLACKBOY, GRASS TREE. A dozen species of palmlike perennials from Australia, occasionally used in landscapes in warm climates. The sap may cause skin rash.

Xeranthemum annuum. 3

IMMORTELLE. Six species of annual flowers from the Mediterranean region, grown in full sun; immortelle is a popular, long-lasting dried flower.

Xylococcus bicolor. 3

MISSION MANZANITA. An evergreen shrub native to California and Baja California, and hardy in zones 7 to 11. It produces clusters of small white or pink flowers followed by small red fruit.

Xylosma. MALES 7, FEMALES 1 ✿

About 100 species of spiny, glossy-leafed, separate-sexed evergreen shrubs or trees from the tropics and subtropics, increasingly used in landscaping in zones 8 to 13. The most common and cold-hardy is *X. congestum*, the shiny Xylosma, a common landscape shrub often used as a tall hedge.

Because Xylosma does not have many commonly used close relatives, possible cross-allergic responses are sharply limited. Nonetheless, male shrubs shed considerable airborne pollen and those living or working where a great deal of Xylosma grows may develop allergy. Female shrubs are identified by their small berries. In California, where *X. congestum* is a very common landscape shrub or small tree, 100 percent of all the plants appear to be clonal males. If any reader should ever happen to find *X. congestum* with any fruit on it (a female plant) I would be delighted to see it.

In areas with very high smog levels, Xylosma often gets heavily infected with whitefly, and subsequently the bushes then almost always become covered with molds and their spores, a very serious allergenic situation.

Xyris. 2 ✿

YELLOW-EYED GRASS. A perennial for zones 5 to 10. Not a true grass, several species of yellow-eyed grass are grown for the small, yellow, three-petaled flowers they produce. Not particular about soil, they grow best with ample water and tolerate wet soil.

Allergy Index Scale: 1 is Best, 10 is Worst.
✪ for 1 and 2   ◗ for 9 and 10
No matter what the ranking, always read the full plant description carefully and take note of any warnings.

YARROW. See *Achillea*.

YARROW GILIA. See *Gilia*.

YATE. See *Eucalyptus*.

YELLOW BACHELOR'S BUTTON. See *Polygala*.

YELLOW FLAX. See *Reinwardtia indica*.

YELLOW IRONWEED. See *Verbesina*.

YELLOW OLEANDER. See *Thevetia*.

YELLOW PALM. See *Chrysalidocarpus*.

YELLOW PARILLA. See *Menispermum*.

YELLOW POPLAR. See *Liriodendron*.

YELLOW POPOLO. See *Solanum*.

YELLOW TRUMPET VINE. See *Anemopaegma chamber-laynii*; *Macfadyena unguis-cati*.

YELLOW-EYED GRASS. See *Xyris*.

YELLOW-FLOWERED DAISY. See *Bidens ferulifolia*.

YELLOWWOOD. See *Cladrastis lutea*; *Rhodosphaera rhodanthema*.

YERBA BUENA. See *Satureja*.

YERBA DE SALVA. See *Whipplea modesta*.

YERBA MANSA. See *Anemopsis californica*.

YESTERDAY-TODAY-AND-TOMORROW. See *Brunfelsia pauciflora calycina*.

YEW. See *Taxus*.

YEW, STINKING. See *Torreya*.

YEW PINE. See *Podocarpus*.

Yucca. 2 ✪

ADAM'S NEEDLE, BANANA YUCCA, BLUE YUCCA, DAGGER PLANT, JOSHUA TREE, NEEDLE PALM, PALM LILY, PALMA PITA, ROMAN CANDLE, SOAP TREE, SOAPWELL, SPANISH BAYONET. A group of about forty species of sharp-spined plants native to the warm areas of North America; some are hardy to zone 4, but few will flower north of zone 4. Yucca flowers are usually creamy white, tinged with pink or purple, and borne on tall, stiff stalks that rise well above the foliage. The flowers are entirely insect-pollinated and do not shed pollen.

The long, daggerlike leaves are dangerous, especially to small children, and placement of these vigorous plants requires good judgment. One species from Florida, *Y. recurvifolia*, lacks the sharp-tipped leaves and makes a better garden plant than most Yuccas. Another species, *Y. elephantipes*, the giant yucca, grows far too large for most gardens and is difficult to remove.

Allergy Index Scale: 1 is Best, 10 is Worst.
✪ for 1 and 2   ☙ for 9 and 10
No matter what the ranking, always read the full plant description carefully and take note of any warnings.

ZABEL LAUREL. *See Prunus laurocerasus.*

Zaluzianskya capensis. 5

NIGHT PHLOX. A shrubby tender perennial for zones 10 to 13, grown for its fragrant tubular flowers that are white on the outside and purple inside. The scent may affect perfume-sensitive individuals. The sap of these plants may occasionally cause skin rash. The sap is poisonous.

Zamia. MALES 6, FEMALES 1 ✪

ARROW ROOT, COMPTIE, COONTIE, FLORIDA ARROWWOOD, SAGO CYCAS, SEMINOLE BREAD. Small, separate-sexed, palmlike plants often used as house-plants, and sometimes as garden plants in zones 10 to 13. An occasional plant should pose little allergy potential, but because they are separate-sexed, the males may trigger allergic response. Female Zamia are identified by their central cone, which is considerably larger than that of the male. Viable seeds may be produced on the female plants.

Zantedeschia. 4

CALLA, CALLA LILY. Tall perennials, with unusually prominent calyxes in white, yellow, pink, or red; they are easy to grow and hardy in zones 8 to 13. In cooler climates, the roots must be lifted and overwintered indoors. They thrive in shade or sun, but require ample water. The pollen, which is prominently displayed on the stiff stamens, may cause allergy if inhaled. The sap of calla lilies has properties similar to that of dumb cane (Dieffenbachia), and it may cause contact rash. All parts of the plant are poisonous if eaten.

Zanthoxylum. MALES 7, FEMALES 1 ✪

HERCULES' CLUB, JAPAN PEPPER, PEPPERWOOD, PRICKLY ASH, SEA ASH, TOOTHACHE TREE, WEST INDIAN SATINWOOD, WILD LIME. Several hundred species of prickly, evergreen or deciduous shrubs and trees native to North and South America, Africa, Asia, and Australia. In California, *Z. piperitum*, Japan pepper, a small evergreen tree, hardy to zone 8, is common. *Z. clava-herculis*, the southern prickly ash, pepperwood, or Hercules' club, is common from Florida to Oklahoma and hardy to zone 7. *Z. fagara*, wild lime, is used in Florida and southern Texas into Mexico. Several species of deciduous Zanthoxylum trees are used in Japan and China. *Z. americanum*, the toothache tree, is used for medicinal purposes and is hardy in zones 5 to 10.

Male plants of this large genus produce airborne pollen, but allergy is uncommon. Female plants produce no pollen and only female plants produce the small fruit. As citrus relatives, some species may cause contact skin rash, and in some fragrant varieties negative odor challenges are possible.

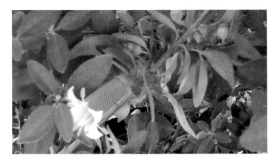

Zauschneria. 2 ✪

CALIFORNIA FUCHSIA, HUMMINGBIRD FLOWER. (Pictured above.) Four species of woody perennials. *Z. californica latifolia* is the hardiest, growing well in zones 6 to 11. It is a small, shrubby, drought-tolerant native plant with small tubular red flowers that resemble those of Fuchsia. Easy to grow in full sun, the flowers are attractive to hummingbirds. *Z. californica* has been reclassified in the Epilobium (fireweed) genus.

Zea mays. 5

CORN. Annual. The tassels at the top of the corn plant are male flowers; the ears of corn themselves are actually female flowers. The pollen only goes airborne early in the morning. Corn pollen is quite large and heavy.

ZEBRA PLANT. See *Calathea*.

ZEBRINA. See *Tradescantia*.

Zelkova. 8

JAPANESE ZELKOVA, SAWLEAF ZELKOVA. Five species of elmlike and elm-related trees native to Japan and China and used throughout most of the United States. The most commonly used is *Z. serrata*, a hardy deciduous tree for zones 3 to 11. Also common is *Z. carpinifolia*, occasionally sold as *Z. ulmoides*, which is hardy to zone 4. Either of these two trees can grow to 50 feet; *Z. serrata* has a slightly wider growth habit and *Z. carpinifolia* forms a classic elmlike vase shape.

Zelkova was little used in the past but has now become popular as a replacement tree for elms killed by Dutch elm disease—Zelkova is resistant to the disease. Little research has been done on allergy caused by Zelkova, but many have recently been planted and are only now starting to mature.

Zelkova is a direct elm relative and, unlike the elms, which have bisexual flowers, Zelkova has separate male flowers. When large and mature, Zelkova is able to put even more pollen into the air than an elm of the same size. Elm pollen is the cause of some

allergy, and reactions are often severe. Pollinosis (asthma and hay fever) to Zelkova will likely grow rapidly in importance in the future as these newly planted trees grow and mature.

Zenobia pulverulenta (Andromeda speciosa). 3

A deciduous shrub native to the southeastern United States and used in landscaping for its clusters of fragrant white flowers. It needs moist, acid soil and grows well in partial shade.

Zephyranthes. 3

FAIRY LILY, RAIN LILY, ZEPHYR FLOWER. A small, hardy bulb, related to Amaryllis, for full sun or light shade in zones 4 to 13. It must be winter-mulched heavily in zones 4 to 8.

Zigadenus. 7

ALKALI GRASS, DEATH CAMAS, STAR LILY, WHITE CAMAS. A bulbous perennial growing wild in fields from Minnesota to California and north to Alaska. It is sometimes used in perennial gardens for its white flowers. All parts are highly poisonous. Contact with the sap or roots may cause skin rash. This plant is sometimes confused with wild onions, with deadly results.

Zingiber officinale. 3

TRUE GINGER. An easy-to-grow tall perennial with greenish yellow flowers, for zones 8 to 13. Tubers of ginger root can be bought at the grocery store and planted in spring. Plants die back with the first frost and regrow in spring. In colder regions, a heavy mulch may carry the tender roots through the winter.

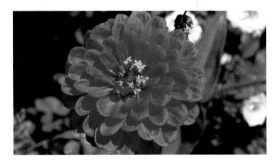

Zinnia. 3

(Pictured above.) Popular garden annuals for full sun, in many different sizes, shapes, and colors. Zinnias are related to the ragweeds and as such, may cause allergy. Zinnia flowers, however, shed very little pollen and in many tests, reaction to Zinnia was neither common nor severe.

Z

ZINNIA, CREEPING. *See Sanvitalia procumbens.*

Zizania. 4

WILD RICE. Rarely implicated in allergy; the pollen has low allergenicity.

Zizia aurea. 5

GOLDEN ALEXANDERS. Tough native perennials for average soils in zones 3 to 8. Bright yellow flowers attract large numbers of native pollinators. It is a member of the carrot family, and none of the carrot family's many members should be used as a cut flower or in floral bouquets, because they may shed more pollen if brought indoors. Outside in the garden these should be fine.

Ziziphus. MALES 6, FEMALES 1 ✪

CHINESE DATE, CHINESE JUJUBE, JUJUBE. More than forty species of deciduous and evergreen shrubs or trees, often with many sharp spines, and most producing small edible, datelike fruits; hardy to zone 5, although the fruits require high summer heat to ripen fully. The fruits have a crunchy texture and a flavor resembling pear and apple; these fruits are sometimes dried and used like dates.

Jujube is related to the buckthorns and its heavy pollen may cause allergy to those in the immediate vicinity of the male trees. The common jujube tree, *Z. jujuba*, may reach 40 feet, although half that size is more common. The cultivar 'Inermis' is thornless. 'Lang' and 'Li' are two common fruiting cultivars; the fruits of 'Li' are slightly larger (to 2 inches long), but 'Lang' is faster to bear after planting.

Zombia antillarum. 1 ✪

ZOMBI PALM. A 10-foot fan palm from Haiti, the zombi palm has a stout trunk sheathed in long fibers. Completely insect-pollinated, it causes no allergy.

Zoysia. 4

Three species of common lawn grass for milder areas of the United States. *Z. japonica* is Korean grass; *Z. matrella* is Japanese carpet or Manila grass; and *Z. tenuifolia* is Mascarene or Korean velvet grass. All three are propagated from plugs or by stolons. Zoysia lawns are popular in parts of zones 9 and 10. The lawns are coarse, thick, and spongy and tend to produce a great deal of thatch. Unlike Bermuda grass, Zoysia does not often flower while it is short, so regular mowing eliminates almost all pollen-producing potential. Zoysia sometimes escapes cultivation to become a problem weed in vacant lots. In these circumstances, it will produce pollen that, while allergenic, is not nearly as potent as that of other lawn grasses. For a similar but superior lawn grass for mild winter areas, see *Stenotaphrum secundatum*, St. Augustine grass, or a female clone of saltgrass, bluegrass, or buffalo grass.

Glossary of Horticultural Terms

Amphiphilous. These are plants that are pollinated by *both* insects and the wind, and many are important in allergy studies. A few examples are olives, acacia, goldenrod, and privet. More than a dozen years ago, frustrated by reading so often that plants were "pollinated by either the wind or by insects," I started to use the term *amphiphilous* to mean "pollinated by both." Consulting with my Latin and Greek language expert, Vicki Leon, I have since added these other similar (linguistically, perhaps more correct) terms: *amphientoanemophily*, or *amphientoanemophilous*, synonym *amphiphilous*.

Anaphylaxis. Anaphylaxis is increased susceptibility to an allergen that one has already had a severe allergic reaction to. When people have a severe allergic reaction they can go into anaphylactic shock.

Androdioecious. Applied to a dioecious species in which male and hermaphrodite (perfect) flowers occur on different plants. This system is a negative, indicating high potential for allergy.

Anemophilous, anemophily. Plants that are completely pollinated only by the wind or by gravity. Such plants are quite likely to be the sources of pollen allergy. Examples are male mulberry trees, ragweed, and male pistache trees.

Annual. A plant that lives, flowers, produces seed, and dies within one year or less. Examples of annuals are corn, beans, and marigolds.

Asexual. No sex; not grown from seed. Asexual propagation (see *propagation*) is growing new plants from cuttings, divisions, runners, budding, grafting, layering, or tissue cultures. An asexually grown plant is essentially a clone; nonetheless, there are sometimes slight variations even among these clones.

Biennial. A plant that lives for more than one year but not more than two years. Biennials usually flower in their second year. Examples of biennials are carrots, cabbage, and many, but not all, foxgloves.

Biogenic allergens. This normally refers to pollen and to mold spores, but it could also mean anything from a plant that triggers allergic response, such as certain odors or the tiny irritating leaf hairs found on sycamore leaves.

Bisexual. A flowering system where both male and female functional parts are found in the same flower. Other names for bisexual are "perfect," "complete," and "hermaphroditic." Bisexual flowers are found in roses, apples, plums, and snapdragons.

Botanical sexism. The predominance of male cloned trees and shrubs in modern urban landscapes is now frequently described as "botanical sexism." Male plants were used because they do not make seeds, fruit, or pods, but they shed large amounts of allergenic pollen and cause widespread allergies. Botanical sexism was first written about by Thomas Leo Ogren. In some cities almost all of the trees and shrubs are now either all-male or mostly male. As botanical sexism continues to increase, so will rates of urban allergies.

Bract. A highly colored leaf that resembles a flower petal. Common plants with colorful bracts are bougainvillea and poinsettia.

Clone, clonal. Clones are totally alike in all ways, including sex. Clonal plants are propagated by asexual methods, usually by cuttings, grafting, layering, division, or tissue culture. A clonal plant that is propagated and given a common name then becomes a "cultivar."

Complete flower. A perfect or bisexual flower, having both male and female functional parts in the same flower. A complete flower also has a full set of petals and sepals.

Conifer. A cone-bearing plant, usually evergreen, often with slender leaves or needles, belonging to the large plant order Coniferales. Examples of conifers are pines, spruce, yew, juniper, cedar, and cypress.

Coniferous. Belonging to the group of conifers.

Cross-allergic reactions. Also called cross-reactive allergy. When people become highly allergic to one particular plant, they may easily become allergic to close relatives of that plant. For example, if you are highly allergic to pollen of the black walnut, it may not take long before you develop a cross-allergic response to the pollen of English walnut. In time you may also become allergic to pollen from butternuts, pecans, and hickories, all relatives of walnut. Likewise, after some time it is quite possible that you will also become allergic to eating these nuts, and to using the oil from them. Sometimes there are cross-allergic responses between plant groups that are not closely related, although this is not as common.

People who are already highly allergic to ragweed pollen often can develop cross-allergic reactions to daisy, coyote bush, marigold, calendula, aster, and sunflower, all of which are in the same large family of plants. Likewise, a person already allergic to poison ivy or poison oak will be at additional risk of developing cross-allergic reactions to their relatives, plants such as lemonade berry, smoke bush, and pepper trees.

Crown. A cluster of vegetative buds. Most hardy perennial plants form crowns at or just under the soil line. If the top part of the plant is killed off by frost, the plant usually resprouts from this crown. Crowns are protected by mulching. In certain plants, like strawberries, it is essential at planting to set the crowns in the soil at just the right depth. Buried too deeply, they rot, and not planted deep enough, they dry out and die.

Cryptically dioecious. A term that means that the dioecy of the plant is hidden, both male and female parts appearing in each flower, but in actuality, only one sex is functional. As often seen in species such as Pittosporum.

Cultivar. A cultivated variety. Using the maple tree *Acer rubrum* 'Red Sunset' as an example, the cultivar is 'Red Sunset'. Cultivar implies that it is a cultivated plant, not just a variation of some species that only grows in the wild. A cultivar can only be duplicated asexually. It will not normally come true (see "Seedling grown," page 232) from seed.

Cytotoxic. Toxic to all living cells.

Deciduous. A tree, shrub, or vine that loses its leaves, usually in the fall, and then grows new leaves in the spring. Common deciduous plants are maples, elms, willows, and apples. The opposite of deciduous is evergreen.

Dicliny. Any plant with unisexual (single-sexed) flowers.

Dicot, dicotyledon. Dicot seeds sprout and emerge from the soil with two first leaves. Examples of dicots are beans, tomatoes, maple trees, marigolds, petunias, junipers, and pines. Dicots typically have their flower parts in sets or multiples of five. Plum flowers, for example, usually have five petals, five sepals, and fifteen stamens. All flowering plants in the world are either dicots or monocots.

Dioecious. A separate-sexed plant, having only male flowers on one plant and only female flowers on another. Many of the most allergenic plants are dioecious males. Examples of dioecious plants are most willows, all box elders, some junipers, all yews, most of the ash and poplars, many palm trees, and all ginkgoes, pepper trees, and hollies.

Dioecy. Complete separation of the sexes.

Dormant. Alive, but not actively growing. Deciduous plants are dormant during the winter, as are many perennials. Many hardy plants go through a dormant period.

Entomogamous. Pollinated only by insects. Plants pollinated only by insects are usually (but not always) less allergenic.

Evergreen. A tree, shrub, or vine that holds its leaves all year long. Common evergreens are pines, yews, lemons, and oranges. The opposite of evergreen is deciduous.

Exserted stamens. In some flowers, the male parts (the stamens) stick out from the flower, or are exserted. On the tips of the stamens are the anthers, and the anthers contain all the pollen. If a flower type has exserted stamens, the pollen is more easily contacted. Not all flowers with exserted stamens cause allergies; it is, however, always one of many factors considered in ranking.

Family. A large group of related genera. In the beech family are found all the tan oaks, beechnuts, chestnuts, and oaks. Family members share common traits. For example, in the beech family, all the members are monoecious. In the study of allergy, we often find that someone who is allergic to a particular plant may later become allergic to different plants in the same family. For example, someone allergic to the pollen of arborvitae may well become allergic to pollen from junipers. Both juniper and arborvitae are in the larger family Cupressaceae, the cypress family.

Foundation shrubs. Permanent bushes planted around a building, often to hide the foundation lines. A good foundation plant is bushy and attractive, does not grow too large or too fast, is generally evergreen, and is easy to grow, pest-free, long-lived, and reliable. A well-landscaped house will always have a good selection of foundation shrubs.

Functional dioecy. This is another term for cryptic dioecy, where each plant and all the flowers on it appear (to the untrained eye) to be perfect-flowered, but are actually only of one sex. The nonfunctioning sexual parts of the flower will often abort and fall off before they are viable. A plant could be either a functional male or a functional female.

Genus. Usually the first part of a plant's scientific name. Using the red maple as an example, the correct name is *Acer rubrum*. Acer is the genus. This system of giving all plants two names, called binomial nomenclature, was created by the great Swedish botanist Carl Linnaeus. It was his intention that genus meant group, and that the next word, the species, meant kind. Genera is plural for genus.

Gynodioecious. A system where some entire plants have perfect flowers and other plants have all-female individuals. This system is a plus, as it indicates less potential for allergy.

Hardy, hardiness. The measure of a plant's ability to withstand frost and cold. This term is confused perhaps more than any other in horticulture. Hardy does not mean that a plant is strong, easy to grow, or tough. A hardy plant is one that can take frost and cold and not suffer. A tomato plant is not hardy; it is tender. A hard frost will quickly kill a tomato plant. A cabbage plant is hardy. Kale is hardier than cabbage, and a sugar maple tree is considerably hardier than either.

Herb, herbaceous. A plant without woody stems. A pepper plant is herbaceous, as is a potato plant. A shrub or tree is not an herb because it has woody stems.

Intergeneric hybrids. Hybrid crosses between two different genera. Some intergeneric hybrids will be male-sterile, and hence often less (or not) allergenic.

Interspecific hybrids. These are hybrid crosses between two different species, but where both are in the same genus. These crosses are sometimes male-sterile and make no viable pollen.

Invasive. Plants that have a tendency to spread from where they are planted into wild areas, where they often become a serious environmental problem. Also, see "naturalize."

Monocarpic. This translates loosely from Latin as "one life." Monocarpic plants (such as *Agave americana* and most bamboo) bloom only once in their lifetime, and then set seed and die.

Monocot, monocotyledon. Monocot seeds sprout and emerge from the soil with one first leaf only. Examples of monocots are all grasses, lilies, onions, corn, wheat, and palm trees. In monocots, the veins run parallel to each other and the flowering parts are usually in threes. All the flowering plants in the world are either dicots or monocots.

Monocots do not form growth rings and they grow altogether differently than dicots. For example, if a slash is made three feet from the ground on the trunk of a young palm tree, ten years later this slash mark might be ten feet up on the tree trunk. If a similar slash were made on the trunk of a young dicot tree, ten years later the tree would be taller and the trunk wider, but the slash mark would still be exactly three feet from the ground.

Monoecious. A flowering system where separate male and female flowers are found on the same plant. In the example of corn, the top of the plant, the tassels, are the male flowers. The actual ears of corn are clusters of female flowers. In the example of a common cattail, a similar system is at work. The tip of the cattail has the male (pollen) flowers and the thicker, fatter, round part is composed of individual female flowers. Monoecious flowering systems are very important in allergy studies because often the pollen will be dispersed not by insects but by the wind. Some examples of monoecious plants are cypress, many of the palms, redwoods, oaks, some of the junipers, hickory, boxwood, pecans, and walnuts.

Naturalize. Some domestic plants naturally spread by runners, corms, or rhizomes, while others drop much viable seed that will quickly sprout and grow. Certain cultivated plants, like daffodils, narcissus, ajuga, Japanese honeysuckle, and Mexican evening primrose, often spread far from their original plantings. Sometimes this spreading, or naturalizing, is welcomed and other times it isn't.

Perennial. A plant that lives longer than two years. Perennial is a term most often used for winter-hardy plants like phlox, poppy, peony, lupine, foxglove, delphinium, and columbine. Trees and shrubs are woody plants, not perennials. The top parts of a perennial plant may die to the ground in late fall, but the plant will resprout from the underground crown in the spring.

Petals. Most flowers have petals, although in some they are totally lacking. Most dicot flowers have five petals (or multiples of five), although some have four. Monocots usually have three petals or multiples of three. Large, colorful, attractive petals are always considered a plus in allergy studies. All of the petals collectively form the corolla.

Photodermatitis. A contact skin condition resulting in a rash or an itch from touching leaves or flowers when the sun is shining. Photodermatitis may also suddenly recur when one is outside in bright sun. Numerous plants can trigger this sort of allergic response; an example is *Dictamnus alba*; citrus may on occasion also trigger photodermatitis.

Pistillate. A term used in botany to mean female.

Poisonous. In this text the word *poisonous* means that the plant, its seeds, leaves, flowers, roots, and so on are toxic if eaten. There are many kinds of poisons in plants, some deadly, but because a plant is poisonous does not mean it causes allergy. Bear in mind, though, that often poisonous plants also produce poisonous pollen. Examples are podocarpus, taxus, and to a lesser degree, rhododendrons.

Pollen. Pollen grains are the male sexual expression of flowering plants.

Pollinosis. This is normally used to mean allergy or "hay fever" triggered by allergenic pollen. Pollinosis is also sometimes used to describe any illness or symptom caused by exposure to pollen.

Propagation. To start a new plant. There are many methods of propagation used, such as seed, cuttings, spores, grafting, and so on. Propagation using seeds is considered sexual propagation. Methods not involving seed are asexual propagation. To propagate cultivars, which do not come true from seed (see "Seedling grown," below), asexual methods must be used. It is not legal to asexually propagate patented plants unless permission has been granted from the license holder.

Proximity pollinosis. Pollen allergy is most often caused by the pollen produced by the plants closest to the individual. Landscape plants growing next to one's house, or where one works or goes to school, are prime examples of plants (if allergenic) that will trigger proximity pollinosis. The closer you are to pollen-producing plants, the greater your exposure. Thus, highly allergenic plants in your own yard expose you to far more pollen than they do your immediate neighbors.

Rhizomes. Thick, spreading, underground roots that are capable of sprouting new plants. Rhizomes are similar to runners, except that runners spread along the top of the soil, and rhizomes usually spread just under the soil line.

Seedling grown. Many plants are grown from seeds, and often these do not come true from seed, meaning that they may not be exactly like the seed's parent plant. For example, a female cultivar of a red maple will set seed if pollinated; however, these seeds will grow maple trees, which will be both male and female. If a female cultivar is desired, it cannot be exactly duplicated from seed. To get an identical plant, it must be grown asexually.

Sepals. Leaflike appendages just below the flower petals. The sepals are usually considered part of the flower. Most dicots produce five sepals, although sometimes four are present in species like evening primrose and poppies. Colorful sepals sometimes take the place of petals as insect attractors for pollination. In allergy studies, the presence of attractive sepals is considered a plus. All of the sepals taken together form the calyx.

Species. The second part of a scientific name. With the common tall marigold, the scientific name is *Tagetes erecta*. The species is *erecta*. The general meaning of *species* is "kind." For example, in the name *Juniperus horizontalis*, *horizontalis* is the species and tells us that this species is a low-growing, spreading (horizontal) kind of juniper.

Spp. Used as in *Salix* spp., spp. is an abbreviation for the word *species*, meaning more than one species. *Salix* spp. translates to willow species.

Stamens. The male parts of a flower. On the tip of the stamen is the anther, which contains the pollen. A flower that is all-male is called a staminate flower.

Staminate. A term used in botany to mean male.

Subshrub. A woody plant that may grow like a big perennial, and sometimes becomes shrublike. A subshrub is not usually considered as permanent a plant as most species described as either shrubs or bushes.

Toxic. In this book the word *toxic* is synonymous with *poisonous*. It is different than allergenic, as an allergenic substance will only affect those with allergies, but a toxic substance will affect anyone. Some plants that are toxic if eaten, such as yew (*Taxus* spp.), will also produce toxic pollen on male plants.

Unisexual. A flowering system where separate-sexed flowers are present. Any flowering plants that are dioecious or monoecious are unisexual. Examples are hickory, walnut, sweet gum, and currants.

Variety. A subdivision of a species. For example, in the tree often called rubber tree, the name is stated as *Ficus elastica* 'Decora'. In this example, the variety is 'Decora'. The difference between a cultivar and a variety is that a cultivar is a variety of only a cultivated species.

Vegetative. Growth that consists of stems and leaves, but not flowers. Often shrubs that are frequently sheared hard grow only vegetatively and do not produce flowers.

Volatile organic compounds (VOCs). Air pollutants (hydrocarbons) released by trees and shrubs, a component of smog. Most trees and shrubs remove huge amounts of air pollutants daily; however, a few trees, such as liquidambar, oak, eucalyptus, and sycamore, produce more VOCs than they absorb, thus adding to industrial-produced smog. VOCs from plants are also often termed BVOCs, as in biologic emissions, or biogenic emissions.

Zones, zones of winter hardiness. Expressed as a number; in this book the new, standard USDA 1 to 13 zone ratings are used. The lower the zone number, the more cold and frost a plant can tolerate. Plants hardy to zone 3, for example, can live where winters may get to -40°F. Plants hardy only in zones 10 to 13 will normally not tolerate any frost, and may not live if the temperature ever gets below 32°F. There are other useful, more sophisticated plant zone systems, such as that used by Sunset's *Western Garden Book*, which uses some twenty-four different plant zones of hardiness. In Europe there are also various zoning systems, and the system used in this book closely correlates European plant hardiness zones to similar U.S. zones.

Recommended Reading

This list of references is in no way complete, but included are a few of the books and articles that I found especially useful in the writing of *The Allergy-Fighting Garden*.

Bailey, Liberty Hyde, Ethel Zoe Bailey, and Cornell University, eds. *Hortus Third*. London, New York: Collier Macmillan Publishers, 1976.

Clark, David, and Elizabeth L. Hogan, eds. *Sunset Western Garden Book*. Menlo Park, CA: Lane Publishing Company, 1986. For the western United States, this is one of the most useful general gardening books.

Flint, Harrison L. *Landscape Plants for Eastern North America*. New York: John Wiley & Sons, 1983.

Jacobson, Arthur Lee. *North American Landscape Trees*. Berkeley, CA: Ten Speed Press, 1996. One of the very best books on hardy landscape trees. Jacobson understands sex systems in trees and always includes this information. Great attention to detail.

Jury, S. L., Cutler Reynolds, and F. J. Evans. *The Euphorbiales*. Great Britian: The Linnean Society of London, The Whitefriars Press, 1987.

Lewis, Walter H. "Airborne Pollen of the Neotropics." *Grana* 25 (March 20, 1986): 75–83.

Lewis, Walter H. *Tropical to Warm Temperate Aerospora of Vascular Plants*. St. Louis, MO: Washington University, 1990. This is a very extensive bibliography of useful sites up to 1990. For the serious allergy researcher, this is a good place to start.

Lewis, Walter H., Anu Dixit, and Walter Ward. "Distribution and Incidence of North American Pollen Aeroallergens." *American Journal of Otolaryngology* 12 (1991): 205–26.

Lewis, Walter H., and Wayne E. Imber. "Aeroallergens in the Midwestern United States: Pollen and Spores Hazardous to Health." Fourth International Palynological Conference, Lucknow, India, vol. 3 (1978): 466–474.

Lewis, Walter H., and Memory Elvin Lewis. *Medical Botany*. New York: John Wiley & Sons, 1977. A fascinating book!

Lewis, Walter H., and Prathibha Vinay. "North American Pollinosis Due to Insect-Pollinated Plants." St. Louis, MO, Washington University Department of Biology, May 1979.

Lewis, Walter H., Prathibha Vinay, and Vincent E. Zenger. *Airborne and Allergenic Pollen of North America*. Baltimore: Johns Hopkins University Press, 1983. From a purely scientific point of view, I consider this the best book ever written on the connections between plants and pollen allergy.

McMinn, Howard E., and Evelyn Maino. *Pacific Coast Trees*. Berkeley, CA: University of California Press, 1981. A fine, easy-to-use book for identifying West Coast trees.

Mortensen, Ernest, and Ervin Bullard. *Handbook of Tropical and Sub-Tropical Horticulture*. Washington, DC: USDA, 1964.

Munz, Philip A., and David D. Keck. *A California Flora and Supplement*. Berkeley, CA: University of California Press, 1968. This is not light reading, but it is nonetheless the bible on native California species.

Nowak, David J., P. J. McHale, M. Ibarra, D. Crane, J. Stevens, and C. Luley. *Modeling the Effects of Urban Vegetation on Air Pollution*. New York: Plenum Press, 1998.

Peattie, Donald Culross. *A Natural History of Trees of Eastern and Central North America*. Boston, MA: Houghton Mifflin Company, 1991.

Peattie, Donald Culross. *A Natural History of Western Trees*. Boston, MA: Houghton Mifflin, 1991. This volume and the one above are two of my favorite books about trees; they are extremely readable and packed full of interesting and important observations that other writers miss.

Sargent, Charles Sprague. *Manual of the Trees of North America*. New York: Dover Publications, Inc., 1965. One of the very best.

Snyder, Leon C. *Gardening in the Upper Midwest*. Minneapolis, MN: University of Minnesota Press, 1978.

Taylor, Norman. *Taylor's Encyclopedia of Gardening*. Boston, MA: Houghton Mifflin, 1948. This is an old but wonderful book. One of my all-time favorites, this is a very useful general gardening book.

Utterback, Christine. *Reliable Roses*. New York: Clarkson Potter, 1997. Good book for picking out roses with extra disease resistance.

Van Gelderen, D. M., P. C. de Jong, and H. J. Oterdoom. *Maples of the World*. Portland, OR: Timber Press, 1994. The very best book I've ever read on maples.

Wodehouse, R. P. *Pollen Grains*. New York: McGraw-Hill, 1935. Wodehouse was one of the first and one of the best. *Pollen Grains* is a classic in allergy literature.

Useful Websites

allallergy.net A highly recommended website from Dr. Harris Steinman, MD, a widely respected allergist and allergy researcher from South Africa. Especially valuable is the Allergy Advisor Digest, a monthly updated link to interesting new research articles on asthma and allergy. Suggest you sign up for monthly email updates from All Allergy Net.

allergyfree-gardening.com This is my own website and it is always a good way to contact me. It has been in existence (advertisement-free) for more than fifteen years. Contains many photos and articles by me and other researchers.

foodsmatter.com This is the best website for food-allergy issues; a new issue comes out each month and I suggest you sign up for their emails. Hundreds of articles and thousands of research reports on allergy, intolerance, sensitivity, and related health problems. Edited by the very knowledgeable Michelle Berriedale-Johnson.

greenlegacyguernsey.org.uk This is the website of educator, horticulturist, and nurseryman Nigel Clarke and is based in Guernsey, in the Channel Islands, UK. Clarke is already growing and selling OPALS-tagged female, allergy-free trees and shrubs.

healthyschoolyards.org This is a Canadian website devoted solely to the promotion of allergy-free schoolyards and public parks. Created by hardworking horticulturist and educator Peter Prakke of Hamilton, Ontario, Healthy Schoolyards has already been successful in getting schools and parks to relandscape their allergenic landscapes.

minnesotalawreview.org/headnotes/regulating-pollen This is a link to an interesting, intelligent, and thought-provoking essay. Published by the *Minnesota Law Journal*, written by attorney Brian Sawers, this is the go-to article on how to use the law to regulate pollen.

safegardening.org This is the website of the Society for Allergy Friendly Environmental (SAFE) Gardening. A nonprofit group formed to promote the concept of allergy-fighting gardens, to change public policy, to promote pollen-control ordinances, and to actually re-landscape highly allergenic elementary schools. I am on the board of directors of SAFE Gardening. SAFE is always looking for volunteers from all areas.

Pollen Calendar

These are approximate dates of bloom periods of some of the most common allergenic trees, grasses, and shrubs. The actual blooming periods will be earlier in southern areas and later in northern climates. Poplars, for example, may start blooming in January in Florida, but in Washington State they may not start until May. Some species of plants, such as cypress, may be in and out of bloom all year long in the areas farthest south.

SPECIES	JAN	FEB	MAR	APR	MAY	JUNE	JULY	AUG	SEPT	OCT	NOV	DEC
Acacia	███	███	███	███	███	███	███	███	███	███	███	
Acer		███	███	███	███							
Ailanthus			███	███	███	███						
Albizia						███	███	███	███	███		
Alder/Alnus		███	███	███	███							███
Almond		███	███	███	███							
Artemisia							███	███	███	███		
Baccharis								███	███	███	███	███
Bermuda Grass			███	███	███	███	███	███	███	███	███	
Betula			███	███	███	███			███	███		
Broussonetia	███	███	███	███	███	███						
Buxus	███	███	███	███	███							
Callistemon	███	███	███	███	███	███	███	███	███	███	███	
Calocedrus			███	███	███	███	███					
Carya		███	███	███	███	███	███					
Casurina	███										███	███
Catalpa					███	███	███					
Ceanothus			███	███	███							
Celtis			███	███								
Chionanthus					███	███	███					

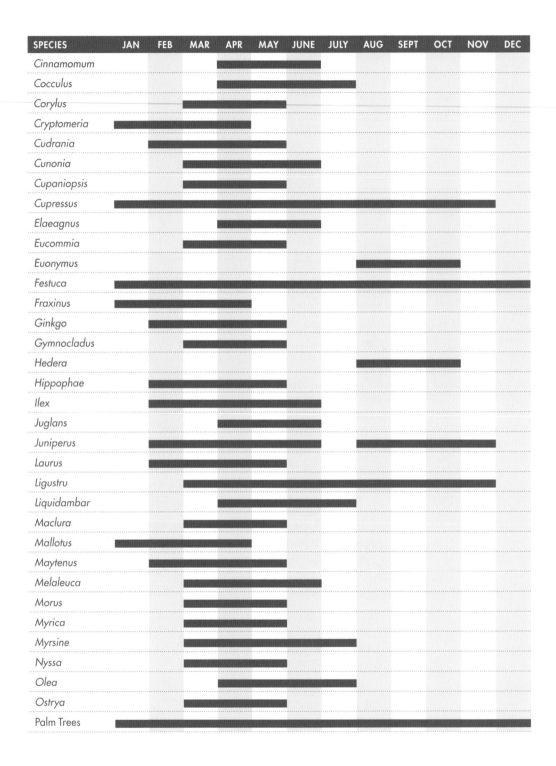

SPECIES	JAN	FEB	MAR	APR	MAY	JUNE	JULY	AUG	SEPT	OCT	NOV	DEC
Cinnamomum				████	████	██						
Cocculus				████	████	████						
Corylus			████	████	██							
Cryptomeria	████	████	████	██								
Cudrania			████	████								
Cunonia				████	████							
Cupaniopsis			████	████								
Cupressus	████	████	████	████	████	████	████	████	████	████	████	████
Elaeagnus				████	████	████						
Eucommia			████	████								
Euonymus								████	████	██		
Festuca	████	████	████	████	████	████	████	████	████	████	████	████
Fraxinus	████	████	████	██								
Ginkgo		████	████	████	██							
Gymnocladus			████	████								
Hedera								████	████	██		
Hippophae		████	████	████								
Ilex		████	████	████	████							
Juglans				████	████	██						
Juniperus		████	████	████				████	████	████		
Laurus		████	████	████								
Ligustru			████	████	████	████	████	████	████	████		
Liquidambar				████	████	████	██					
Maclura			████	████	██							
Mallotus	████	████	████	██								
Maytenus		████	████	██								
Melaleuca			████	████	████	██						
Morus			████	████								
Myrica			████	████								
Myrsine			████	████	████	████						
Nyssa			████	████	██							
Olea				████	████	████						
Ostrya			████	████								
Palm Trees	████	████	████	████	████	████	████	████	████	████	████	████

SPECIES	JAN	FEB	MAR	APR	MAY	JUNE	JULY	AUG	SEPT	OCT	NOV	DEC
Pennisetum	X	X	X	X	X	X	X	X	X	X	X	X
Phellodendron			X	X	X	X						
Pistache			X	X	X							
Planera									X	X	X	
Platanus			X	X	X							
Platycarya												X
Platycladus			X	X	X	X						
Poa	X	X	X	X	X	X	X	X	X	X	X	X
Podocarpus		X	X	X	X	X	X	X				
Populus			X	X	X	X	X					
Prosopis			X	X	X	X	X					
Quercus		X	X	X	X	X	X					
Ragweed								X	X	X	X	
Rhamnus		X	X	X	X	X	X					
Rhus			X	X	X	X	X					
Ribes			X	X	X	X						
Ricinus				X	X	X	X	X	X			
Salix	X	X	X	X	X	X						
Sapindus							X	X	X	X		
Sapium							X	X	X			
Schinus					X	X	X	X	X			
Senecio								X	X	X	X	
Solidago								X	X	X		
Syringa				X	X	X						
Tamarix	X	X	X	X							X	X
Taxodium	X	X										X
Taxus		X	X	X	X							
Thujopsis			X	X								X
Tilia						X	X	X				
Ulmus	X	X	X	X								
Umbellularia	X	X	X	X	X							
Xylosma									X	X	X	X
Zanthoxylum	X	X	X	X	X	X						
Zelkova	X	X	X	X	X							X

USDA Plant Hardiness Zone Map

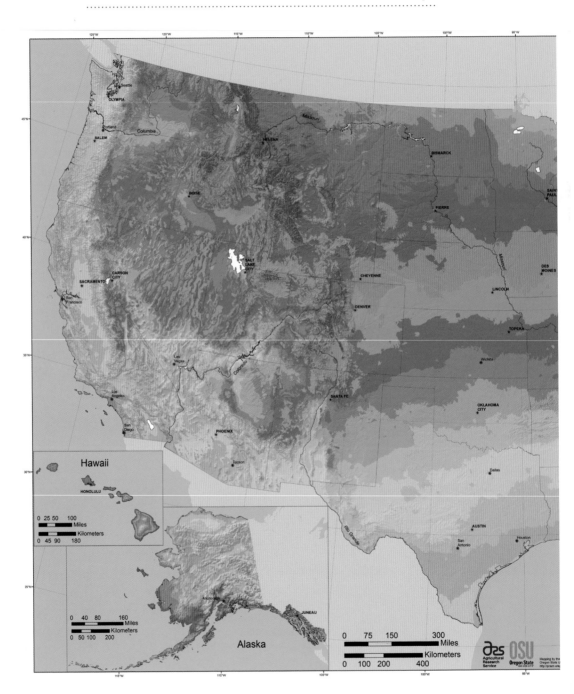

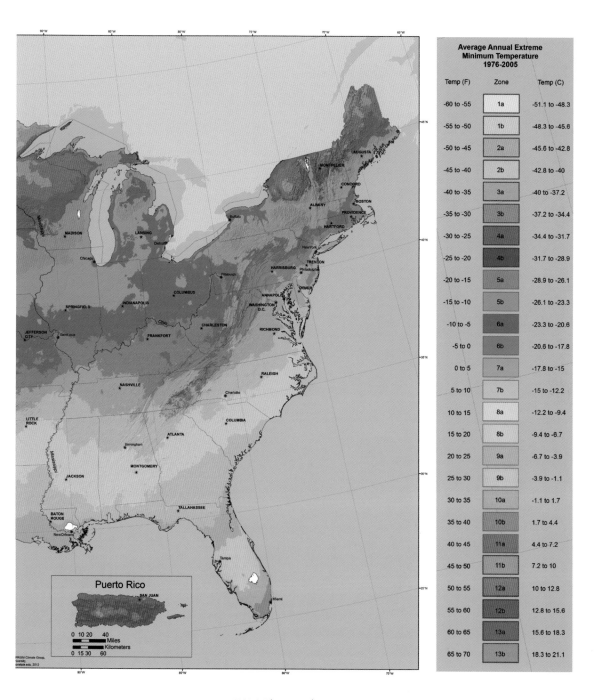

Average Annual Extreme
Minimum Temperature
1976-2005

Temp (F)	Zone	Temp (C)
-60 to -55	1a	-51.1 to -48.3
-55 to -50	1b	-48.3 to -45.6
-50 to -45	2a	-45.6 to -42.8
-45 to -40	2b	-42.8 to -40
-40 to -35	3a	-40 to -37.2
-35 to -30	3b	-37.2 to -34.4
-30 to -25	4a	-34.4 to -31.7
-25 to -20	4b	-31.7 to -28.9
-20 to -15	5a	-28.9 to -26.1
-15 to -10	5b	-26.1 to -23.3
-10 to -5	6a	-23.3 to -20.6
-5 to 0	6b	-20.6 to -17.8
0 to 5	7a	-17.8 to -15
5 to 10	7b	-15 to -12.2
10 to 15	8a	-12.2 to -9.4
15 to 20	8b	-9.4 to -6.7
20 to 25	9a	-6.7 to -3.9
25 to 30	9b	-3.9 to -1.1
30 to 35	10a	-1.1 to 1.7
35 to 40	10b	1.7 to 4.4
40 to 45	11a	4.4 to 7.2
45 to 50	11b	7.2 to 10
50 to 55	12a	10 to 12.8
55 to 60	12b	12.8 to 15.6
60 to 65	13a	15.6 to 18.3
65 to 70	13b	18.3 to 21.1

USDA Plant Hardiness Zone Map

Acknowledgments

The Allergy-Fighting Garden has been a long time in the making, and a good many people have helped me with research for this new book. My literary agents, Sheree Bykofsky and Janice Rosen, have been a great deal of help in making this happen. My wonderful and savvy editor at Ten Speed Press, Lisa Regul, has done a masterful job of editing and keeping me on task.

Harris Steinman, MD, world-traveling allergist, speaker, and researcher, has always been quick to answer my questions on a host of subjects. Peter Prakke from Hamilton, Ontario, has been pushing me for years to get this project off the ground, and I am indebted to him for his hard work, energy, guidance, and friendship. Dr. Vicki Stover, a former university VP and good friend, has been great at keeping me organized and on track. John Banks, a close friend for many years, serves on the board of SAFE Gardening and is always free with good advice. My thanks go to Rachele Melious, nurserywoman, registered pollen counter, and dedicated worker, for considerable help and advice.

In the UK I am indebted to Michelle Berriedale-Johnson from Foods Matter, who took me to the Chelsea Garden Show and treated me like a king in London. I am most appreciative of my close friend Nigel Clarke, a dedicated and responsible nurseryman and environmentalist from Guernsey who has been working with me for years now. In New Zealand I am indebted to the head arborist of the city of Christchurch, Dieter Steinegg. Dieter and his family treated me like family when I stayed with them while doing allergy research in New Zealand. In Israel I wish to thank Esti and Yuval Lior, who put up with me as I roamed for weeks searching for new plants and new birds.

I would like to thank the hundreds of garden clubs and Master Gardener groups who have hosted me to speak. These people know and love gardening and they are always a pleasure to spend some quality time with. From their multitude of questions I have learned a great deal. Likewise, to the thousands of folks who have bought my books and sent me emails over the years, I appreciate every one of you, and I've learned many a new thing from our correspondence. Often you've pointed me in directions that otherwise I might well have missed.

I am also very grateful for the constant encouragement over the years to keep doing this research from my parents, Bud and Paula Ogren. They're both gone now, alas, and I sure do miss them. Also gone now, but still deserving of thanks, is Dr. David Stadner, a marvelous old-school allergist from Stockton, California, who provided much-needed advice.

For their friendship and the wealth of information in their incredible books, I am always grateful to Dr. Walter H. Lewis and Dr. Memory Lewis.

Special thanks, too, goes to my son-in-law, David Bush, who helps me track down unusual plants and who took many of the photos for this book. Last, and certainly not least, a profound thank-you to my wonderful wife, Yvonne Marie Bradshaw Ogren.

About the Author

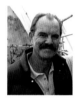Thomas Leo Ogren has a master's degree in agricultural science, with an emphasis on plant flowering systems and their relationship to allergy. He is a horticulturist and allergy researcher as well as a former nursery owner, landscape gardening instructor, and gardening radio-show host. Ogren is the creator of the Ogren Plant Allergy Scale (OPALS), the first plant-allergy ranking system, now used by the United States Department of Agriculture. He has done consulting for the American Lung Association; the city of Christchurch, New Zealand; the USDA; the California Department of Public Health; Allegra; and Johnson & Johnson. His work on allergies has been seen on TV shows, including the Canadian Discovery Channel. He has been a guest on many radio shows, including twice on National Public Radio. He writes for *New Scientist*, *Grandiflora*, *Alternative Medicine*, *Landscape Architecture*, and many other publications. Ogren lives with his family in San Luis Obispo, California. His email address is tloallergyfree@earthlink.net.

Index

This book is dedicated to my wife, Yvonne Marie Bradshaw Ogren.

Published in the United States by Ten Speed Press, an imprint of the Crown Publishing Group,
a division of Random House LLC, a Penguin Random House Company, New York.
www.crownpublishing.com
www.tenspeed.com

Ten Speed Press and the Ten Speed Press colophon are registered trademarks of Random House LLC.

Much of this work is composed of material, revised and reworked, previously published in
Allergy-Free Gardening, in 2000, and in *Safe Sex in the Garden*, in 2003, by Ten Speed Press, Berkeley.

Library of Congress Cataloging-in-Publication Data
Ogren, Thomas Leo.
 The allergy-fighting garden : stop asthma and allergies with smart landscaping /
Thomas Leo Ogren. — First edition.
     pages cm
 Portions of this book were previously published in a different form in *Allergy-Free Gardening*
in 2000 and in *Safe Sex in the Garden* in 2003.
 Includes index.
 1. Low-allergen gardens. 2. Low-allergen plants. 3. Plants, Sex in. I. Title.
 SB433.4.O46 2015
 635.9—dc23

2014023777

Trade Paperback ISBN: 978-1-60774-491-7
eBook ISBN: 978-1-60774-492-4

Printed in China

Design by Chloe Rawlins
All photographs by Thomas Leo Ogren, except for:
Front cover by ballycroy
Pages ii, iv, vi, 3, 39, 70, 100, 128 (right), 147, 186, (right), 190, 193, 204, 217, spine,
    and back cover (except second from top) by Ildiko Laszlo
Pages 101 (left), 114 (right), 129, 183 (left), and 187 by Lisa Regul
Page 135 by Nigel Clarke
Illustrations on page 10 by Shelby Stover
Illustration on page 14 by Paquerette

10 9 8 7 6 5 4 3 2 1

First Edition

Page ii: Low-pollen Petunia
Page iv: Aeonium